GUIDEBOOK FOR DRUG REGULATORY SUBMISSIONS

GUIDEBOOK FOR DRUG REGULATORY SUBMISSIONS

Sandy Weinberg, PhD
Clayton State University

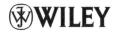

A JOHN WILEY & SONS, INC., PUBLICATION

Published by John Wiley & Sons, Inc., Hoboken, New Jersey
Published simultaneously in Canada

For general information on our other products and services or for technical support, please contact our Customer Care Department within the United States at (800) 762-2974, outside the United States at (317) 572-3993 or fax (317) 572-4002.

Wiley also publishes its books in a variety of electronic formats. Some content that appears in print may not be available in electronic formats. For more information about Wiley products, visit our web site at www.wiley.com.

Library of Congress Cataloging-in-Publication Data:

Weinberg, Sandy, 1950–
    Guidebook for drug regulatory submissions / Sandy Weinberg.
       p. cm.
    Includes bibliographical references and index.
    ISBN 978-0-470-37138-1 (cloth)
    1. Drugs–Law and legislation–United States. 2. Drug approval–United States. I. Title.
    [DNLM: 1. Drug Approval–United States. 2. Drugs,
Investigational–United States. QV 771 W423g 2009]
    KF3885W45 2009
    344.7304′233–dc22

                                                                                    2008044679

10 9 8 7 6 5 4 3 2 1

For Ronnie, whose threat or promise of a book-signing party kept me going.

◼◼◼ CONTENTS

A formal submission to the United States Food and Drug Administration is a professionally frightening proposition. There is a great deal at stake: the submission can lead to permission to move forward with a drug development project, with the promise of patient improvement and corporate profits. The submission represents the tightest of bottlenecks in that development process: delays affect every other part of the operation, leading to criticism from clinical medical; chemistry, manufacturing, and control testing; and all other departments. And the submission response itself is open, with blunt comments from a heartless agency widely distributed. Many a regulatory professional has lost sleep over the prospect of a major submission.

This book is intended as a (nonprescription, not reviewed by the FDA) sleep remedy for those regulatory professionals. Each chapter features a description of the submission and a discussion of the key elements. To help in the internal quality review of the document, a Checklist for Submissions has been prepared, providing guidance in content, format, and direction. An FDA Review Checklist, replicating the criteria utilized by the agency in evaluating the submission, is provided to avoid unpleasant surprises and to provide further aid in focusing the document. And, accessible for easy reference, the key FDA guidelines, interpretations, and documents are provided.

After an introductory chapter providing general principles for submissions, seven chapters focus on the most common types of submissions:

FDA Meeting Requests
Orphan Drug Applications
Investigational New Drug Applications (INDs)
New Drug Applications (NDAs)
505(b)2 NDAs
Abbreviated New Drug Applications (ANDAs)
Annual Reports

A ninth chapter, guest-authored by Carl A. Rockburne, a retired Canadian trade console and regulatory consultant, compares the FDA process with those in Canada, the European Union, Japan, and Australia, the four other major regulatory environments. He has included FDA documents describing the regulatory harmonization process in his chapter.

A final chapter, more speculative in nature, focuses on the future of drug regulatory submissions. As the FDA's role is expanded and its budget is not, as an increasing number of companies introduce a growing list of new products, what is likely to "give"? How will the agency cope? What other pressures are affecting the industry and the general public? And how will all of these pressures change the general nature and specific aspects of the submissions process over the near future?

The *Guidebook for Drug Regulatory Submissions* is intended as a reference book to sit, dog-eared, worn, and filled with paper slips and margin notes, on the corner of the desk of every regulatory director, submissions manager, VP of Regulatory Affairs—and FDA reviewer—responsible for the process of drug regulatory submissions. I hope it will prove a useful tool in controlling a complex and frightening process leading ultimately to the industry and agency's common altruistic goal: to bring safe and effective drugs to the patients who need them.

SANDY WEINBERG

CHAPTER 1

Ten Rules for Drug Regulatory Submissions

INTRODUCTION

The drug discovery, development, and commercialization process is marked by a number of important milestones. Some of these key points are delineated by scientific observations; some by legal issuance of patents; some by marketing events. But most process milestones seem to involve the submission to, and approval by, the FDA. The granting of permission to conduct clinical studies [the Investigational New Drug Application (IND) approval], the New Drug Application (NDA), which carries permission to market, and the interim steps leading to these major approvals stand out as the most important steps in the process and are tracked by investors, stock analysts, and the industry.

Each major and minor regulatory approval step is characterized by a submission, a regulatory review, and a decision. When that decision is contrary to expectations, it may be followed by a revision and, in rare cases, an appeal.

This process can be intimidating, particularly for the inexperienced regulatory professional charged with preparing a major regulatory submission. A significant chapter in the company's history depends upon the success of the submission. The result can make or break a career. And altruistically, the result can seem to determine if large numbers of patients or potential patients receive life-changing medication.

While the stakes may seem overwhelming and while some companies may maximize the pressure, the reality is much less threatening. While the FDA has an important safety role that results in barriers blocking drug approval until strong evidence is presented, the Agency has a balancing responsibility to provide the public with access to safe drug products. As a result, regulatory professionals inside the FDA are prepared to assist in the process with guidance documents, controlled conferences, and (often) informal advice.

Think of the submissions process as a major exam but one for which you have the questions in advance, can use your notes, and—on hopefully rare occasions—can retake the test if necessary.

Guidebook for Drug Regulatory Submissions, by Sandy Weinberg
Copyright © 2009 John Wiley & Sons, Inc.

To try and explain the process and to minimize those rare retake necessities, here are 10 summary rules for regulatory submissions.

TEN RULES

1. **Seek guidance.** Most things in life are easier the second time around; regulatory submissions are no exception. The first time you file an IND, orphan-drug application, or NDA can be confusing and intimidating. By the time you have filed your second or third submission, though, the process begins to approach the routine. Of course, everything you do has to be accomplished for a first time, but you can minimize that inexperience by seeking guidance from others. In effect, partner your first time with someone who has experience and can advise you.

   One source of that advice is the FDA itself. There are formal FDA meetings, which require a written meeting request and briefing book (see Chapters 2 and 3), most appropriate before development and submission of an IND or an NDA. Less formally, FDA spokespersons often make presentations at local and national conferences. Their presentations are often available on the FDA Web site (http://www.fda.gov) as well as through the specific conference. Finally, some individuals from the FDA will respond directly to telephone or e-mail questions. All three of these sources can be effective information conduits and can help build strong contracts and relationships within the FDA.

   If circumstances exclude the possibility of FDA advice, or if you want to hedge your bets with additional assistance, consider the use of a consulting group. It is possible, of course, to use a consultant to completely and independently prepare a submission. Such a strategy may be tempting for a one-time submission but carries a risk: When your company makes a submission, it assumes full responsibility and liability for the content, regardless of who prepared it. It is much safer and generally better for long-term corporate information culture growth to use a consulting group as guidance and assistance in preparing the submission. Let the consulting group provide help with format, recommendations for wording, the publishing and delivery services that may be onerous, and even an initial draft for review. But make certain that the final draft is a result of your company's careful revisions and acceptance. Fine-tune the document, assume responsibility, and learn the process to streamline the next submission, with or without outside assistance.

   Finally, make certain that your first effort and all submissions are team affairs. Do not put all the responsibility on the director of regulatory affairs, although that person may ultimately pull together the effort, sign the submission, and lead the team. Involve input from Quality

Assurance (QA), Clinical, Marketing, and all other parts of the organization. In-house experience and diverse expertise will allow you to prevent or solve problems when they arise.

2. **Focus on format (in addition to content).** The first hurdle your submission faces is generally a format review: Until an administrative review indicates that the submission is complete and appropriately formatted, no further review can take place. So while content may be most important, do not neglect the importance of proper organization, pagination, referencing, headings, bibliography, and other formatting requirements.

   These formatting issues vary from one submission type to another and sometimes from one submission recipient to another. A CNS review team may have different criteria or preferences from a Metabolic team; INDs have different requirements than orphan applications. As above (1), get some guidance and follow the preferred format.

   The widest difference between FDA groups and submission types is in referencing preferences. Some groups recommend numerical referencing, tying to a numbered bibliography. Others use the American Psychological Association editorial style (author name, date), linked to an alphabetical bibliography. Most applications and most teams require that actual copies of the reference be included in the submission. Barring other statements of formatting, the default is a numerical list of articles (text copies included), with numbered references to those articles inserted in the body of the submission text.

   Some submissions require two copies; some three; some even more exact duplicates. Check the submission guidance documents included here in each chapter for the specific requirements.

   Cover letters are required for most submissions. Every cover letter should be dated, should carry a reference line (referring by number, IND, or other submission reference if available), and should contain complete contact information for a company spokesperson (see 7), including company name, address, contact name, title, telephone numbers, and e-mail address.

   Formatting problems will delay your application and may affect the reputation and impression you are working to build. Checking the specific requirements and preferences of the group to which you are submitting can make this much easier. While content is principal, do not neglect the submission format.

3. **Document everything.** A major submission may take weeks—sometimes even months—to assemble. During that time, the writing team reviews and revises draft after draft.

   When the same material is reviewed over and over, there is a natural tendency to begin subconsciously thinking of some statements as self-obvious and hence not needing documentary support. The result may be a submission in which some key issues and assumptions are not sufficiently referenced, weakening the entire document.

To avoid the problem, identify all claims and assumptions in the first draft and have a different, independent reviewer (presumably from QA) periodically reexamine to make certain that all important points are appropriately referenced. That independence can overcome the problem even as the reviewer serves as a gadfly, challenging any controversial or unsupported assumptions.

Incidentally, most FDA submissions permit unpublished as well as published references. Supporting letters, studies not yet in print, copies of speeches and papers, and other unpublished references can be included. Refer as with any other document and include a copy in the reference section.

Web site information can also be included; reference to include the specific site and page and the date of review. And, again, include a printed copy of the site page in the reference materials.

When in doubt, remember that it is better to have too much than too little documentation. Every reference is potentially adding credibility to your submission.

4. **Self-regulate.** The FDA considers the pharmaceutical industry to be self-regulated; FDA people perceive their job as checking that you have appropriately self-regulated. That is why a technical process, even if appropriate and successful, is considered inadequate if lacking a validation and QA or control review. The double-check, self-regulation step is always required.

Counting on the FDA as your primary submission reviewer is as inappropriate as neglecting QA on the production line on the assumption that a visit from FDA investigators will serve the purpose. In any FDA submission, your QA group has an important role well beyond a proofing function.

Each of the submission documents described in this book includes two checklists. The first is a checklist intended to assist in the preparation of the document; it outlines the requirements, organizational structure, and format. The second is a checklist derived from the FDA's review and guidance documents, discussions with FDA reviewers, and with professionals experienced in the development of type submissions. It is intended to be a checklist that might be used by the FDA reviewer of the final submissions document (in many cases, these checklists have been adopted by FDA personnel and are in actual use).

The FDA Review Checklists can be used by your internal QA team to self-regulate. Acting as FDA reviewers, they can confirm that your submission conforms to all format, content, and support requirements. And, of course, should the QA team find a weakness, you can correct and rereview prior to actual submission.

Self-regulation through an appropriate QA review allows your company to take control of the process and to assume appropriate responsibility.

5. **Examine electronic submission options.** Most FDA submissions can be made manually (paper) or electronically. Obviously, the electronic submission process is more efficient, particularly when delivering large documents (INDs routinely run over 5,000 pages; NDAs may be even larger). However, there are some additional considerations.

Electronic submission standards are evolving and may not be clearly established for all FDA groups and divisions. The common electronic submission gateway (ESG, see Chapter 1 FDA Documents) is sometimes problematic.

Consider also the possibility of providing a paper submission with an accompanying hyperlinked CD-ROM disk, allowing reviewers to move between electronic and paper versions. Some FDA groups may offer other suggestions as well.

6. **Schedule the submission.** Not only does the submission take some lead time planning (perhaps as much as six months for the development of an NDA—much less for other submissions), but there are other considerations as well.

An orphan-drug application and an IND both receive responses in about 30 days. Try to schedule submissions so that the response date will not fall within planned vacations or critical international travel. And both submissions (and many others) require an annual update report; it is best to stagger report due dates to avoid complications in the future.

But most important, to avoid submission bottlenecks, a clear schedule allows other team members—proofers, printers, collators, IT, QA, etc.—to make certain they are prepared. If QA needs a three-day period to review, count back a week (their three days, and two more to correct any problems they find) from the planned duplication, assembly, and submission dates.

7. **Designate contacts.** FDA submissions require a designated contact person, identified in the cover letter and (generally) in the submission itself. The contact person should be identified by name and title, with telephone (office and cell) and e-mail contact information provided.

But what if the contact person is ill, on vacation, traveling in Asia, or otherwise inaccessible? Rather than delay important FDA inquiries or information until the contact returns, most companies develop an alternate contact responsibility. The FDA wants a single name, but you can arrange to have other people monitor that person's e-mail account and telephone.

Some companies involved with a steady stream of multiple submissions establish a special e-mail address and telephone number exclusively for FDA contacts. That box and number can be monitored by any company employee, who can then pass information on to the designated contact person.

Particularly in a time-critical environment, do not miss a message from FDA personnel. Because of their busy schedule, it may be several days before they try to make contact again.

8. **Keep the FDA informed.** Once a file has been opened through a meeting request, inquiry, or submission, the project is assigned to an FDA contact. That designated individual can serve as a conduit to appropriate directors, committees, review boards, and divisions.

Communication with the FDA contact can take a variety of forms; most will accept telephone calls and e-mails and will request formal, written communications when significant issues arise. But regardless of the format, keep your contact in the loop if schedules or plans change.

Remember, though, that all contacts—even contact reports of telephone conversations—will be appended to the file. Keep all questions clear and direct and avoid speculative questions. Use the contact to keep the FDA informed of all official issues, but nothing is "off the record."

9. **Make appeal and legal action as very last possible steps.** Regulatory decisions on submissions are communicated to applicants through a variety of channels, including verbal (telephone calls), e-mails, and formal letters. With careful self-regulation through a thorough QA review prior to submission, you should gain some control over the process, avoiding many but not all unpleasant surprises.

If the review result is not what was anticipated or expected, there are several levels of response that are possible. The first, and generally most successful, is a conversation to pinpoint the problem, followed by a clarification (if the adverse result is due to a simple misunderstanding), submission amendment (if more detail or support is requested), or resubmission (if significant issues need to be addressed). These informal requests for reconsideration are often successful, particularly if approached in a cooperative framework.

The next steps are clearly confrontation in varying degrees of severity. For most divisions and groups to which a submission is directed, there is a formal appeals process (see Chapter 6). If not, or as a step beyond that appeals channel, the FDA Office of the Ombudsman has a dispute-resolution procedure. Finally, it is possible to bring suit against the FDA in Federal Court.

While these formal appeal processes are available, and while careful mechanisms are built into the procedures to avoid any spirit of retaliation, there is likely to be an adverse effect on the cooperative atmosphere that ought to prevail in FDA interactions. While it is certainly appropriate to follow through on all available and appropriate avenues of appeal, these formal steps should be considered as the last possible steps, to be followed only when other informal and nonconfrontational procedures are exhausted.

10. **Build a partnership.** In an appropriately self-regulated environment, the working relationship between the FDA and a submitting organization should be one of cautious partnership, working together within a carefully designed legal and administrative framework to achieve common goals. Both parties share the same general objective: to bring proven safe and effective drug products to a public in need of the potential treatment, therapy, or preventive.

Not-for-profit organizations, including universities and research institutes, have a natural affinity for such partnership arrangements since they avoid the natural skepticism that comes from a profit motivation. But, even for profit, companies can create a virtual partnership by communicating clearly to the FDA—in action as well as words—a willingness to put public health and safety above short-term revenue goals.

In all FDA interactions—verbal, face-to-face, and in submissions—keep this principle of primary, genuine concern for public health and safety as an underlying theme. The result will be slow building of mutual trust into a true partnership. And, if concern for public health and safety is not your true primary purpose, you are in the wrong business.

SUMMARY

The submissions process can be traumatic. Whether you are a start-up company filing your first meeting request or a major pharmaceutical organization with an NDA for the latest blockbuster, there is a great deal resting on the process and the result.

A good portion of that trauma flows from a perception of loss of control: the submission is delivered and seems to enter a black box of FDA review with no clearly predictable outcome.

But that sense of control can be regained and the result made rational and predictable through a careful QA process that checks the submission against FDA established criteria and through the use of an internal, self-regulating review process that applies the checklist criteria used by the FDA to the submission development process.

For meeting requests, orphan-drug applications, INDs, NDAs, 505b(2) NDAs, Abbreviated New Drug Applications (ANDAs), Orphan Annual Reports, and Annual Reports, the tools, checklists, and FDA guidelines are provided. With this tool kit, your organization can regain control of a rational, predictable submissions process.

FDA GUIDELINES

Three general submission guidelines are provided:

Federal Regulations: This document provides a summary of (and links to) the relevant sections of the Federal Food, Drug, and Cosmetic Act, including 21 Code of Federal Regulations (CFR) part 210 (CMPs for Manufacturing; 21 CFR Part 211 (GMS for Finished Pharmaceuticals); and Guidance Documents for NDAs, ANDAs, and Out of Specification (OOS) Test Result Reporting.

FDA ESG: This document provides an overview of the process of electronic submissions and provides registration and confirmation processes as well as links to electronic submission requirements of the Center for Biologics Evaluation and Research (CBER), the Center for Drug Evaluation and Research (CDER), the Center for Veterinary Medicine (CVM), the Adverse Events Reporting System (AERS), and the Center for Devices and Radiological Health (CDRH).

Electronic Regulatory Submissions and Review (CDER): This document (from http://www.fda.gov/cder/regulatory/ersr/default.htm) provides specific ESG guidance for CDER submissions, including NDAs, INDs, and DMFs.

Federal Regulations

CFR. The final regulations published in the Federal Register (daily published record of proposed rules, final rules, meeting notices, etc.) are collected in the CFR. The CFR is divided into 50 titles, which represent broad areas subject to Federal regulations. The FDA's portion of the CFR interprets the Federal Food, Drug and Cosmetic Act and related statutes. Section 21 of the CFR contains most regulations pertaining to food and drugs. The regulations document the actions of drug sponsors that are required under Federal law.

- 21 CFR Part 210. Current Good Manufacturing Practice (CGMP) in Manufacturing Processing, Packing, or Holding of Drugs
- 21 CFR Part 211. CGMP for Finished Pharmaceuticals
- Federal Register Notices for Proposed Changes and Final Changes to CGMP. The Office of Compliance, Division of Manufacturing and Product Quality Web page provides links to in-process changes in CGMP regulations announced in the Federal Register.

Guidance Documents

Guidance documents represent the FDA's current thinking on a particular subject. These documents are prepared for FDA review staff and drug sponsors to provide guidelines for the processing, content, and evaluation of applications, and for the design, production, manufacturing, and testing of regulated products. They also provide consistency in the Agency's regulation, inspection, and enforcement procedures. Because guidances are not regulations or laws, they are not enforceable. An alternative approach may be used if it satisfies the requirements of the applicable statute, regulations, or both.

- Guideline on the Preparation of Investigational New Drug Products (Human and Animal) (Issued November 1992, posted March 2, 1998). This guidance provides practices and procedures for preparing investigational new drug products that comply with certain section of the CGMP regulations for finished pharmaceuticals (Title 21 of the CFR, Parts 210 and 211.)
- Draft Guidance for Industry: Investigating OOS Test Results for Pharmaceutical Production. September 30, 1998 This guidance provides the Agency's current thinking on how to evaluate suspect, or OOS test results. For purposes of this document, the term *OOS results* includes **all** suspect results that fall outside the specifications or acceptance criteria established in new drug applications.
- Draft Guidance for Industry: ANDAs: Blend Uniformity Analysis. This guidance provides recommendations on when and how blend uniformity analysis should be performed. The recommendations apply to original ANDAs and supplemental ANDAs for formulation and process changes. The Federal Register notice for this draft is also available.

CDER Manual of Policies and Procedures (MaPPs)

MaPPs are approved instructions for internal practices and procedures followed by CDER staff to help standardize the new drug review process and other activities. MaPPs define external activities as well. All MaPPs are available for the public to review to acquire a better understanding of office policies, definitions, staff responsibilities, and procedures.

- 4723.1 Standing Operating Procedures for NDA/ANDA Field Alert Reports. (Issued October 30, 1998, posted November 2, 1998). This MaPP establishes a system for evaluating NDA and ANDA Field Alert Reports and provides instructions to the responsible CDER units for handling those reports.

Compliance Policy Programs and Guidelines

- Compliance References. This Web site from the Office of Regulatory Affairs provides links to compliance policy guides, regulatory procedures manuals, and other compliance-related information. Chapter 4 of the Compliance Policy Guide covers human drugs.

- Compliance Program Guidance Manual. These programs and instructions are for FDA field inspectors.
- Consistent Application of CGMP Determinations. The FDA cannot approve applications to market new drugs from companies that have been cited for CGMP violations. Similarly, disapproval of any drug marketing application based upon CGMP deficiencies must also lead to regulatory and/or administrative action against other products produced under the same conditions.

Compliance Questions and Answers

- Human Drug CGMP Notes. These memos are intended to enhance field/ headquarters communications on CGMP issues in a timely manner. The document is a forum to hear and address CGMP questions, provide updates on CGMP projects, and clarify and help apply existing policy to day-to-day activities of FDA staff.

FDA ESG USER GUIDE

July 25, 2007

Introduction

The business of the FDA is extremely information intensive. In recognition of this fact and of the potential benefits offered by information technology for assisting with the management of information, the FDA has undertaken a number of projects supporting the electronic submission of text and data from the industries it regulates.

One of these projects entails the establishment of an Agency-wide solution (referred to as the FDA ESG) for accepting electronic regulatory submissions. The FDA ESG enables the submission of regulatory information for review. The overall purpose of the FDA ESG is to provide a centralized, Agency-wide communications point for receiving electronic regulatory submissions, securely. The new Agency Gateway will enable the FDA to process regulatory information through automated mechanisms while it enables

- a single point of entry for the receipt and processing of all electronic submissions in a highly secure environment;
- automating current electronic processes such as the electronic acknowledgment of submissions; and
- supporting the electronic common technical document (eCTD).

The electronic submission process is defined as the receipt, acknowledgment, routing, and notification to a receiving center of the receipt of an electronic submission. In this definition,

- "receipt" means transfer of a submission from a sender's system to a temporary storage area in the FDA ESG;
- "acknowledgment" to the sender means the submission was sent from the sender's system and received by the Gateway;
- "routing" means delivering a submission to a center-level storage area and initiating a load process to place a submission into a center receiving system; and
- "notification" of a submission's arrival is made to those individuals responsible for the Center's receiving system.

Each of these terms denotes a step in the process of electronic submission delivery, and together, these steps comprise the whole scope of electronic submission delivery.

The FDA ESG is the central transmission point for sending information electronically to the FDA. Within that context, the FDA ESG is a conduit, or a "highway," along which submissions travel to reach their final destination. It does not open or review submissions; it merely routes them to the proper destination.

The FDA ESG uses a software application certified to comply with secure messaging standards. The screen graphics provided in the FDA ESG Web Interface sections of this User Guide are from the application.

The objective of this User Guide is to provide industry participants with information and guidance on how to prepare and send documents through the FDA ESG. A list of submissions that the FDA ESG will accept is given in Table 1.2. This document provides a high level description of the electronic submission process via the FDA ESG.

Overview of the Registration Process

Registering to use the FDA ESG involves a set of sequential steps that are to be conducted for all submitters and types of submissions. The first steps in the process are designed to ensure that the FDA ESG can successfully receive electronic submissions and that the electronic submissions are prepared according to published guidelines. The testing phase is done using the FDA ESG test system. Once the sender has passed the testing phase, an account will be set up, allowing the submissions to be sent to the FDA ESG production system.

Figure 1.1 illustrates the steps in the process. The remaining subsections in this section will explain each of the steps in turn.

Apply for a Test Account. Organizations that wish to submit electronically to the FDA must apply for an account to establish themselves as Transaction Partners. The term "Transaction Partner" refers to

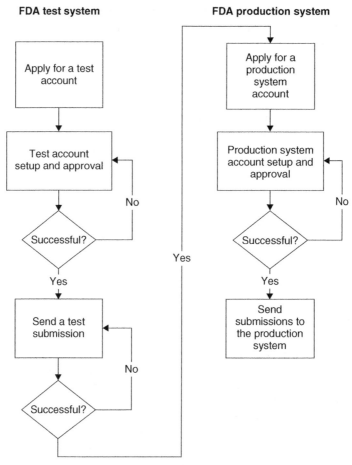

Figure 1.1   Overview of the registration process

an external entity authorized by the FDA to submit electronic submissions. Authorization includes agreement to regulatory conditions, successful completion of a certification process, and FDA administrative inclusion as a Transaction Partner.

Application for a test account must be initially requested for the FDA ESG. This is done to enable Transaction Partners to send a test submission to the FDA ESG.

Applying for an account involves information-sharing activities between the Transaction Partner and the FDA to set up transmission, receipt, and identification parameters. This ensures the correct identification of the Transaction Partner to the FDA. Digital certificate information is provided to the FDA as part of the application.

Test Account Setup and Approval. The account application is reviewed by the FDA ESG Administrator. The Administrator verifies that a letter of nonrepudiation agreement is on file, that the digital certificate conforms to the X.509 version 3 standard, and that all data fields in the **Issuer** and **Subject** fields are completed (see *Appendix A, Digital Certificates* for more information). The Administrator will also communicate with the Transaction Partner to confirm the application information. If these conditions are met, a test account is set up, and connections to the FDA ESG test system are established before the submitting organization is approved as a Transaction Partner.

Send a Test Submission. By sending a test submission, the Transaction Partner ensures the following conditions are met.

- The test submission is received by the FDA ESG. A notification is sent by the FDA ESG, confirming that the submission was successfully received.
- The submission is routed to the correct Center Holding Area.
- The submission is prepared according to regulatory guidelines. The Center sends an acknowledgment confirming that the submission was prepared correctly.

During the testing process, Transaction Partners who will be sending submissions larger than 1 GB will be asked to send a 7.5-GB test submission. This test will allow Transaction Partners to identify and resolve network limitations that will impact the speed of delivery. Send 7.5-GB test submissions to the GW TEST Center and select "SIZE TEST" as the submission type.

When testing connectivity, do not send the submission to the actual Center. Instead, send all connectivity test submissions to the GW TEST Center with the submission type "CONNECTION TEST." Only guidance compliance test submissions should be sent to the FDA Center.

Apply for a Production System Account. Applying for a Production System Account in the FDA ESG follows the same process as applying for a test account. (see "Apply for a Test Account")

Production System Account Setup and Approval. The same process is followed to setup a Production System Account as for a Test Account (see "Test Account Setup and Approval").

Send Submissions to the Production System. After completion of these steps, the Transaction Partner is enabled and approved to send submissions to the FDA ESG. The Production System Account allows the Transaction Partner to send any of the supported submission types to the FDA. **However, the FDA**

will process those submission types only for which the Transaction Partner has received prior approval.

NOTE: It is the responsibility of the Transaction Partner to consult the appropriate FDA Center for information on formats, deadlines, and other information or procedures for submissions.

Preparatory Activities

There are a number of preparatory activities that need to be completed before beginning the registration process. This section describes these preparatory activities and presents system and protocol issues for FDA ESG users to consider.

Submit Letter of Nonrepudiation Agreement. A letter of nonrepudiation agreement **must** be submitted to the FDA. See *Appendix B, Sample Letters of Nonrepudiation Agreement*, for letter examples.

The nonrepudiation agreement allows the FDA to receive electronically signed submissions in compliance with 21CFR Part 11.100.

Obtain Digital Certificate. A digital certificate must be obtained.

Digital certificates ensure private and secure submission of electronic documents. The digital certificate binds together the owner's name and a pair of electronic keys (a public key and a private key) that can be used to encrypt and sign documents.

Digital certificates can be obtained from either a public or a private Certificate Authority. It must be an X.509 version 3 certificate, and all data fields in the **Issuer** and **Subject** fields must be completed. See *Appendix A, Digital Certificates* for more information on digital certificates.

Understand Submission Guidelines. Each FDA Center has specific guidelines that must be followed for successful submission. Table 1.1 contains links to Center-specific preparation guidelines and contacts. Table 1.2 lists electronic submissions supported by the FDA ESG. Important information on the use of digital/electronic signatures on FDA forms can be found in *Appendix C, Digital Signatures*.

The submission acronyms or names listed in Table 1.2 are not to be used as attributes in the submission header. See Table G-1 in *Appendix D, AS2 Header Attributes*, for a list of allowed attributes for the different submission types.

Naming Conventions. A special consideration applies to the naming convention for files and directories. The following characters are not recommended for use when naming submission files and directories.

/—forward slash
\—backslash

TABLE 1.1 FDA links to submission preparation guidelines

Center	Link
Center for Biologics Evaluation and Research (CBER)	http://www.fda.gov/cber/esub/esub.htm
Center for Drug Evaluation and Research (CDER)	http://www.fda.gov/cder/regulatory/ersr/default.htm
Center for Devices and Radiological Health (CDRH)	http://www.fda.gov/cdrh/cesub.html
Adverse Event Reporting System (AERS)	http://www.fda.gov/cder/aerssub/default.htm
Center for Veterinary Medicine (CVM)	http://www.fda.gov/cvm/esubstoc.html

Note: Meeting the requirements for using the FDA ESG to route submissions does not mean that these submissions automatically meet FDA Center-specific submission requirements.

For each test submission type, a test submission must be validated by the Center before sending submissions to the Production System.

It is the responsibility of the Transaction Partner to consult the appropriate FDA Center for information on formats, deadlines, and other information or procedures for submissions.

TABLE 1.2 Electronic submissions supported by the FDAESG

Center	Submissions
CBER	AERS—Adverse Event Reports
	AERS—Attachments
	BLA—Biologics License Application (eCTD and eBLA format)
	eCTD—Electronic Common Technical Document
	IDE—Investigational Device Exemption
	IND—Investigational New Drug Application (eCTD and eIND format)
	DMF—Drug Master File
	Promotional Materials
	Lot Distribution Data
CDER	AERS—Adverse Event Reports
	AERS Attachments
	ANDA—Abbreviated New Drug Application
	BLA—Biologics License Application (eCTD and eBLA format)
	eCTD—Electronic Common Technical Document
	NDA—New Drug Application (eCTD and eNDA format)
	IND—Investigational New Drug Application
CDRH	Adverse Events
	Electronic Submissions
CVM	Electronic Submissions
GW TEST[a]	CONNECTION TEST
	SIZE TEST

[a]These submission types are supported in the test environment only and are intended solely for testing.

:—colon

?—question mark

"—quotation marks

<—less than sign

>—greater than sign

|—vertical bar,

space—If you need to use a space, use_an_underscore_instead or SeparateWordsWithCapitalLetters.

Note: Directories and subdirectories cannot begin with the "." (dot) character.

Determine Submission Method. There are three options for sending FDA ESG submissions.

1. FDA ESG Web Interface sends submissions via Hyper Text Transfer Protocol Secure (HTTPS) through a web browser according to Applicability Statement 2 (AS2) standards.
2. Applicability Statement 1 (AS1) Gateway-to-Gateway is an electronic submission protocol that uses secure e-mail for communications.
3. Applicability Statement 2 (AS2) Gateway-to-Gateway is an electronic submission protocol that uses HTTP/HTTPS for communications.

Determining the best of these options for your organization will be influenced by the types of submissions to be transmitted, infrastructure capabilities, and business requirements.

One or more of these options can be selected to submit electronic documents to the FDA. However, a separate registration will be required for each option selected.

Considerations for each option are shown in Table 1.3.

A factor that determines how quickly a submission can be sent to the FDA ESG is the Transaction Partner's network connection to the Internet. Table 1.4 lists the maximum transmission rates for a variety of network connections and the optimal time it would take to send a 1-GB submission.

Actual times will be greater than those listed in the table due to factors such as network configuration and the amount of traffic coming in and going out through the line. For example, submissions sent in the middle of the day typically take 1.5–2 times longer to send than those sent after business hours. Pilot testing with selected Industry Transaction Partners has shown that it takes approximately 24h for submissions 15GB to 25GB in total size to be transmitted and processed by the FDA ESG. These companies had T3 network connections or better. FDA recommends that submissions of this size be sent overnight, starting at 4:30 p.m. EST, for the submission to be received by the target Center before the end of the next business day.

TABLE 1.3   Considerations for submission protocol choice

Transaction partner considerations	FDA ESG Web Interface	AS1 Gateway-to-Gateway	AS2 Gateway-to-Gateway
Cost	None	High setup and support costs	High setup and support costs
Setup	Minimal	Need to install and configure Gateway	Need to install and configure Gateway
User-friendly Web interface	Yes	No	No
Submission types supported	All, including AERS reports	AERS Reports and AERS Attachments only	All, including AERS reports
Long-term support by FDA	Yes	This particular protocol will be phased out in May 2007	Yes
Preparation of multifile submissions[a]	Occurs automatically	Not applicable	Multifile submissions need to be archived and compressed by using a tar and gzip utility prior to submission
Custom attributes for submission routing[b]	Automatically adds custom attributes to the AS2 header	Not applicable	Need to add custom attributes to the AS2 header
Integration to back-end systems	No	Can be automated	Can be automated
Tracking of submission activity by Transaction Partner	Manual tracking	Can be automated	Can be automated
Automation of submission process	No	Yes	Yes

[a]See *Appendix E, Creating tar Files and Compressing Files for Submission.*
[b]See *Appendix D, AS2 Header Attributes.*

During the testing process, Transaction Partners who will be sending submissions larger than 1 GB in total size will be asked to send a 7.5-GB test submission. This test will allow Transaction Partners to identify and resolve network limitations that will impact the speed of delivery.

TABLE 1.4   Transmission rates for network connections and optimal times for transmission

Network connection	Max. transmission rate (Mbps)	Time (min) 1 GB
T1	1.54	83
T2	6.31	21
T3	44.7	3
OC1	51.8	2.5
OC3	155.4	0.8
T4	274.8	0.5
OC12	621.6	0.2

Mbps = Megabits per second.
1 GB (Gigabyte) = 8,590 Megabits.

Connection Requirements. FDA ESG Web Interface users need the following:

- A high-speed Internet connection
- A web browser, either Internet Explorer 6 (or later) or Mozilla Firefox 1.0 (or later)
- Hard disk space of at least three times the size of the submission. For instance, if the submission is 1 MB in size, then at least 3 MB of hard disk space is required.
- Sun's Java Runtime Edition (JRE) 1.5.10, for the browser plug-in files

See *Appendix F, Java Runtime Edition Installation* for more information on obtaining and installing JRE.

Gateway functionality is optimized with JRE version 1.5.10 installed. It is recommended that the automatic Java update option on the computer be disabled to avoid the automatic installation of a different version of JRE. The steps to do this are as follows:

1. Select Control Panel from the Start menu.
2. Double-click on the Java (or Java Plug-In) icon.
3. Click on the "Update" tab.
4. Uncheck the "Check for Updates Automatically" checkbox.
5. Click OK.

Gateway-to-Gateway users need the following:

- A high-speed Internet connection
- An AS1- and AS2-compliant Gateway product
- Hard disk space of at least three times the size of the submission

TABLE 1.5 Submission process aspects and help and information contacts

Submission process aspect	Contact
Preparation/Registration/Policy Questions	e-mail: esgprep@fda.gov
Technical Issues with Submissions after becoming a Production System Transaction Partner	FURLS Help Desk: 1-800-216-7331, available from 7:30 a.m. to 11:00 p.m., EST www.cfsan.fda.gov/~furls/helpf2.html (This Web site also contains an e-mail link.)
Center-specific Submission Guidance	See "Understand Submission Guidelines."

NOTE: AERS submissions can be sent by using the AS1 protocol. All other types of submissions, including AERS, can be sent by using the AS2 protocol.

Help and Information. There are resources that can be contacted if you need assistance with various aspects of the submission process. These are provided in Table 1.5.

FDA ESG Web Interface Electronic Submissions

The steps for the electronic submission process for FDA ESG Web Interface users are provided in the following sections.

Apply for a Test Account. Applying for an FDA ESG Web Interface Test account is a multistep process. Before beginning the process, the following information should be known:

- Company and contact information
- Digital certificate file location

The FDA ESG Web Interface address and a temporary Login ID and password can be obtained from the FDA ESG Administrator by sending an e-mail to esgprep@fda.gov indicating intent to register for the FDA ESG.

The remainder of this section describes the FDA ESG Test Account Application process using screen shots from the FDA ESG Web Interface.

1. Using the address provided by the FDA, access the FDA ESG Web Interface.

The **Login** page is displayed. Note the test environment warning on the **Login** page. If the **Login** page does not have this warning, do not continue. Exit the browser and contact the FDA ESG Administrator at esgprep@fda.gov to request access to the test environment.

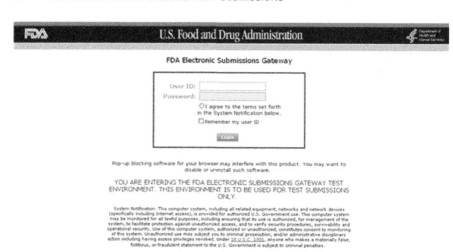

2. Enter the **User ID** and **Password** that was provided by the FDA and click the **Login** button.

The **Welcome to the WebTrader registration wizard** page is displayed. This wizard guides the Transaction Partner through the remainder of the application process.

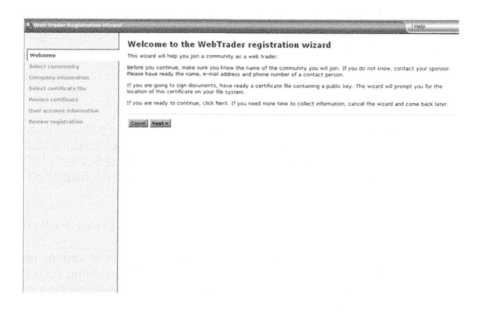

3. Click the **Next** button.

> The **Pick a community** page is displayed
>
> The community represents where submissions will be sent for logging, verification, and ultimately routing to the appropriate FDA Center. The only community will be "FDA VM."
>
> See *Appendix G, Glossary of Terms*, for more information about the community.

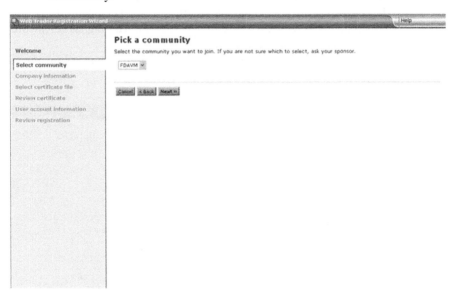

4. Click the **Next** button.

> The **Enter company information** page is displayed.
>
> This page records your company's name for identification purposes.

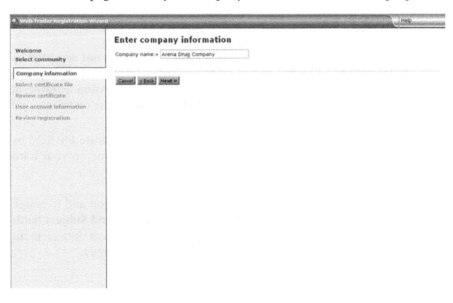

NOTE: Partners who have an existing account, whether it is AS1, AS2, or WebTrader, must enter a unique string (different from the one used when registering for their first account) in the "Company name" field. This is to ensure that this account is treated as a separate identity in the database.

5. Click the **Next** button.

   The **Locate the certificate file** page is displayed.

   This page is used to specify the location of the certificate file. Each submission must be accompanied by a certificate. The digital certificate must be an X.509 version 3 certificate.

   See *Appendix A, Digital Certificates* for more information about digital certificates.

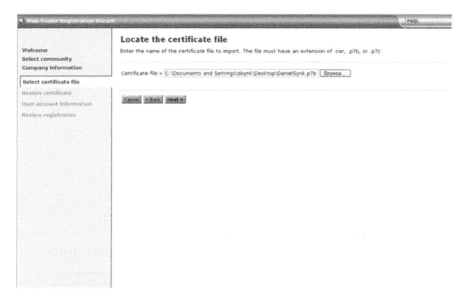

NOTE: There are situations where a valid certificate is not accepted by the registration module and an error message is returned. If this occurs, zip the certificate file and e-mail it to FDA ESG Administrator at esgprep@fda.gov. Once received, the FDA will assess the certificate and send a response.

6. Provide the desired digital certificate file in the **Certificate file** field by entering the name of the certificate or browsing for one on your hard drive by clicking on the **Browse** ... button.

   The **View certificate details** page is displayed.

   This page is used to review the certificate information and to assign a name to the certificate. Carefully review the **Issuer** and **Subject** fields to be sure that all data fields are completed (i.e., for each data element such as "CN," there is a value that follows the equal sign).

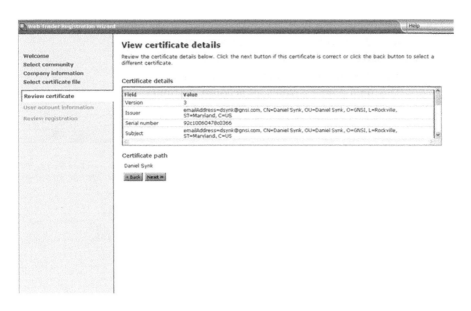

7. Click **Next**.

The **Enter user account information** page is displayed.

This page is used to specify the user ID, password, and contact information selected by the Transaction Partner. After registration is complete, this user ID and password will be used by the Transaction Partner to log on to the FDA ESG Web Interface.

8. Enter a new login user ID and password. Remember this user ID and password—it will be used for subsequent logins.
9. Click **Next**.
   The **Registration summary** page is displayed.
   This final page provides an account summary.

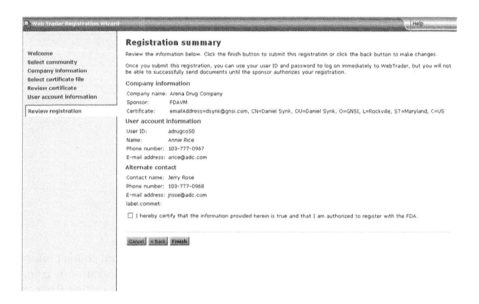

10. Check the box to certify the accuracy of your information.
11. Click the **Finish** button to return to the **Login** page, or close the browser window.

Test Account Setup and Approval. After a successful Test Account setup, the FDA sends an e-mail to the e-mail address provided for the contact, indicating approval as a Transaction Partner and authorization to send a test submission. Typically, the approval notification is sent on the next business day.

The test submission cannot be sent until this notification has been received.

JRE must be installed to send a submission. See *Appendix F, Java Runtime Edition Installation* for the installation procedures.

Once you have fulfilled these criteria, proceed to the next section for instructions on sending a test submission.

Send a Test Submission. After Test Account Setup and Transaction Partner approval, a test submission must be sent to ensure that the submission "conduit" is working properly from end to end. To do this, follow the steps below.

Confirm that the correct version of the JRE is installed before you begin. See *Appendix F, Java Runtime Edition Installation* for the version information and installation procedures.

1. Using the address provided by the FDA, access the FDA ESG Web Interface application.

    The **Login** page is displayed.

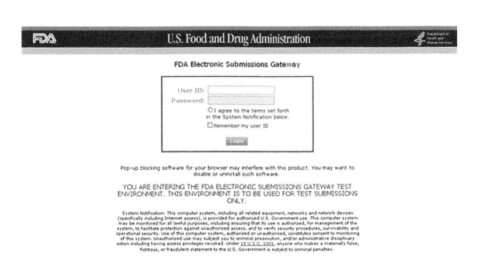

    Note the test environment warning on the **Login** page. If the **Login** page does not have this warning, do not send a test submission. Exit the browser and contact the FDA ESG Administrator at esgprep@fda.gov to request access to the test environment.

2. Enter the **user ID** and **password** that were set up in the registration wizard (see "Apply for a Test Account").

3. Click the **Login** button.

    After a successful login, the **My FDA submissions** page is displayed. This page lists all messages received from the FDA ESG.

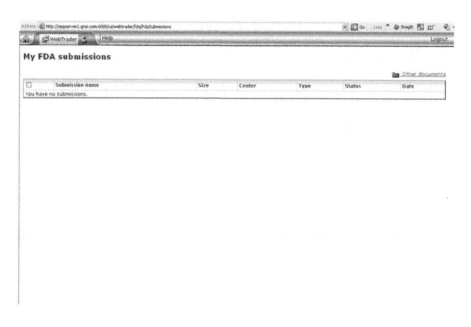

4. Click the **WebTrader** icon.
   The **WebTrader** drop-down menu is displayed.

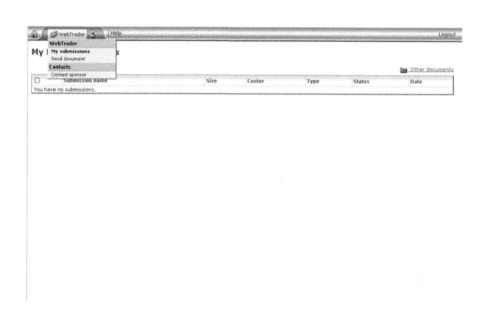

5. Select the **Send document** menu item.
   The **Send document** page is displayed.

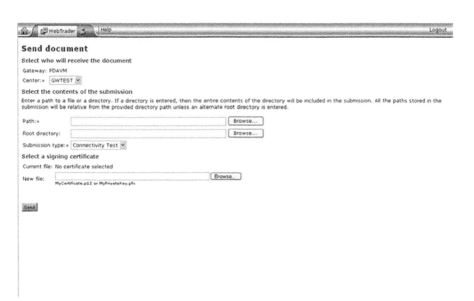

6. Select an FDA Center from the **Center** drop-down box. The Centers that can be selected at present are CBER, CDER, CDRH, CFSAN, CVM, or TESTING. Upon choosing a Center, the **Submission type** drop-down box will be populated with the correct submission types for that Center.

7. For single-file submissions, click the **Browse** button associated with the **Path** text box to select the test submission.

8. For multifile submissions, click the **Browse** button associated with the **Root Directory** text box to select the directory that contains all the files in the test submission. Make sure that the name of any file or subdirectory does not start with "." (dot). **Note:** The **Path** field is still required for multifile submissions. Make sure you have entered a path as well as a root directory.

9. Select a test submission type from the **Submission type** drop-down box. **About submission types:**

   • **Connectivity tests** ensure that your connection to the ESG is up and running. They should be sent to the "Testing" Center.

   • **Load tests** ensure that you are able to send large submissions through the ESG; you should perform a load test if you are planning on sending submissions larger than 100 MB. Load tests should be sent to the "Testing" Center. See "Sending Large (>7.5 GB) Submissions" section.

> • **Guidance-compliant submission tests** are reviewed by your Center so it can clear you for a production account. Guidance-compliant submissions should be sent to your Center.

10. Select a signing certificate by clicking the associated **Browse** button and selecting the signing certificate. All submissions require a certificate to digitally sign and encrypt the submission.

    Note that connectivity tests should only be sent to TESTING, not actual centers.

    The completed **Send document** page should be populated similar to the page below.

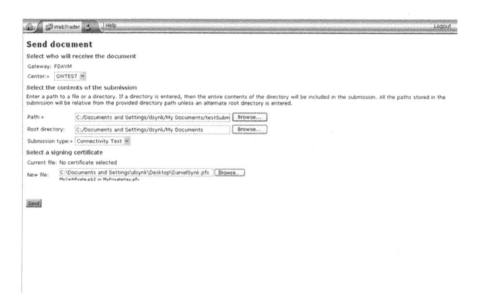

11. Click the **Send** button on the **Send document** page.

    The **Enter password** dialog box is displayed on top of the **Send document** page.

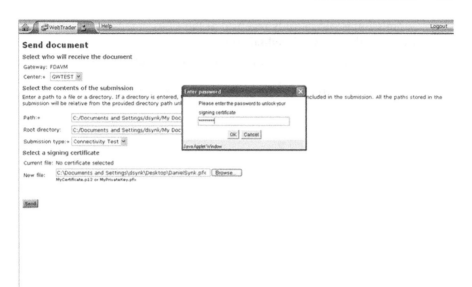

12. Enter the certificate password and click **OK** in this dialog box.

   The **Upload Progress** dialog box is displayed on the **Send document** page:

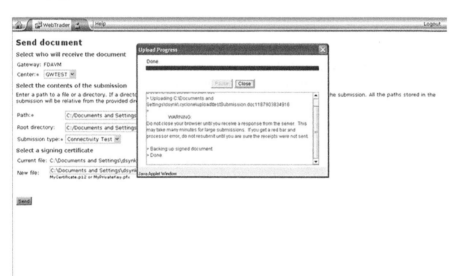

13. When the upload is complete (indicated by the display of **Done**), click the **Close** button in the **Upload Progress** dialog box.

   At this point, the test submission is sent. The FDA ESG logs the submission and verifies submission destination and type. When the submission is successfully received at the FDA, a receipt e-mail will be listed on the **My FDA Submissions** page.

14. To access the receipt, click on the **WebTrader** icon to access the Inbox.

The **WebTrader** drop-down menu is displayed.

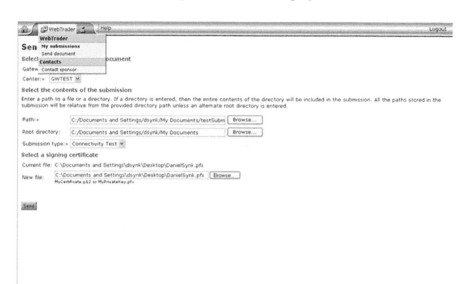

15. Select the **My Submissions** menu item.

The **My FDA submissions** page is displayed.

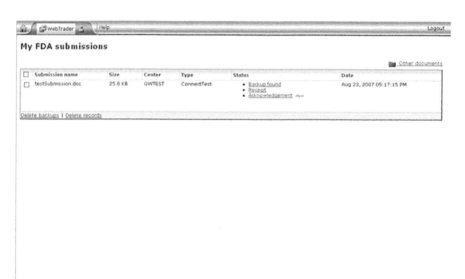

The receipt for the test submission should be displayed here. This first receipt confirms that the submission was received by the FDA ESG. Click on the **Details** link to access the receipt contents.

If there are any errors in the submission, the receipt will not appear on the **My FDA submissions** page but will be sent to the Documents in the Inbox page. The receipt will contain information about why the submission failed.

The FDA ESG will then route the test submission to the Center Holding Area. When the Center system successfully receives the submission, a second acknowledgment will be sent confirming that the Center has received the submission. The Center will then validate the test submission.

Contact the FDA ESG testing representative at esgprep@fda.gov if the receipt for the test submission or the Center acknowledgement is not received.

The next step is to apply for an FDA ESG Production System Account. This process is described in the following section.

Sending Large (>7.5 GB) Submissions   The FDA ESG is able to receive and process regulatory submissions up to 100 GB. The major consideration in determining how quickly large submissions are transmitted to the FDA ESG is the bandwidth available to the Transaction Partner between their company and the FDA ESG. The FDA has the following recommendations concerning the transmission of large regulatory submissions.

- During the testing phase, send a 7.5-GB test submission. This test will allow Transaction Partners to evaluate bandwidth availability and to adjust their network configuration as necessary. This test submission should be sent to the "Testing" Center with "7.5 GB Submission" as the submission type.
- Send a 7.5 GB test submission that is representative of an actual submission. The Web Interface archives and compresses the submission into a single file prior to transmission. Submissions that consist of text files will compress to a greater extent than portable document format (PDF) files, will transmit faster, and thus give an inaccurate assessment of the time it takes for submissions to be sent and processed by the FDA ESG.
- Send submissions greater than 7.5 GB overnight. Pilot testing with selected Industry Transaction Partners has shown that it takes approximately 24 h for submissions 15–25 GB in total size to be transmitted and processed by the FDA ESG. These companies had T3 network connections or better. FDA recommends that large submissions be sent overnight, starting at 4:30 p.m. EST, for the submission to be received by the target Center before the end of the next business day.

Sending large submissions may result in the FDA ESG Web interface erroneously reporting that the transmission was not successful, even though the

FDA ESG has successfully received the transmission. This is a known bug, and the FDA has asked Axway to provide an update to the Web interface that fixes this error.

When the FDA ESG has received a complete submission, a backup copy is made before the Java applet receives a reply from the server confirming the submission is complete. For large submissions (>7.5 GB), this can take many minutes. Since there is no network activity for such a long time, the session has time-outs and the Java applet never receives the response. The FDA ESG has received the submission successfully, but the Java applet returns an error and indicates that the submission needs to be resumed. Receipt of the first acknowledgment [Message Delivery Notification (MDN)] confirms that the submission was successfully received by the FDA ESG and that it is okay to cancel the resume request. Since this is a large submission, it will take several hours before the first acknowledgment is received.

If you receive this error and it has clearly occurred at the end of the transmission, do not resend the submission right away. Wait for several hours (or longer, depending on the size of the submissions) and see if the MDN is sent before attempting to resend the submission.

Apply for a Production System Account. The steps for applying for an FDA ESG Production System Account are the same as those described in "Apply for a Test Account" section.

However, there is a difference in the **Login** page. The **Login** page *should not* have the test environment warning that it has when sending a test submission; it should look like the **Login** page shown below:

FDA — U.S. Food and Drug Administration — Department of Health and Human Services

FDA Electronic Submissions Gateway

User ID

Password

☐ Remember my user ID

Login

Licensed to: FDA

Pop-up blocking software for your browser may interfere with this product. You may want to disable or uninstall such software.

If the **Login** page does have the warning, do not send a submission. Exit the browser, contact the FDA ESG Administrator at esgprep@fda.gov, and obtain the correct address for the FDA ESG **Login** page.

Production System Account Setup and Approval. After successful completion of the Production System Account setup, the FDA sends an e-mail to the e-mail address provided for the primary contact, indicating approval as a Transaction Partner and authorization to send submissions to the FDA ESG. Typically, the approval notification is sent on the next business day.

Submissions cannot be sent to the FDA ESG until this notification has been received.

Send Submissions to the Production System. The steps to send a Submission to the FDA ESG are the same as those in the "Send a Test Submission" section.

However, there is a difference in the **Login** page. The **Login** page *should not* have the test environment warning that it has when sending a test submission; it should look like the **Login** page shown in the "Apply for a Production System Account" section.

If the **Login** page does have the warning, do not send a submission. Exit the browser, contact the FDA ESG Administrator at esgprep@fda.gov, and obtain the correct address for the FDA ESG **Login** page.

Tracking Submissions. Once a submission has been sent by using the FDA ESG Web Interface, the Transaction Partner can track the submission to ensure that it was received by the FDA ESG and the Center.

The Submission Process   When a submission is sent by using the FDA ESG Web Interface, it goes through the following steps.

1. The submission is transmitted by using the FDA ESG Web Interface to the Gateway. When the FDA ESG receives this submission, it sends a receipt known as an MDN to the Inbox of the account from which the submission was received.
2. The submission is delivered from the FDA ESG to a central holding area for all the Centers.
3. The submission is then delivered from the holding area to the appropriate Center. When a Center receives a submission, it sends an acknowledgment to the Inbox of the account from which the submission was sent.

MDNs and Acknowledgments   When a submission is sent by using the FDA ESG Web Interface, the following two messages are delivered to the Inbox of the account from which the submission was sent.

1. A receipt from the FDA ESG, also known as an MDN. This message denotes that the submission has been delivered to the FDA ESG. The name of the receipt message includes the file name of the submission that was sent. If a directory of files was submitted, the file name of the submission will be the name of the directory followed by the extension ".tar.gz". The MDN message contains the message ID of the submission and a date stamp for when the submission was received by the FDA ESG. These items may be used to track a submission.

2. An acknowledgment from the Center to which the submission was sent. This file is named with a unique alphanumeric string known as the Core ID. The Core ID is also used by the FDA ESG to track a submission.

A sample Inbox looks similar to this, once submissions have been sent:

My FDA submissions

📖 Other documents

Submission name	Size	Center	Type	Status	Date
testSubmission.doc	25.8 KB	GWTEST	ConnectTest	• Backup found • Receipt • Acknowledgement *New*	Aug 23, 2007 05:17:15 PM

Delete backups | Delete records

Message IDs and Core IDs   Among other information, the MDN contains a Message ID and a time stamp denoting the time the submission was received. The Message ID is a unique alphanumeric string that identifies each submission. This Message ID can also be used to track a submission and to correlate a submission to its Center acknowledgment.

A sample MDN looks similar to the file shown below. The Message ID and date stamp in this MDN are highlighted.

```
Message-ID: <1140124426654.2852@11nap01>
Date: Thu, 16 Feb 2006 21:13:46 GMT
From: esgprep@fda.gov
Subject: AcmeDrugCompany;ZZFDA
Mime-Version: 1.0
Content-Type: multipart/signed; micalg=sha1; protocol="application/pkcs7-
signature"; boundary="----=_Part_65_16583928.1140124426654"
X-Cyclone-From: ZZFDA
X-Cyclone-To: AcmeDrugCompany
Content-Length: 1952

------=_Part_65_16583928.1140124426654
Content-Type: multipart/report; report-type=disposition-notification;
        boundary="----=_Part_64_17446017.1140124426654"

------=_Part_64_17446017.1140124426654
Content-Type: text/plain; charset=us-ascii

This MDN (Message Disposition Notification) was automatically built on
Thu, 16 Feb 2006 21:13:46 GMT in response to a message with id
<12689343.1140124473009.JavaMail.sacharya@pvenkat> received from
ZZFDA on Thu, 16 Feb 2006 21:13:46 GMT.
Unless stated otherwise, the message to which this MDN applies
was successfully processed.

------=_Part_64_17446017.1140124426654
Content-Type: message/disposition-notification

Original-Message-ID: <12689343.1140124473009.JavaMail.sacharya@pvenkat>
Disposition: automatic-action/MDN-sent-automatically; processed
Received-Content-MIC: Jkm19bjOa6J8JBn/pv87oYIBnTA=, sha1
```

When a Center receives a submission, it associates the submission's Message ID with a Core ID. This Core ID can be used along with the Message ID generated as part of the MDN to track a submission on the FDA ESG. A sample acknowledgment message with the Core ID highlighted is shown below:

```
MessageId: <12689343.1140124473009.JavaMail.sacharya@pvenkat>

CoreId: 1140124426155.2844@11nap01

DateTime Receipt Generated: 02-16-2006, 16:17:11

The date and time stamp contained in this message conveys when CBER
received your submission from the Electronic Submission Gateway.  If
your submission was received at CBER after 4:30 PM EST, the official
receipt date for the submission is the next government business day.
```

Accessing MDNs and Acknowledgments   To access an MDN after sending a submission, follow the steps below.

1. Log on to the ESG using the user name and password for the account from which you sent the submissions.

2. From the **WebTrader** menu, select the "Check inbox" option. The receipts that are displayed specify the name of the submission file as part of their name.

3. Click the **Details** link next to the name of the required receipt to see its details.

To access an acknowledgment after sending a submission, follow the steps below.

1. Log on to the ESG using the user name and password for the account from which you sent the submissions.

2. From the **WebTrader** menu, select the "Check inbox" option. The messages with ".ack" or ".txt" extensions are the acknowledgments from Centers for submissions. The message name before the extension denotes the Core ID generated by the Center for the submission.

3. Click on the name of the required acknowledgment to see its details.

ELECTRONIC REGULATORY SUBMISSIONS AND REVIEW (ERSR)

The ERSR Web page (http://www.fda.gov/cder/regulatory/ersr) provides information about the electronic submission of regulatory information to the Center and its review by CDER staff. Additional guidance documents, when available in draft or final form, will be added to the Web page.

Submission of Electronic Documents (June 7, 2004)

- Send all electronic submissions (except ANDAs) to
  5901-B Ammendale Road
  Beltsville, MD 20705
- Send ANDA submissions to
  7500 Standish Place, E-150
  Rockville, MD 20855

Electronic Regulatory Submissions

General Considerations. CDER and CBER have copublished a guidance document called *Guidance for Industry: Providing Regulatory Submissions in Electronic Format–General Considerations* (http://www.fda.gov/cder/guidance/6719.fnl.htm). This document provides general information about the electronic submissions process.

Note: In the general considerations guidance, we recommend the following: Digital Tape–Digital Equipment Corp. DLT 20/40 and 10/20-GB format using OPENVMS with VMS backup or NT server 4.0 with NT backup or backup exec.

Since the release of this guidance, there have been some changes in CDER. First, we are currently not able to accept tapes using OPENVMS with VMS backup. Second, we are able to use 35/70 DLT tapes. We are not, however, able to handle 40/80 DLT tapes. We are working on an update to this guidance and are planning to add this information accordingly. (Posted March 1, 2001)Since the above posting on March 1, 2001, CDER has now been able to handle 40/80 DLT tapes, although we prefer 35/70. CDER cannot process DLT tapes that have been prepared by using the backup applet included with the Windows 2000 operating system. It is recommended that systems running Windows 2000 use backup exec to produce the DLT transport tape for CDER. (Posted September 28, 2001)

For more information on ERSR guidance documents, please contact Randy Levin at randy.levin@fda.hhs.gov.

ANDAs. Information on electronic data sets that accompany an ANDA submission:

You may now submit ANDAs in electronic format in place of paper. We have placed the ANDA on public docket 92S-0251 as a submission acceptable in electronic format as allowed under 21 CFR Part 11. It should be noted that Part 11 requires that data sets provided in electronic format and used in the review process meet the requirements for archiving, i.e., protection of those records to enable their accurate and ready retrieval throughout the records retention period.

Electronic data sets, including those accompanying a paper submission, cannot be considered as official and used to support the application if they are submitted in a file format that is not archivable. As FDA and industry progress in meeting the goals of use of electronic submissions, compliance with electronic submission regulations will be expected. Typically, electronic data sets accompany an ANDA to support the review of bioequivalence studies. With the implementation of the guidance for industry Providing Regulatory Submissions in Electronic Format–ANDAs (June 2002), the submission of these data set records for use in the review should be in archivable format. At this time, the archival data set format is SAS Transport. (Posted July 15, 2002)

NDAs. Please refer to Providing Regulatory Submissions in Electronic Format–Human Pharmaceutical Product Applications and Related Submissions.

Carcinogenicity Data. An example of a SAS transport file for carcinogenicity data set is available. This is a self-extracting ZIP file that will be loaded to your C drive. If you download this file, the path to the example is: C:\WINDOWS\TEMP\example\N123456\pharmtox\datasets\101.

For more information on carcinogenicity data, please contact Karl Lin at karl.lin@fda.hhs.gov.

Providing Digital Electrocardiogram (ECG) Data

Why   The FDA is interested in having access to ECG waveform data collected during the course of "definitive" studies on drug effects on ventricular repolarization and annotated for interval measurements. The basis for this interest is described in detail in the concept paper "The Clinical Evaluation of QT Interval Prolongation and Proarrhythmic Potential for Non-antiarrhythmic Drugs," jointly authored by the U.S. and Canadian regulatory authorities and discussed at a joint FDA/DIA meeting in January 2003.

How   In 2004, the FDA announced its intent to accept annotated ECG waveform data in electronic format [extensible markup language (XML)] following the Health Level Seven (HL7) Annotated ECG Waveform Data Standard (aECG) accredited by the American National Standards Institute. You can find more detailed information on the aECG message standard and supporting materials by visiting the HL7 Version 3 ECG page and following the "Link to ECG Annotation Message Review Material." To facilitate access to the aECG data, FDA has entered into a Cooperative Research and Development Agreement with Mortara Instruments to develop and implement a digital data warehouse to collect, store, and archive aECG data from controlled clinical trials. FDA reviewers have access to this data warehouse to support their assessment of the risk of new drugs.

You can upload data to the warehouse for FDA access at the Mortara ECG Warehouse. For questions, contact the project manager in the appropriate review division.

Drug Master File (DMF).

Drug Master File (DMF).   Refer to the Guidance for Industry "Providing Regulatory Submissions in Electronic Format–Human Pharmaceutical Product Applications and Related Submissions Using the eCTD Specifications" for information on the submission of electronic DMFs.

For more information on electronic submissions for DMF, please contact CDER at esub@fda.hhs.gov. General DMF questions may be sent to dmfquestion@cder.fda.gov.

INDs.

INDs.   On March 26, 2002, the FDA published final guidance on the submission of INDs in electronic format to the CBER (http://www.fda.gov/cber/gdlns/eind.pdf). Once the IND submission to CBER is posted on public docket 92S-0251, we will be capable of accepting INDs submitted to CBER in electronic format without paper copies. At this time, we are not extending this to INDs submitted to CDER.

The electronic IND guidance leverages the current Biologics License Application /NDA guidances and the experience set from CBER's eIND pilot program. This guidance features PDF tables of contents, road-map files, and a folder structure that enables the reviewer to easily access and review documents. We expect the experience of receiving the IND applications and amendments with or without media, featuring an electronic signature, as well as the review of these electronic INDs submissions to help the FDA further other electronic submission initiatives.

In the future, we plan on upgrading the electronic IND filing and review process to include the use of XML-based technology. We are currently working toward accepting the electronic CTD using XML for marketing applications and will build on this to accept XML-based electronic INDs. Once this is completed, we will then issue draft guidance that incorporates the XML-based technology for all INDs including those submitted to CDER. We hope to have XML specifications for electronic INDs available in 2003.

- Federal Register notice for the public meeting to discuss the cumulative table of contents for the IND. Optional format: PDF. (Posted December 29, 2000)
- Agenda for the *Electronic Investigational New Drug Application: Cumulative Table of Contents (CTOC) Public Meeting.* (Posted January 22, 2001)
- *Electronic Investigational New Drug Application: Cumulative Table of Contents (CTOC)* (Posted December 6, 2000). This Web page provides technical information for an upcoming public meeting to discuss the possibility of a cumulative table of contents in XML for the electronic IND.

Launch Material and Other Submissions to the Division of Drug Marketing, Advertising, and Communications (DDMAC)

- *Draft Guidance: Providing Regulatory Submissions in Electronic Format– Prescription Drug Advertising and Promotional Labeling.* Optional format: PDF. (Issued January 2001, Posted January 30, 2001)

NDAs

- *Regulatory Submissions in Electronic Format; General Considerations.* (Issued January 1999, Posted January 27, 1999)
- MaPP 7600.7 Processing an Electronic NDA (Issued May 31, 2000, Posted June 5, 2000)
- Sample Electronic NDA Submission

Postmarketing Adverse Events Reporting

- *Guidance for Industry Providing Regulatory Submissions in Electronic Format–Postmarketing Expedited Safety Reports.* Optional format: PDF. This guidance document assists applicants making regulatory submissions in electronic format to CDER and CBER. (Issued May 2001, Posted May 25, 2001).

- *Postmarketing Expedited and Periodic Individual Case Safety Reports.* This allows for voluntary electronic submission of all postmarketing individual case safety reports, whether expedited or periodic, in electronic format in place of paper.
- AERS. A pilot program for electronic submission of individual case safety reports is now being conducted with pharmaceutical manufacturers with approved products. The format follows the International Conference on Harmonization (ICH) standards. For more information on the ICH, please contact Timothy Mahoney at mahoneyt@cder.fda.gov.
- For more information on the proposed electronic submission of individual case safety reports, see 63 *FR* 59746, Advanced Notice of Proposed Rulemaking for *Electronic Reporting of Postmarketing Adverse Drug Reactions*, published on November 5, 1998.

Electronic Review

Electronic Document Room (EDR)

- The EDR is an extension of the central document room. We perform a check on each submission sent to the EDR for file formats used and for integrity of bookmarks and hypertext links.
- NDA Conformance Checklist (February 22, 2000)

Secure e-Mail and the FDA ESG. e-Mail is in widespread use within CDER and industry. Secure e-mail between CDER and industry is useful for informal communications when confidential information may be included in the message (for example, trade secrets or patient information). Secure e-mails should not be used for formal regulatory submissions (for example, NDAs, INDs, amendments, and supplements).

Formal regulatory submissions can be securely submitted to CDER via the FDA ESG. For more information on the FDA ESG, see http://www.fda.gov/esg/default.htm.

For more information on establishing a secure e-mail link with CDER, contact Wendy Lee at wendy.lee@fda.hhs.gov.

Division Files System (DFS). DFS is the cornerstone of the administrative management of files initiative. It provides document management, tracking, archiving, and electronic signature capabilities for internally generated review documents. It also provides search and retrieval capabilities for final versions of internally generated review documents.

DFS is being developed incrementally. The first phase focuses on building an electronic repository for final review documents and for capturing signature information. The review documents tracked and saved by DFS are associated with regulatory submissions in the Centerwide Oracle Management Information System (COMIS). Future phases of DFS will include an update of COMIS assignments when the author signs the review in DFS. Reviewers use DFS to check in final review documents, to route them for sign-off, to sign off on them electronically, to automatically store review documents in the electronic repository, and to find and view documents stored in the DFS electronic repository.

The DFS is a graphical user interface software application that has the look and feel of most Windows-based applications. DFS uses standard Windows features, such as icons, drop-down menus, buttons, scroll bars, and dialog boxes.

Reviewer Training

- Electronic Submissions Training. Instructs reviewers on how to search for a specific NDA via the EDR Intranet site and to map the drive path of the folder. Acrobat Exchange is then used to open, navigate, view, follow links, create electronic notes, and copy and paste text, tables, and graphics into other applications from a sample electronic NDA.
- Electronic Data Analysis Training. Instructs reviewers on how to access NDA data in SAS Transport format via the EDR and to convert the files to formats that can be used with a variety of software packages. **NDA Electronic Data Analysis Training (NEDAT)** incorporates the use of the SAS System Viewer, Stat/Transfer, and JMP to convert the data and perform basic analysis. Additional introduction to JMP courses that discuss analysis of adverse events, exposure, efficacy, lab, and demographic data are also available.
- Creating PDF Reviewer Documents. Instructs reviewers on how to create a PDF version of a review document that maintains the formatting of the original MS Word document. Instruction covers fonts, paragraph, page, and section formatting are needed prior to converting an MS Word review document to the PDF archiving standard used in the DFS. Adobe Acrobat 4.0 is then used to convert the document to PDF and to open, view, and enhance the PDF review document.
- JMP. An introduction to JMP teaches reviewers how to use JMP to review electronic data. Users learn how to use a variety of JMP functions to analyze electronic data, with a specific focus on adverse event, laboratory, exposure, and efficacy data. Basic functions of summary tables, graphs, statistical tests, and the formula calculator are covered. The course is taught in the computer lab with hands-on instruction. Prior completion of the **NEDAT** course or familiarity with electronic data sets or both are recommended. Although primarily geared toward the clinical reviewer, the course provides useful instruction for reviewers of all disciplines.

Helpful Links

Docket. The Agency established the Electronic Submissions Public Docket number 92-0251 to provide a permanent location for a list of the Agency units that are prepared to receive electronic submissions, as well as a list of the specific types of regulatory records that can be accepted in electronic format (62 FR 13467, March 20, 1997).

PDF Format. PDF is an open format developed by Adobe Systems. Additional information is available at http://www.adobe.com.

SAS Transport File Format. We are able to archive data sets in SAS XPORT transport format, also called version 5 SAS transport format. This is an open, published file format developed by SAS Institute. For additional information, see the SAS Institute's Standards for Electronic Submissions and SAS XPORT transport format Web site.

Technical Assistance. For more general information regarding the preparation of submissions in electronic format, please contact the Electronic Submissions Coordinator at esub@fda.hhs.gov.

Recent Presentations

- 42nd Annual Meeting of the Drug Information Association, June 18–22, 2006, Philadelphia, PA
  - Gensinger, Gary, MBA, Director, Regulatory Review Support Staff, Office of Business Process Support; *Standards and Successful Document Creation*
  - Ventura, Virginia, Regulatory Information Specialist, FDA Office of Business Process Support; *eSUBS and eCTDs: Practical Advice and Pitfalls to Avoid*
- eCTD Tutorial, April 22, 2005, Rockville, MD, Agenda and Presentations (April 26, 2005)
- Electronic Submissions and Data Standards Quarterly Update, March 4, 2004, Rockville, MD, FDA
  - Update on Standard for Exchange of Nonclinical Data, Thomas Papoian, PhD, CDER
  - Overview of the eCTD Guidance and Its Implementation, Gary M. Gensinger, MBA, CDER
  - Introduction to SDTM v3.1, Norman Stockbridge, CDER
- Study Tagging File Workshop Thomas Selnekovic, CDER, February 26, 2004
- eCTD Workshop, February 26, 2004, Randy Levin, MD. CDER
- Public Meeting on Clinical Data Interchange Standard Consortium Version 3 Submission Data Standards and Electronic Case Report Tabulations, October 2, 2003, Rockville, MD (Posted October 7, 2003)

- Future of Case Report Tabulation Submissions, Randy Levin, MD,
- Web Submission Data Manager: Demonstration, Steve Wilson, DrPH.
- 2003 Annual DIA Meeting, June 2003, San Antonio TX (Posted July 15, 2003)
- DIA Annual Clinical Data Management Meeting in Philadelphia held on March 31, 2003.
  - Data Standards Update, Randy Levin, MD
- DIA Electronic Document Management Meeting, February 13, 2003 (Posted February 24, 2003)
  - DailyMed Initiative: Enhancing Patient Safety Through Accessible Medication Information, Randy Levin, MD
  - FDA Data Council Initiatives, Randy Levin, MD
- *Electronic Submissions to the FDA*, Randy Levin, MD, Fifth Annual Electronic Document Management Conference, September 23, 2002 (Posted November 14, 2002)
- *Impact of Regulations on Data Management Practice*, Randy Levin, MD, DIA Twelfth Annual European Clinical Data Management Conference, November 5, 2002 (Posted November 14, 2002)

Other ERSR Links

- CDER Electronic Records; Electronic Signature Regulations. This page provides links to pertinent *Code of Federal Regulations* and Federal Register documents.
- ERSR Agency Charter. Federal Register–Electronic Records; Electronic Signatures, Final Rule, March 20, 1997.

CHAPTER 2

FDA Meeting Requests

In the 1980s and 1990s, the FDA generally refused all requests for meetings with individual companies. In the words of one FDA official, "We are not your consultants."

Early in the twenty-first century, that policy changed. More slowly, the attitude is changing to meet the same policy. Sometimes reluctantly, the FDA will now meet to discuss Investigational New Drug (IND) plans, New Drugs Application (NDA) plans, and other drug development landmarks. These meetings are formal, generally proceed with a briefing document that defines for the Agency the specific issues to be discussed and provides detailed background information, and generally conclude with an official FDA letter outlining the Agency's responses and clarifying requirements.

On first pass, a letter requesting a meeting may seem insufficiently complex as to require a guidance chapter. This letter, however, has hidden dimensions. First, it is another important initial contact, setting the tone for Agency interactions. Second, it establishes the agenda for the pre-IND meeting, identifying the questions for discussion and (often) obtaining FDA buy-in on issues that are identified as noncontroversial. Finally, while the purpose of the document is to request a meeting, it is possible that the FDA will decline on the grounds that the questions raised are all noncontroversial. In such a situation, the meeting request serves to replace the Briefing Book and pre-IND meeting and significantly grows in importance.

Whether the meeting requested is to discuss an initial program of clinical research (the pre-IND meeting), to outline the intended IND or Abbreviated New Drug Application (ANDA), or to obtain feedback on an interim step or issue, the key to an effective meeting request letter lies in the questions posed. These questions are not the result of casual listing but rather are carefully crafted to obtain the results you are seeking.

First, avoid asking questions to which you do not know the answer. This is not an opportunity for research or general education. Make certain you thoroughly understand the requirements and guidance relevant to your product, and craft questions that do not merely seek factual summary.

Guidebook for Drug Regulatory Submissions, by Sandy Weinberg
Copyright © 2009 John Wiley & Sons, Inc.

Second, provide the Agency with sufficient background and details to obtain a targeted, applicable response to your questions. That background information is summarized in the Meeting Request Letter and is detailed and documented in the Briefing Book that follows the FDA's setting of a meeting date but precedes the meeting (usually by two or more weeks). Purely hypothetical questions may elicit positive responses, but, without context, those responses are of little use in planning and decision making. The FDA will not be held to a general response applied to a tightly defined specific situation. To get good answers, place questions in a clear and exact context.

Third, phrase questions to obtain, whenever possible, the answers your organization desires. Instead of "What does the agency require?" try "Based on the following rationale, we have determined the appropriate testing will be ... Does the agency agree?" Negative responses from the FDA will be accompanied by its interpretation of the requirements, but positives can be considered clear endorsements of your position, with an opportunity to argue your rationale (with appropriate supporting evidence) in advance of an Agency decision.

Avoid questions in which you try to tie the Agency to a position based upon a precedent. The FDA is not required to consistently follow a historical position as conditions evolve, and prior actions of one part of the FDA do not create inviolate precedents incumbent on other parts. While there is an attempt by the Agency to maintain fairness and consistency, the fundamental issue always is human health and safety. Concerns emerging from differing conditions or from advances in the field will always trump consistency.

Finally, consider including in your meeting request a dangerous but potentially very valuable open-ended question: "Is there anything else the Agency will require ... ." If the response is in the negative, or if the meeting is declined on the grounds that none of the questions are controversial, you will obtain a clear agreement on the extent and design of the clinical program. Of course, there is the risk that the FDA will take the opportunity to suggest additional studies or significant design changes, but, generally, it is best to have this information in advance and not at the conclusion of the clinical program.

Once the questions are formulated, the background context is explained and referenced, and the request is formulated, it is time to begin developing the Briefing Book. In fact, since the request may result in a meeting in a relatively short period (as early as a month from request) and since the Briefing Book may take several weeks to prepare, it may be prudent to overlap the two preparations. And, of course, the research and preparation of the Briefing Book can provide the contextual references to place the meeting questions in the appropriate context.

The Briefing Book repeats the key questions and is organized around those issues. It then provides a narrative summary of the question context, a bibliography of references relevant to those issues, and an indexed copy of those actual references.

The Meeting Request, Briefing Book, actual meeting, and FDA Summary Memo will provide important context and reaction to the planned IND, NDA, or ANDA. Careful design and careful management of the process can go far to a successful conclusion to the final NDA.

FDA MEETING REQUEST REVIEW CHECKLIST

Perhaps uniquely, the FDA has developed and distributed its own checklist for meeting requests, used internally to evaluate requests when they are received. Presumably, this unusual inclusion is a result of the relatively mundane—administrative only—review. The checklist can be found in the second FDA document included here: "How to Submit a Request for a Meeting or Teleconference in Electronic Format to CVM"—"Checklist."

Remember that after accepting or rejecting the Meeting Request Document, using the FDA's Checklist, the Agency makes a separate decision based on the content of the submitted document. Each question raised is considered. If all of the questions are considered noncontroversial (i.e., if the submitter's answers are all in agreement with Agency thinking), the request will be rejected as unnecessary, and approval to move ahead will be granted.

Meeting Request Submission Checklist

This checklist is intended for use in the preparation and submission of Meeting Requests. It is recommended that, prior to transmission to the FDA, a second internal review be conducted by an individual or department not involved (presumably Quality Assurance) in the preparation of the submission.

The checklist was developed through discussions with consultants and Quality Assurance directors and has been field-tested in final form with five successful requests.

- Request is addressed to current head of appropriate division or group.
- Cover letter includes
  - name and address of sponsor
  - name and address, title, telephone, e-mail of contact person
  - generic and trade name of drug or drug product
- Request conforms to style requirements as specified in FDA Guidance.
- Meeting request begins with a brief—approximately one-page—summary of developmental plan (i.e., in a request for a pre-IND meeting, summary describes planned IND process; a pre-NDA meeting describes the intended NDA procedures).
- Summary provides sufficient background to provide context for questions.
- Integrated references: All referenced articles are included in the final section, internally referenced in text.

- Request identifies 5 to 10 key questions for discussion.
- Each question provides a one-paragraph context, proposes the expected (desired) response, and is in the "Does the Agency agree?" formulation.
- Request includes final open-ended question in the "Does the Agency anticipate any additional requirements or areas of concern?" formulation.

GUIDANCE FOR INDUSTRY[1]—IND MEETINGS FOR HUMAN DRUGS AND BIOLOGICS. CHEMISTRY, MANUFACTURING, AND CONTROLS (CMC) INFORMATION

Contains Nonbinding Recommendations
Additional copies are available from:
Office of Training and Communication
Division of Drug Information (HFD-240)
Center for Drug Evaluation and Research
Food and Drug Administration
5600 Fishers Lane
Rockville, MD 20857
Tel: 301-827-4573
http://www.fda.gov/cder/guidance/index.htm
or

Office of Communication, Training and Manufacturers Assistance (HFM-40)
Center for Biologics Evaluation and Research
Food and Drug Administration
1401 Rockville Pike
Rockville, MD 20852-1448
http://www.fda.gov/cber/guidelines.htm
Fax: 1-888-CBERFAX or 301-827-3844
Phone: The Voice Information System at 800-835-4709 or 301-827-1800

U.S. Department of Health and Human Services
Food and Drug Administration
Center for Drug Evaluation and Research (CDER)
Center for Biologics Evaluation and Research (CBER)
May 2001
CMC

---

[1]This guidance was prepared by the IND Reform Committee of the Chemistry, Manufacturing, and Controls Coordinating Committee in CDER in cooperation with CBER at the FDA.

This guidance represents the FDA's current thinking on this topic. It does not create or confer any rights for or on any person and does not operate to bind the FDA or the public. An alternative approach may be used if such approach satisfies the requirements of the applicable statutes and regulations.

Introduction

This document provides guidance to industry on formal meetings between sponsors of IND applications and CDER or CBER on CMC information. This guidance applies to INDs for human drugs and biologics (referred to as *drugs*[2]).

This guidance covers three kinds of meetings that may be held between sponsors and the Agency: (1) pre-IND application, (2) end-of-phase 2 (EOP2), and (3) pre-NDA or prebiologics license application (pre-BLA). These meetings may be requested by the sponsor to address outstanding questions and scientific issues that arise during the course of a clinical investigation, to aid in the resolution of problems, and to facilitate evaluation of drugs. The meetings, which often coincide with critical points in the drug development and/or regulatory process, are recommended but not mandatory. Additional meetings may be requested at other times, if warranted. This guidance is intended to assist in making these meetings more efficient and effective by providing information on the (1) purpose, (2) meeting request, (3) information package, (4) format, and (5) focus of the meeting when the meeting addresses CMC information.

General information about meetings can be found in the following documents.

- Section 119 of the FDA Modernization Act (Pub. L. 105-115)
- Regulations applicable to meetings on investigational products in 21 Code of Federal Regulations (CFR) 312.47
- FDA guidance for industry on *Formal Meetings with Sponsors and Applicants for Prescription Drug User Fee Act (PDUFA) Products* (February 2000)
- FDA guidance for industry on *XFast Track Drug Development Programs Designation, Development, and Application Review* (November 1998)
- FDA policies and procedures for formal meetings with external constituents described in CDER's Manual of Policy and Procedures (MAPP 4512.1) and CBER Standard Operating Procedures and Policies (SOPP) 8101.1

---

[2]The term *investigational new drug* or *drug* as used in this guidance refers to the drug and/or biological substance and/or product.

General Aspects

The general aspects of pre-IND, EOP2, and pre-NDA meetings provided in this guidance summarize the information discussed in the formal meetings and fast-track drug development guidances listed in the "Introduction," and supplement this information with respect to CMC.

Purpose of Meeting. The purpose of meetings between sponsors and CDER or CBER on CMC information varies with the phase of the investigational study. For pre-IND meetings, the purpose is to discuss CMC issues as they relate to the safety of an IND proposed for use in initial clinical studies. The purpose of EOP2 meetings is to evaluate CMC plans and protocols to ensure that meaningful data will be generated during phase 3 studies to support a planned marketing application. Safety issues, nevertheless, will remain an important consideration during all phases of the study. The purpose of pre-NDA or pre-BLA meetings is to discuss filing and format issues. Under certain circumstances, other types of meetings may be appropriate, such as EOP1 meetings for fast-track drugs or meetings to discuss new protocols or changes during phase 3 studies that affect previously agreed upon strategies (see "EOP 2 Meetings").

Meeting Request. For general information on procedures for written meeting requests, sponsors should refer to the regulations, guidances, and policies and procedures listed in the "Introduction." The request should contain a list of the specific objectives and/or desired outcomes of the meeting, including a draft list of CMC-related questions.

Information Package. Sponsors should prepare an information package that includes a brief summary of the relevant CMC information, the developmental status, and the plan and time line for future development of the drug. The CMC-related questions should be presented in the information package in final form, grouped together, and identified. The questions should be as specific, comprehensive, and precise as possible to identify the critical issues. The questions should be presented in the same relative subject matter order as a typical CMC section of an application or as otherwise appropriate to aid in the review of the information. Sufficient CMC background information on the drug should be provided by the sponsor in the information package to allow the Agency to address the specific questions. Sponsors should coordinate the agenda and the content of the information package to expedite review of the material and discussion at the meeting. Where data presentation is appropriate, sponsors should present a summary of the data (e.g., tables, charts, graphs).

Format of Meeting
Multidisciplinary Meeting   Usually, the format of meetings prior to and during the IND stage is multidisciplinary, involving Agency personnel in clinical, pharmacology, pharmacokinetics, chemistry, microbiology, statistics, and other

disciplines. Sufficient time should be allotted during multidisciplinary meetings to discuss CMC issues. Of particular importance are CMC-related issues that affect other disciplines. The sponsor can provide a brief introductory presentation of CMC information; however, the majority of the meeting time allotted to CMC should be used to discuss specific CMC issues. Appropriate technical experts (e.g., chemists, microbiologists, biologists) representing the sponsor and the Agency should be present during all discussions of CMC-related issues.

CMC-Specific Meeting   Under appropriate circumstances, a separate CMC-specific meeting can be held in addition to, or as an alternative to, the multidisciplinary format. For example, a CMC-specific meeting is encouraged to discuss CMC issues that are too extensive or detailed to be adequately addressed in a multidisciplinary meeting or that are otherwise beyond the scope of a multidisciplinary meeting.

Focus of Meeting.   Meetings should focus primarily on addressing the specific questions listed in the information package. The Agency may also wish to discuss relevant questions on safety issues or various scientific and/or regulatory aspects of the drug (see "Pre-IND Meeting," "EOP2 Meeting," and "Pre-NDA or Pre-BLA Meeting"). These can arise from Agency guidance documents, the reviewing division's experience, the manufacturing industry's experience, or scientific literature. The actual questions, issues, and/or problems discussed at a given meeting will be specific to the sponsor, drug, route of synthesis or isolation, dosage form, formulation, stability, route of administration, dosing frequency, or duration.

The following sections provide specific guidance and more detailed information on each of the three basic types of meetings—pre-IND, EOP2, and pre-NDA or pre-BLA—as well as examples of the CMC issues typically addressed in each of these meetings.

Pre-IND Meeting

Purpose of Meeting.   With respect to CMC information, the purpose of pre-IND meetings for phase 1/phase 2 is to discuss safety issues related to the proper identification, strength, quality, purity, or potency of the investigational drug, as well as to identify potential clinical hold issues. Meetings at the pre-IND stage regarding CMC information are often unnecessary when the project is straightforward.

Meeting Request, Information Package, and Format.   See "General Aspects" regarding the meeting request, information package, and format of the meeting.

Focus of Meeting.   The pre-IND meeting should focus on the specific questions related to the planned clinical trials. The meeting should also include a discussion of various scientific and regulatory aspects of the drug as they relate to safety and/or potential clinical hold issues. Examples of the CMC issues that could be discussed in pre-IND meetings include, but are not limited to

- physical, chemical, and/or biological characteristics;
- manufacturers;
- source and method of preparation;
- removal of toxic reagents;
- quality controls (e.g., identity, assay, purity, impurities profile)
- formulation;
- sterility (e.g., sterilization process, release sterility, and endotoxin testing, if applicable);
- linkage of pharmacological and/or toxicity batches to clinical trial batches; and
- stability information.

The discussion of safety issues for conventional synthetic drugs is typically brief. For certain types of drugs, such as biotechnological drugs, biological drugs, natural products, complex dosage forms, and drug–device combinations, it may be appropriate to discuss the CMC information in more detail. Examples where detailed discussion may be appropriate include, but are not limited to

- drugs from human sources (e.g., appropriate donor screening procedures for tissues, blood, or other fluids; removal or inactivation of adventitious agents, e.g., viruses, bacteria, fungi, mycoplasma);
- drugs from animal sources (e.g., removal or inactivation of adventitious agents, transmissible spongiform encephalopathy-free certification);
- biotechnology drugs, particularly rDNA proteins from cell line sources (e.g., adequacy of characterization of cell banks, potential contamination of cell lines, removal or inactivation of adventitious agents, potential antigenicity of the product);
- botanical drugs (e.g., raw material sources, absence of adulteration);
- reagents from animal or cell line sources (same considerations as for drugs derived from animal cell or cell line sources);
- novel excipients;
- novel dosage forms (e.g., characteristics, potential for overly rapid release of dose, if applicable); and
- drug–device delivery systems (e.g., demonstration of device and its characteristics, potential for overly rapid release of dose, particle size distribution considerations, where applicable).

EOP 2 Meetings

Purpose of Meeting. The purpose of the EOP2 meeting, with respect to CMC information, is to provide an opportunity for the sponsor and reviewing division to (1) evaluate the results of the drug development program to date, (2) discuss the sponsor's plans and protocols relative to regulations, guidances, and Agency policy, (3) identify safety issues, scientific issues, and/or potential problems and resolve these, if possible, prior to initiation of phase 3 studies, and (4) identify additional information important to support a marketing application. The CMC portion of the EOP2 meeting is a critical interaction between the sponsor and the chemistry review team to ensure that meaningful data will be generated during phase 3 studies. The goal is to identify potential impediments to further progress at an early stage, thus reducing the number of review cycles for the proposed marketing application. Although the EOP2 meeting is important for all drugs, it is particularly important for new molecular entities, biotechnology drugs, biological drugs, natural products, complex dosage forms, and/or drug-device delivery systems.

Meeting Request, Information Package, and Format. See "General Aspects" for general aspects of the meeting request, information package, and format for the meeting. A multidisciplinary or separate CMC-specific EOP2 meeting can be held. If a CMC-specific meeting is held, it is preferred that it be scheduled to take place immediately prior to or after the meeting on clinical issues. Under appropriate circumstances, such CMC-specific meetings can occur during phase 3 trials, but prior to phase 3-associated scale-up and manufacturing changes.

Focus of Meeting. The EOP2 meeting should focus on the CMC-specific questions on the planned phase 3 studies. Typically, the meeting will also include a discussion identifying additional information to support a marketing application. Examples of the CMC issues that can be addressed in EOP2 meetings include, but are not limited to the following:

All Drugs

- Unique physicochemical (e.g., polymorphic forms, enantiomers) and biological properties
- Adequacy of physicochemical characterization studies
- Starting material designation
- Coordination of all activities, including full cooperation of Drug Master File holders and other contractors and suppliers in support of the planned NDA or BLA
- Qualification of impurities (update from phase 1/phase 2)

- Removal or inactivation of adventitious agents (update from phase 1/ phase 2, where applicable)
- Approach to specifications (i.e., tests, analytical procedures, and acceptance criteria)
- Coordination between sponsor and Agency chemists and pharmacokineticists to establish proper dissolution test procedures (particularly because dissolution testing will be included in the stability protocols, where applicable)
- Link between formulations and dosage forms used in preclinical, clinical, pharmacokinetic/pharmacodynamic studies, and formulations planned for the NDA or BLA
- Specific considerations for container/closure system components for specialized delivery systems such as metered dose inhalers, dry-powder inhalers, disposable pen injectors, transdermal patches, or other novel dosage forms
- Approach to sterilization process validation and/or container closure challenge testing, where applicable
- Devices (e.g., pumps, valves, cartridge injectors, actuators), where applicable
- Appropriateness of the stability protocols to support phase 3 studies and the planned NDA or BLA
- Major CMC changes, including site changes, anticipated from phase 2 through the proposed NDA or BLA, ramifications of such changes, and appropriateness of planned comparability and/or bridging studies, if applicable
- Environmental impact considerations, if pertinent
- Identification of any other CMC issues, including manufacturing site, which pose novel policy issues or concerns, or any other questions, issues, or problems that should be brought to the attention of the Agency or sponsor

rDNA Protein Biotechnology Drugs   In addition to the items listed in this section CMC issues that can be addressed in EOP2 meetings for rDNA protein biotechnology drugs include, but are not limited to

- adequacy of physicochemical and biological characterization (e.g., peptide map, amino acid sequence, disulfide linkages, higher order structure, glycosylation sites and structures, other post-translational modifications, and plans for completion, if still incomplete);
- bioassay (e.g., appropriateness of method, specificity, precision);
- adequacy of cell bank characterization (e.g., update from phase 1/phase 2, plans for completion, if still incomplete);

- removal of product- and process-related impurities (e.g., misfolded proteins, aggregates, host cell proteins, nucleic acid); and
- bioactivity of product-related substances and product-related impurities relative to desired product.

Conventional Biologics In addition to the items listed in this section, CMC issues that could be addressed in EOP2 meetings for conventional biologics (e.g., nonrecombinant vaccines and blood products) include, but are not limited to

- coordination of facility design,
- process validation considerations, and
- potency assay.

Follow-Up Meeting. In the event that new issues arise during phase 3 studies that affect the drug development program, a follow-up meeting may be warranted. The meeting can be used to address major changes in plans from those previously discussed in the EOP2 meeting or to resolve potential problems and/or refuse-to-file issues.

Pre-NDA or Pre-BLA Meeting

Purpose of Meeting. The purpose of the pre-NDA or pre-BLA meeting is to discuss filing and format issues. The CMC portion of the pre-NDA or pre-BLA meeting is a critical interaction between the CMC review team and the sponsor to ensure the submission of a well-organized and complete NDA or BLA.

Meeting Request, Information Package, and Format. See "General Aspects" for general guidance on the meeting request, information package, and format for the meeting. A pre-NDA or pre-BLA meeting should be held about six months prior to the planned NDA or BLA submission date.

Focus of Meeting. The pre-NDA or pre-BLA meeting should focus on addressing the specific questions related to filing and format issues. Typically, the meeting also includes a discussion to identify problems that can cause a refuse-to-file recommendation or hinder the review process. Examples of CMC issues that could be addressed in pre-NDA or pre-BLA meetings include, but are not limited to

- discussion of the format of the proposed NDA or BLA submission, including whether an electronic submission will be provided;

- confirmation that all outstanding issues discussed at the EOP2 meeting or raised subsequently will be adequately addressed in the proposed NDA or BLA;
- assurance that all activities in support of the proposed NDA or BLA have been coordinated, including the full and timely cooperation of Drug Master File holders or other contractors and suppliers;
- discussion of the relationship between the manufacturing, formulation, and packaging of the drug product used in the phase 3 studies and the final drug product intended for marketing, and assurance that any comparability or bridging studies agreed upon at the EOP2 meeting have been appropriately completed;
- assurance that the submission will contain adequate stability data in accordance with stability protocols agreed upon at the EOP2 meeting;
- confirmation that all facilities (e.g., manufacturing, testing, packaging) will be ready for inspection by the time of the NDA or BLA submission; and
- identification of any other issues, potential problems, or regulatory issues that should be brought to the attention of the Agency or sponsor.

GUIDANCE FOR INDUSTRY—HOW TO SUBMIT A REQUEST FOR A MEETING OR TELECONFERENCE IN ELECTRONIC FORMAT TO CVM[3] (Guideline No. 88)

Contains nonbinding recommendations guidance for industry[4]

Revised January 15, 2008
U.S. Department of Health and Human Services
Food and Drug Administration
Center for Veterinary Medicine

This guidance represents the Agency's current thinking on how to submit a request for a meeting or teleconference in electronic format to the Office of New Animal Drug Evaluation (ONADE). It does not create or confer any rights for or on any person and does not operate to bind the FDA or the public. You can use an alternative approach if the approach satisfies the requirements of the applicable statue and regulations. If you want to discuss an alternative

---

[3]This version of the guidance replaces the version made available in June 2007.
[4]This guidance was prepared by the CVM at the FDA. For additional copies, access the document on the CVM home page (http://www.fda.gov/cvm/default.html), or send a request to the Communications Staff, HFV-12, 7519 Standish Place, Rockville, MD 20855.

approach, contact the FDA staff responsible for implementing this guidance. If you cannot identify the appropriate FDA staff, call 1-888-INFO-FDA (1-888-463-6332).

This guidance document is intended to provide instruction on how to submit a request for a meeting or teleconference in electronic format to ONADE at the CVM (or the Center). The guidance was revised to update the phone number for the Electronic Document Control Unit and to replace the Web site to submit electronic comments.

Comments and suggestions regarding this document should be sent to Division of Dockets Management (HFA-305), Food and Drug Administration, 5630 Fishers Lane, Rm. 1061, Rockville, MD 20852. Submit electronic comments to http://www.regulations.gov. All comments should be identified with the exact title of the document. Please note that on January 15, 2008, the FDA Web site transitioned to the Federal Dockets Management System (FDMS). FDMS is a governmentwide, electronic docket management system. Electronic submissions will be accepted by the FDA through FDMS only.

For questions regarding this document, contact Margaret Zabriski, Center for Veterinary Medicine (HFV-016), Food and Drug Administration, 7519 Standish Place, Rockville, MD 20855, 240-276-9143, e-mail: margaret.zabriski@ fda.hhs.gov.

According to the Paperwork Reduction Act of 1995, a collection of information should display a valid OMB control number. The valid OMB control number for this information collection is 0910-0452. The time required to complete this information collection is estimated to vary from 15 min to 2 h per response, including the time to review instructions, search existing data resources, gather the data needed, and complete and review the information collection.

Introduction

This guidance provides advice to industry regarding the procedures to submit a request for a meeting or teleconference in electronic format to ONADE.

The FDA's guidance documents, including this guidance, do not establish legally enforceable responsibilities. Instead, guidances describe the Agency's current thinking on a topic and should be viewed only as recommendations, unless specific regulatory or statutory requirements are cited. The use of the word "should" in Agency guidances means that something is suggested or recommended, but not required.

Any person intending to file a new animal drug application or abbreviated new animal drug application is entitled to request meetings and/or teleconferences to reach agreement regarding a submission or investigational requirement [21 U.S.C. 3606(b)(3)]. Every person outside the Federal Government may request a meeting with representative(s) of the FDA to discuss a matter [21 CFR 10.65(c)]. This guidance document describes the procedures that should be followed by persons who submit a request for a meeting or teleconference to ONADE in electronic format. The procedures are designed to ensure compliance with FDA regulations governing Electronic Records found in 21 CFR Part 11, taking into account the CVM's current information technology capability and its ability to ensure the confidentiality, integrity, security, and authentication of data submitted to the Center in electronic format.

To submit electronically a request for a meeting or teleconference, the sponsor should use the Request for a Meeting or Teleconference form provided by the CVM (Form FDA 3489[5] OMB No. 0910-0452). The sponsor should enter the data directly into an Adobe Acrobat form, attach the Agenda for the meeting, and submit the form to CVM as an Adobe portable document format (PDF) file (compatible with Adobe Acrobat 6.0).[6] The electronic submission of a request for meeting or teleconference is part of the Center's ongoing initiative to provide a method for paperless submissions.

The meeting and teleconference requests should be submitted by the applicant to the CVM. For reasons of security and verifying the sender's identity, the applicant should register each individual participant, including a coordinator, and all individuals who will be submitting electronic submissions with the Center as outlined in Guidance for Industry #108 "How to Submit Information in Electronic Format to CVM using the FDA Electronic Submission Gateway," available at the Center's Guidance Page (http://www.fda.gov/cvm/guidance/published.htm).

Electronic records may be submitted instead of paper records, provided the requirements of Part 11 are met (21 CFR 11.2). The procedures in this guidance are designed to provide for a means of electronic submission that meets the requirements of Part 11. If an applicant does not follow this guidance to submit a meeting request electronically, the applicant should consult with the CVM regarding alternative methods for electronic submission that meet the requirements of Part 11 or submit the request in paper.

Request for a Meeting or Teleconference Form

A copy of Form FDA 3489 Request for a Meeting or Teleconference (for use with electronic submissions) is available on the CVM Electronic Submission Page at http://www.fda.gov/cvm/esubstoc.html.

Checklist for Electronic Submission of a Request for a Meeting or Teleconference Using Form FDA 3489

An applicant submitting an electronic request for a meeting or teleconference should create an agenda as a single PDF file. This file will be attached to Form FDA 3489. This checklist describes the process applicants should follow to fill out the form, attach the agenda, and submit the information.

---

[5] A copy of the form, along with instructions for completing it, can be found on the CVM Electronic Submissions Project Page, http://www.fda.gov/cvm/esubstoc.html.

[6] FDA use of specific products does not constitute an endorsement of those products.

1. Open the Meeting Request Form FDA 3489.
2. Fill in all of the applicable fields of Form FDA 3489.
3. If the "Multiple Documents" box in A2 is selected, up to 20 documents can be entered into the fields provided. If you are amending a pending meeting request involving multiple documents, then you must enter all pending documents being amended in the fields provided. If the "Multiple Documents" box is not selected, enter the single-document information in A3.
4. Select the "Insert Comments" button to add a PDF file containing any comments regarding the meeting request.
5. Select the "Insert Agenda" to add the PDF file containing the Agenda. The form cannot be successfully validated until an agenda has been attached.
6. Once the form is completed, select the "Validate" button to verify that all the required fields are completed. Those fields that are required will be highlighted and must be completed before the form can be sent to CVM.
7. Select the "Save" button to save all changes in the form.
8. Select the "Signature" button to digitally sign the form. Once the form is digitally signed, you cannot make any changes because all the fields will be locked for editing.
9. If you do not receive an acknowledgment receipt from the CVM by the third business day after you have sent the submission, call the Electronic Document Control Unit at 301-827-8277 to report the problem and find out what happened to your submission. After review of the agenda and proposed dates, the CVM will contact the sponsor to finalize details of the meeting.

After review of the agenda and proposed dates, CVM will contact the applicant to finalize details of the meeting

FREQUENTLY ASKED QUESTIONS ON THE PRE-IND MEETING

The pre-IND meeting can be very valuable in planning a drug development program, especially if sponsors' questions are not fully answered by guidances and other information provided by the FDA. Early interactions with FDA staff can help to prevent clinical hold issues from arising. A pre-IND meeting can also provide sponsors with information that will assist them in preparing to submit complete IND applications. Efficient use of FDA resources can lead to more efficient drug development. These questions and answers can be especially helpful to small businesses that may have limited experience interacting with the Agency, or are unfamiliar with pre-IND meetings.

What are the definitions of the terms used in these questions and answers?

IND—The IND application is the vehicle through which a sponsor advances to the next stage of drug development known as clinical trials (human trials). Information on the IND application process is available at http://www.fda.gov/cder/regulatory/applications/ind_page_1.htm.

Active Pharmaceutical Ingredient—This is any substance or mixture of substances intended to be used in the manufacture of a drug (medicinal) product and that, when used in the production of a drug, becomes an active ingredient of the drug product.

Good Clinical Practice—

Good Clinical Practice (GCP) is a standard for the design, conduct, performance, monitoring, auditing, recording, analysis, and reporting of clinical trials. For more information on the FDA's GCP program, go to http://www.fda.gov/oc/gcp.

Orphan Drug—The term refers to a product that treats a rare disease affecting fewer than 200,000 Americans. For additional information, go to http://www.fda.gov/orphan/index.htm.

Fast Track—Fast-track programs are designed to facilitate the development and expedite the review of new drugs or biologics that are intended to treat serious or life-threatening conditions and that demonstrate the potential to address unmet medical needs. For additional information, go to http://www.fda.gov/cder/guidance/5645fnl.htm.

Accelerated Approval—This is a program that the FDA developed to make new drug products available for life-threatening diseases when they appear to provide a benefit over available therapy (which could mean that there was no existing effective treatment). This guidance provides additional information: http://www.fda.gov/cder/guidance/5645fnl.htm.

505(b)(1) Application—A 505(b)(1) application is an application that contains full reports of investigations of safety and effectiveness. The investigations the applicant relied on for approval were conducted by or for the applicant, or the applicant has obtained a right of reference or use for the investigations.

505(b)(2) Application—A 505(b)(2) application is an application submitted under section 505(b) for which

- some or all of the investigations the applicant relied on for approval were not conducted by or for the applicant; and
- the applicant has not obtained a right of reference or use for the investigations [21 U.S.C. 355(b)(2)]

Section 505(b)(2) expressly permits the FDA to rely, for approval of an NDA, on data not developed by the applicant, such as published literature or the Agency's finding of safety and/or effectiveness of a previously approved drug product.

> *Animal Efficacy Rule*—The animal efficacy rule permits the FDA to rely on animal evidence when (1) the agent's mechanism of toxicity is well understood; (2) the end points in the animal trials are clearly related to benefit in humans; (3) the drug's effect is demonstrated in a species expected to react similarly to humans; and (4) data allow selection of an effective human dose.

Can pre-IND meetings reduce time to market? Yes, time can be reduced by the following:

- Identifying and avoiding unnecessary studies
- Ensuring that necessary studies are designed to provide useful information
- Gaining FDA support for a proposed strategy
- Potentially minimizing potential for clinical hold
- Providing opportunity for creative exchange of ideas
- obtaining regulatory insight
- Minimizing costs
- Clearly defining end points and goals of the development program
- Allowing early interactions/negotiations with the FDA

In the process of drug development, when can a pre-IND meeting be very important?

- When the product is intended to treat a serious or life-threatening disease
- When there is a novel indication
- When there are no current guidance documents
- When there are sponsors new to drug development
- When there are questions from the sponsor
- When there are pharmacological or toxicological signals of concern
- When the drug is a new molecular entity

Can pre-IND meetings be helpful in developing a strategy for drug development? Yes. The following can be helpful in developing a strategy.

- Identifying studies that will support the initiation of clinical trials
- Discussing available methods to enhance development, for example:
  - Orphan-Drug Designation
  - Fast Track Designation

- Accelerated Approval
- Animal Efficacy Rule
- Discussing the differences between submitting a 505(b)(1) and 505(b)(2) application

What information should be included in the meeting request? Sponsors should review the guidance on meetings at http://www.fda.gov/cder/guidance/2125fnl. pdf. Adequate information in the meeting request is an important part of having a successful outcome of a pre-IND meeting and should include the following information.

- Meeting objective
- Proposed agenda, including estimated times needed for each agenda item
- Listing of specific questions categorized and grouped by discipline, i.e., CMC, pharmacology/toxicology, clinical pharmacology and biopharmaceutics, and clinical investigations
- List of sponsor participants
- List of requested participants from CDER
- Quantitative composition (all ingredients by percent composition) of the drug proposed for use in the study to be discussed
- Proposed indication
- Dosing regimen, including concentration, amount dosed, and frequency and duration of dosing if known
- Proposed meeting date (propose six to eight weeks in the future)
- When the background packet will be available (at least four weeks before the proposed meeting date)

What is the purpose of the pre-IND meeting packet?

- Provides the historical background information on the chemical development concept
- Provides information on the active ingredient
- Provides an initial clinical and preclinical development strategy
- Provides future development strategy including product scale-up and final formulation, and animal and clinical studies proposed in support of an NDA
- Provides the FDA with a clear and concise overview of the planned development program
- Allows the FDA the opportunity to comment on a proposed program of development

What do you include in a pre-IND meeting packet?

- Overall program synopsis
- Whether the animal efficacy rule is being considered
- Clinical study synopsis to obtain FDA input on inclusion, exclusion, and end points
- Results for *in vitro* and early *in vivo* toxicology
- Rationale for safety, based on toxicological profile and safety margin using dose regimen and exposure
- Brief description of the manufacturing scheme for the active pharmaceutical ingredient and formulation for clinical study
- Brief assay descriptions
- Full description of the development plan
- Copy of the meeting request with updates to reflect the most current information

Is communication important in a pre-IND meeting? Yes, be sure to

- ask specific, well-phrased questions;
- prioritize questions;
- stay focused on the agenda;
- disclose all concerns;
- present only data included in the meeting packet; and
- obtain clear and concise information through clear questions and listening.

Are there recurrent problems at pre-IND meetings? Yes, the following have been identified in pre-IND meetings.

- Inadequate CMC information
- Insufficient preclinical support
- Unacceptable clinical trial design
- Noncompliance with GCPs
- Lack of information on selection of dosage

In addition to the above, what else can be helpful?

- Make the best use of allotted time.
- Agree with the FDA on timing and required attendees.
- Identify questions to ask the FDA.
- Make sure that a pre-IND meeting is necessary; answers to your questions may be available in the guidances.

- Make sure that issues support good use of industry and FDA time.
- Present data clearly and consistently.

Additional information (regulations, guidances, MAPPs, and Web sites)

- 21 CFR 312.47 (meetings)
- 21 CFR 312.82 (early consultation)
- MAPP 4512.1: Formal Meetings between CDER and CDER's External Constituents at http://www.fda.gov/cder/mapp/4512-1.pdf
- Guidance for Industry: Formal Meetings with Sponsors and Applicants for PDUFA Products at http://www.fda.gov/cder/guidance/2125fnl.pdf
- M3 Nonclinical Safety Studies for the Conduct of Human Clinical Trials for Pharmaceutical Products http://www.fda.gov/cder/guidance/1855fnl.pdf
- E6 GCP: Consolidated Guideline http://www.fda.gov/cder/guidance/959fnl.pdf
- Small Business Assistance Web site http://www.fda.gov/cder/about/smallbiz/default.htm

REFERENCES

FDA guidance for industry on *Content and Format of Phase 1 Investigational New Drug Applications (INDs) for Phase I Studies of Drugs, Including Well-Characterized, Therapeutic, Biotechnology-Derived Products* (November 1995).

FDA, *CDER Manual of Policies and Procedures (MAPP) 4512.1, Training and Communications, Formal Meetings between CDER and External Constituents*, March 1996 (http://www.fda.gov/cder/).

FDA, *Scheduling and Conduct of Regulatory Review Meetings with Sponsors and Applicants*, CBER Standard Operating Procedures and Policies (SOPP) 8101.1 (http://www.fda.gov/cber/).

FDA guidance for industry on *Formal Meetings with Sponsors and Applicants for PDUFA Products* (February 2000).

FDA guidance for industry on *Fast Track Drug Development Programs: Designation, Development and Application Review* (November 1998).

FDA guidance for industry on *CMC Content and Format of Investigational New Drug Applications (INDs) for Phase 2 and 3 Studies of Drugs, Including Specified Therapeutic Biotechnology-Derived Products* (Draft, February 1999).

CHAPTER 3

Orphan-Drug Applications

Basic economic forces encourage pharmaceutical companies to actively pursue potential blockbuster drugs than can significantly improve the lives or longevity of a large number of persons suffering from widespread diseases. If you have a viable cure or treatment for cancers, heart diseases, diabetes, or other diseases that affect large segments for the population, the potential sales provide incentive to invest in the clinical testing and development processes.

But if pharmaceutical companies focused exclusively on these major diseases, millions of people with very serious but less widespread conditions would be left without help or hope. The solution, of course, is for the government to provide incentives that supplement the potential sales value of an important treatment for a relatively obscure disease, thus encouraging development in the absence of market blockbuster potential. In the United States, the mechanism for that encouragement is orphan-drug designation.

The Orphan-Drug Act (ODA) was signed into law on January 4, 1983, to encourage the development of drugs and therapies for conditions that might not represent economically attractive commercial markets. Since 1983, more than 100 orphan drugs have been brought to market, each designed to treat conditions affecting fewer than 200,000 Americans.

A drug qualifies for orphan status if credible documentation, with authoritative references, is submitted to prove that

"(i) the disease or condition for which the drug is intended affects fewer than 200,000 people in the United States, or, if the drug is a vaccine, diagnostic drug, or preventive drug, the persons to whom the drug will be administered in the United States are fewer than 200,000 per year as specified in Sec 316.21(b); or

(ii) for a drug intended for diseases or conditions affecting 200,000 or more people or for a vaccine, diagnostic drug, or preventive drug to be administered to 200,000 or more persons per year in the United States, there is no reasonable expectation that the costs of research and development of the drug for the indication can be recovered by sales of the drug in the United States as specified in Sec. 316.21(c)."

Designation as an orphan drug carries a number of incentives, designed to encourage development, specifically the following:

1. Orphan designation carries a seven-year market exclusivity.
2. Orphan designation provides developmental tax incentives.
3. Orphan designation permits application (but does not guarantee) for orphan grants to fund all or part of the costs of clinical trials.
4. Orphan-drug applications for prescription drug products are not subject to a fee, unless the human drug application includes an indication other than the rare disease. In addition, Orphan designation permits application (but does not guarantee) for exemption from FDA annual product and establishment fees under a section 736(d)(1) of the Federal Food, Drug, and Cosmetic Act waiver.

These incentives are obviously designed to encourage the development of drugs for rare diseases and conditions and often lead drug development companies to pursue initial orphan indications in advance of seeking approval for more widespread conditions. While an orphan-drug application can be submitted any time prior to the filing of a marketing application, it is often the first regulatory submission of a new company or new drug program.

Review of an orphan-drug application is generally completed within 30 days of submission. The process begins with an administrative review to assure the application is complete, conforms to the required format, and clearly designates the proposed drug and disease or condition.

Once this administrative hurdle is successfully negotiated, a reviewer examines the application in detail to make certain that four basic criteria are met.

1. Clear and credible evidence is presented to support the contention that the disease or condition affects fewer than 200,000 people in the United States (see above);
2. A credible scientific rationale is presented in support of the contention that the proposed drug or therapeutic represents a promising treatment or preventive for the disease or condition.
3. A review of previous US and worldwide experience with the drug or therapeutic indicates reasonable expectation of minimal or controllable risk.
4. Assurances from the sponsor or applicant provide reasonable expectation that the drug or therapeutic will be appropriately tested and, if proven safe and effective, will be brought to market.

The Office of OPD is generally very helpful and cooperative in preparing and submitting applications, and reviews are thorough and rigorous but not onerous.

Orphan status is often an important first step in the development of a promising compound with multiple indications. By focusing initially on an indication with limited market size, the sponsoring organization gains inexpensive credibility, market exclusivity, and (possibly) funding. The subsequent marketing of the orphan indication can provide funding and can attract outside investors for the more expensive testing of wider application indications.

Submission of an orphan application does not require a formal FDA preapplication meeting, though the Office of Orphan Products Development will generally be helpful in responding to clarification questions via telephone. The application—generally a notebook tabbed to separate the application sections and the enclosed references—is submitted in duplicate, with an accompanying cover letter.

Since review focuses largely on the four key criteria, the process is predictable. Postreview clarification and additional documentation may be necessary to further support a contention, but process appeals are very rare.

ORPHAN-DRUG APPLICATION SUBMISSION CHECKLIST

This checklist is intended for use in the preparation and submission of orphan-drug applications. It is recommended that, prior to transmission to the FDA, a second internal review should be conducted by an individual or department not involved in the preparation of the submission (presumably Quality Assurance).

The checklist was developed through discussions with consultants and Quality Assurance directors and has been field-tested in final form with five successful Orphan-Drug Application submissions.

- ☐ Cover letter
    - ☐ Name and address of sponsor
    - ☐ Name and address, title, telephone, e-mail of contact person
    - ☐ Generic and trade name of drug or drug product
    - ☐ Description of rare diseases
- ☐ Two copies of application in indexed binders
- ☐ Statement requesting Orphan-Drug designation for specific rare disease
- ☐ Name and address of sponsor
- ☐ Name, address, title, telephone, e-mail of contact person
- ☐ Generic and trade name of drug or drug product
- ☐ Description of rate disease or condition, proposed indication, reasons why therapy is needed
- ☐ Scientific rationale for the drug including data from nonclinical and clinical investigations
- ☐ Copies of published and unpublished papers included

- ☐ Statement of superiority of proposed therapy to other available treatments
- ☐ If drug is intended for subset of persons with a specific disease or condition, evidence that the subset is medically plausible
- ☐ Summary of regulatory status and marketing history in the United States and foreign countries
- ☐ Summary of adverse reactions to proposed drug in any country
- ☐ Documentation demonstrating disease or condition affects fewer than 200,000 people in the United States
- ☐ Statement as to whether the sponsor is the real party intending to produce and sell the drug
- ☐ Bibliography cited numerically to text, separated by tabbed dividers

FDA ORPHAN-DRUG REVIEW CHECKLIST

This FDA Orphan-Drug Review checklist has been designed in consultation with FDA reviewers, industry consultants, and regulatory professionals to serve as a summary tool indicating the evaluative criteria used by the Office of Orphan-Drug Development to critique and assess applications received. It can be used internally as a part of the Quality Assurance process, as a guideline for regulatory development of an application, and/or as a self-assessment tool to predict likely FDA response to an application.

- ☐ **Logistics:** Submission conforms to FDA guideline 21 Code of Federal Regulations (CFR) Part 316.20.
  - ☐ **Receipt:** Application was received in the FDA mail room.
  - ☐ **Identification of rare disease or condition:** Application clearly defines a rare disease or condition.
  - ☐ **Contact information:** Application provides contact information including corporate name, contact name, address, telephone number, name and address of drug source, and generic and trade name of drug.
  - ☐ **Dual copies:** Two copies of the application are included.
  - ☐ **Cover letter:** A cover letter indicates disease and therapy names.
- ☐ **Format:** Submission conforms to FDA guideline 21 CFR Part 316.20(b) and to FDA norm standards
  - ☐ **Pagination:** All pages are included and properly numbered.
  - ☐ **Headings:** Section headings conform to submission subparagraphs.
  - ☐ **Integrated references:** Copies of all referenced articles, with references integrated into the body of text.
  - ☐ **Bibliography:** Standard format bibliography is complete as referenced in text.

- ☐ **Qualification:** Submission meets criteria of ODA 21 CFR Part 316.
  - ☐ **Patient population:** Evidence of patient population of 200,000 in the United States
  - ☐ **Evidence of viable therapy:** Evidence of scientific rationale for the product drug or vaccine
  - ☐ **Advantage over existing therapies:** Evidence of clinical superiority over existing therapies
  - ☐ **Unique therapy:** Qualification as first proposed orphan use of the drug
- ☐ **Support:** Evaluation of the referent support is provided.
  - ☐ **Key issues:** All key issues are appropriately referenced, including:
    - ☐ Size of patient population
    - ☐ Scientific rationale for therapy
    - ☐ Clinical effectiveness/superiority of therapy
  - ☐ **Credible:** References are from credible scientific journals and/or sources.
  - ☐**Organized:** References are organized and tied to text.

COMMENTS:
DISPOSITION:
  Receipt date:
  Response due date:
  Disposition:
  Notification date:

FDA DOCUMENTS

Original copies of four FDA documents related to orphan drugs are provided in this section.

How to Apply for Designation as an Orphan Product is an FDA guideline providing useful definitions of a rare disease, of a scientific rationale for a therapy, and of the standard of potential clinical superiority. It also provides a detailed application outline and developmental procedure. The document's final section describes the unusual situation in which a nonorphan indication may qualify if there is no reasonable expectation of recovering development costs.

Tips for Submitting an Application for Orphan Designation updates the "How to Apply ..." guideline and offers specific suggestions for formatting and referencing. The document is in effect a very useful summary of submission problems encountered over the years, with suggestions for avoiding these errors.

Draft Guidance for Industry: Providing Regulatory Submissions in Electronic Format for Orphan Drug and Humanitarian Use Device Designation

Requests and Related Submissions outlines the evolving requirements for electronic submission of orphan-drug applications using the (still pending) ESG and physical media (CD-ROM).

The **ODA (as amended)** provides an actual copy of the current law 21CFR Part 316 for review and reference.

How to Apply for Designation as an Orphan Product

This information has been extracted from:

(December 29, 1992, 57 FR 62076)
Department of Health and Human Services
Food and Drug Administration
21 CFR Part 316
(Docket NO. 85N-0483)
RIN 0905-AB55 Orphan-Drug Regulations
Agency: Food and Drug Administration, HHS
Action: Final Rule

Subpart C Designation of an Orphan Drug. § 316.20 Content and Format of a Request for Orphan-Drug Designation

(a) A sponsor that submits a request for orphan-drug designation of a drug for a specified rare disease or condition shall submit each request in the form and containing the information required in paragraph (b) of this section. A sponsor may request orphan-drug designation of a previously unapproved drug or of a new orphan indication for an already marketed drug. In addition, a sponsor of a drug that is otherwise the same drug as an already approved orphan drug may seek and obtain orphan-drug designation for the subsequent drug for the same rare disease or condition if it can present a plausible hypothesis that its drug may be clinically superior to the first drug. More than one sponsor may receive orphan-drug designation of the same drug for the same rare disease or condition, but each sponsor seeking orphan-drug designation must file a complete request for designation as provided in paragraph (b) of this section.

(b) A sponsor shall submit two copies of a completed, dated, and signed request for designation that contains the following:

(1) A statement that the sponsor requests orphan-drug designation for a rare disease or condition, which shall be identified with specificity

(2) The name and address of the sponsor; the name of the sponsor's primary contact person and/or resident agent including title, address, and telephone number; the generic and trade name, if any, of the drug or drug product; and the name and address of the source of the drug if it is not manufactured by the sponsor.

(3) A description of the rare disease or condition for which the drug is being or will be investigated, the proposed indication or indications for use of the drug, and the reasons why such therapy is needed

(4) A description of the drug and a discussion of the scientific rationale for the use of the drug for the rare disease or condition, including all data from nonclinical laboratory studies, clinical investigations, and other relevant data that are available to the sponsor, whether positive, negative, or inconclusive. Copies of pertinent unpublished and published papers are also required.

(5) Where the sponsor of a drug that is otherwise the same drug as an already approved orphan drug seeks orphan-drug designation for the subsequent drug for the same rare disease or condition, an explanation of why the proposed variation may be clinically superior to the first drug

(6) Where a drug is under development for only a subset of persons with a particular disease or condition, a demonstration that the subset is medically plausible

(7) A summary of the regulatory status and marketing history of the drug in the United States and in foreign countries, e.g., IND and marketing application status and dispositions; what uses are under investigation and in what countries; for what indication is the drug approved in foreign countries; what adverse regulatory actions have been taken against the drug in any country

(8) Documentation, with appended authoritative references, to demonstrate that

   (i) the disease or condition for which the drug is intended affects fewer than 200,000 people in the United States or, if the drug is a vaccine, diagnostic drug, or preventive drug, the persons to whom the drug will be administered in the United States are fewer than 200,000 per year as specified in § 316.21(b); or

   (ii) for a drug intended for diseases or conditions affecting 200,000 or more people or for a vaccine, diagnostic drug, or preventive drug to be administered to 200,000 or more persons per year in the United States, there is no reasonable expectation that costs of research and development of the drug for the indication can be recovered by sales of the drug in the United States as specified in § 316.21(c)

(9) A statement as to whether the sponsor submitting the request is the real party in interest of the development and the intended or actual production and sales of the product

(c) Any of the information previously provided by the sponsor to FDA under Subpart B of this part may be referenced by specific page or location if it duplicates information required elsewhere in this section.

Tips for Submitting an Application for Orphan Designation

1. The required information to be included in the application is found under 21 CFR 316.20(b), shown as (9) items. Number the items in your application 1 though 9 and respond to the nine items as described. Creative numbering is not helpful.

   21 CFR 316.20(b) is easily accessed through the Internet at http://www.fda.gov/orphan. **Click on "Orphan Product Designations," then click on "How to Apply for Orphan Product Designation."**

2. While all nine items will be reviewed, the application will be reviewed most critically in two areas: scientific rationale (Item 4) and population prevalence (Item 8). Do not confuse prevalence with incidence. They are different entities and cannot be substituted for one another.

   The application must contain a copy of every reference used in the application to document prevalence. While most references are from published sources, this also includes information obtained from Web sites. Provide a hard copy of the reference obtained from the Internet, plus the Web site address.

   It will facilitate the review process if the application contains a copy of every reference used to support the scientific rationale for the use of the drug/biological in the treatment of the rare disease.

3. Information provided by the sponsor relating to Item 7 is often incomplete. Provide the Investigational New Drug Application (IND) or New Drug Application/Biologics License Application (NDA/BLA) numbers if they are available to you.

   Sometimes sponsors submit an NDA/BLA after they have requested orphan designation but before the Office of OPD has made a determination on their application. In that case, amend the application for orphan designation by providing a copy of the NDA/BLA (or supplement) acknowledgment letter that you received from the FDA Reviewing Division.

   In the event that the product is approved abroad, list the countries where it is approved and for how long. In this case, it is helpful to provide copies of the package insert(s) under a separate tab. (Tabs are discussed in tip 4.)

4. Format your application so that it is user friendly. After addressing the nine required items, provide a bibliography displayed in a related fashion as shown in the text of your document. This is described below. Usually, references within the application are cited numerically with superscripts. In this case, provide the bibliography with the corresponding numeric superscripts, 1 through "n." References need to be separated by a tabbed divider—colored sheets of paper placed between references are not functional. Place a copy of the first reference cited behind tab "1," and so on.

Some sponsors prefer to mention their references by author directly after the cited work, for example (Abel E, Shaw FG, Elder GF, et al. 1997). An advantage of this method is that, as the text of the application is being developed, renumbering of the references is not necessary. Provide the bibliography (listed alphabetically) directly after the application, followed by the tabbed references. In this case, the references will be arranged alphabetically. In the example used above, the first tab will read, "Abel et al. 1997."

In the event that there are additional documents included in the application, such as the investigator's brochure, provide the document behind a tab, in this case, labeled "Investigator's Brochure."

Proper formatting of your application is very important. The reviewer of the application needs to be able to "walk through" your application with ease.

5. Submit the original and one photocopy of the application in separate binders or report covers to the Office of OPD. The photocopy needs to be an exact duplicate of the original application. If there is a cover letter with the original, there needs to be a copy of the cover letter with the duplicate. Also, no correspondence should arrive loose, or out of the binder or report cover. An example of a useful type of report cover is the "ACCO 25973" with metal fasteners. They are inexpensive and readily available, plus they fit in standard filing cabinets nicely. It helps to label the front of each report cover or binder with the name of the sponsor, drug/biological, indication, and date of application.

6. Submit the application (one original and one photocopy) for orphan designation to:

Marlene E. Haffner, MD, MPH, Director, Office of Orphan Products Development Food and Drug Administration, HF-35 5600 Fishers Lane, Room 6A55 Rockville, MD 20857

If you have any questions, please call Jeff Fritsch R. Ph. at (301) 827-0989.

Draft Guidance for Industry: Providing Regulatory Submissions in Electronic Format for Orphan-Drug and Humanitarian Use Device Designation Requests and Related Submissions

NOTE: On April 1, 2006, OPD will begin accepting orphan-drug and humanitarian use device designation requests and related submissions in electronic format only through the use of physical media (e.g., CD-ROMs) as described in the guidance document Providing Regulatory Submissions in Electronic Format—Orphan-Drug and Humanitarian Use Device Designation Requests and Related Submissions. This guidance is available on the FDA website at http://www.fda.gov/OHRMS/DOCKETS/98fr/06d-0128-gdl0001.pdf.

Summary. The FDA is announcing the availability of a draft guidance for industry entitled "Providing Regulatory Submissions in Electronic Format—Orphan-Drug and Humanitarian Use Device Designation Requests and Related Submissions." This is one in a series of guidance documents on providing regulatory submissions to FDA in electronic format. This guidance discusses issues related to the electronic submission of orphan-drug and humanitarian use device (HUD) designation requests and related submissions to the Office of OPD. The submission of these documents in electronic format should improve the Agency's efficiency in processing, archiving, and reviewing them.

Electronic submissions will eventually be made to OPD in one of two ways: totally electronic through the FDA Electronic Submission Gateway (ESG) pathway or directly to OPD through the use of physical media (e.g., CD-ROMs). However, the ESG pathway has not been cleared to begin receiving submissions and cannot be utilized at this point in time. Instructions on each procedure and on formatting of submissions are included in the Guidance. Questions regarding electronic submissions to OPD can be made to: desigesub@fda.hhs.gov for orphan-drug designation requests or hudesub@fda.hhs.gov for HUD designation requests.

Dates. Submit written or electronic comments on the draft guidance by May 30, 2006. General comments on Agency guidance documents are welcome at any time.

Addresses. Submit written requests for single copies of the draft guidance to the Electronic Submissions Coordinator, Office of OPD (HF–35), FDA, 5600 Fishers Lane, Rm. 6A–55, Rockville, MD 20857. Send one self-addressed adhesive label to assist that office in processing your requests. Submit written comments on the draft guidance to the Division of Dockets Management (HFA–305), FDA, 5630 Fishers Lane, Rm. 1061, Rockville, MD 20852. Submit electronic comments to http://www.fda.gov/dockets/ecomments. See "Supplementary Information" for electronic access to the draft guidance document.

For further information, contact:

James D. Bona, Office of Orphan Products Development (HF–35), Food and Drug Administration, 5600 Fishers Lane, Rockville, MD 20857, 301–827–3666.

Supplementary Information

Background FDA is announcing the availability of a draft guidance for industry entitled "Providing Regulatory Submissions in Electronic Format—Orphan-Drug and Humanitarian Use Device Designation Requests and Related Submissions." This draft document provides guidance to industry regarding submissions of designation requests and related submissions to OPD in electronic format. It describes the two methods by which submissions can be made electronically to OPD. The first is totally electronic through use of the FDA's electronic submission gateway pathway, and the second is directly to OPD through the use of physical media (e.g., CD–ROMs). Recommendations are described for the formatting and organization of these submissions. A listing of Agency contacts for assistance is also provided. This draft guidance is being issued consistent with the FDA's good guidance practices regulation (21 CFR 10.115). The draft guidance, when finalized, will represent the agency's current thinking on providing designation requests and related submissions in electronic format. It does not create or confer any rights for or on any person and does not operate to bind FDA or the public. An alternative approach may be used if such approach satisfies the requirements of the applicable statutes and regulations.

Comments   Interested persons may submit to the Division of Dockets Management (see "Addresses") written or electronic comments on the draft guidance. Submit a single copy of electronic comments or two paper copies of any mailed comments, except that individuals may submit one paper copy. Comments are to be identified with the docket number found in brackets in the heading of this document. The draft guidance and received comments may be seen in the Division of Dockets Management between 9:00 a.m. and 4:00 p.m., Monday through Friday.

Paperwork Reduction Act of 1995   This notice contains no new collections of information. The information requested for designation requests and related submissions is already covered by the regulations for orphan-drugs under 21 CFR 316.20 and for HUDs under 21 CFR 814.102. This notice announces the availability of a guidance that provides applicants with an alternative mechanism for submitting designation requests and related submissions to the Agency. Therefore, clearance by the Office of Management and Budget under the Paperwork Reduction Act of 1995 is not required.

Electronic Access   Persons with access to the Internet may obtain the document at http://www.fda.gov/orphan/esub/esub.htm or at http://www.fda.gov/ohrms/dockets/default.htm.

Dated: March 24, 2006. Jeffrey Shuren, Assistant Commissioner for Policy. [FR Doc. E6–4709 Filed 3–30–06; 8:45 am] BILLING CODE 4160–01–S

ODA (AS AMENDED)

Congressional Findings for the ODA

The Congress finds that

(1) there are many diseases and conditions such as Huntington's disease, myoclonus, ALS (Lou Gehrig's disease), Tourette syndrome, and muscular dystrophy that affect such small numbers of individuals residing

in the United States that the diseases and conditions are considered rare in the United States;

(2) adequate drugs for many of such diseases and conditions have not been developed;

(3) drugs for these diseases and conditions are commonly referred to as "orphan drugs";

(4) because so few individuals are affected by any one rare disease or condition, a pharmaceutical company that develops an orphan drug may reasonably expect the drug to generate relatively small sales in comparison to the cost of developing the drug and consequently to incur a financial loss;

(5) there is reason to believe that some promising orphan drugs will not be developed unless changes are made in the applicable Federal laws to reduce the costs of developing such drugs and to provide financial incentives to develop such drugs; and

(6) it is in the public interest to provide such changes and incentives for the development of orphan drugs.

Recommendations for Investigations of Drugs for Rare Diseases or Conditions

SEC. 525 [360aa].

(a) The sponsor of a drug for a disease or condition that is rare in the United States may request the Secretary to provide written recommendations for the nonclinical and clinical investigations that must be conducted with the drug before

(1) it may be approved for such disease or condition under section 505;

(2) if the drug is an antibiotic, it may be certified for such disease or condition under section 507; or

(3) if the drug is a biological product, it may be licensed for such disease or condition under section 351 of the Public Health Service Act.

If the Secretary has reason to believe that a drug for which a request is made under this section is a drug for a disease or condition that is rare in the United States, the Secretary shall provide the person making the request written recommendations for the nonclinical and clinical investigations which the Secretary believes, on the basis of information available to the Secretary at the time of the request under this section, would be necessary for approval of such drug for such disease or condition under section 505, certification of such drug for such disease or condition under section 507, or licensing of such drug for such disease or condition under section 351 of the Public Health Service Act.

1. The Secretary shall by regulation promulgate procedures for the implementation of subsection (a).

Designation of Drugs for Rare Diseases or Conditions

SEC. 526 [360bb].

(a)

    (1) The manufacturer or the sponsor of a drug may request the Secretary to designate the drug as a drug for a rare disease or condition. A request for designation of a drug shall be made before the submission of an application under section 505(b) for the drug, the submission of an application for certification of the drug under section 507, or the submission of an application for licensing of the drug under section 351 of the Public Health Service Act. If the Secretary finds that a drug for which a request is submitted under this subsection is being or will be investigated for a rare disease or condition and

    (A) if an application for such drug is approved under section 505;

    (B) if a certification for such drug is issued under section 507; or

    (C) if a license for such drug is issued under section 351 of the Public Health Service Act, the approval, certification, or license would be for use for such disease or condition, the Secretary shall designate the drug as a drug for such disease or condition. A request for a designation of a drug under this subsection shall contain the consent of the applicant to notice being given by the Secretary under subsection (b) respecting the designation of the drug.

    (2) For purposes of paragraph (1), the term "rare disease or condition" means any disease or condition that (A) affects fewer than 200,000 persons in the United States; or (B) affects more than 200,000 in the United States and for which there is no reasonable expectation that the cost of developing and making available in the United States a drug for such disease or condition will be recovered from sales in the United States of such drug. Determinations under the preceding sentence with respect to any drug shall be made on the basis of the facts and circumstances as of the date the request for designation of the drug under this subsection is made.

(b) A designation of a drug under subsection (a) shall be subject to the condition that

    (1) if an application was approved for the drug under section 505(b), a certificate was issued for the drug under section 507, or a license was issued for the drug under section 351 of the Public Health Service Act, the manufacturer of the drug will notify the Secretary of any discontinuance of the production of the drug at least one year before discontinuance; and

(2) if an application has not been approved for the drug under section 505(b), a certificate has not been issued for the drug under section 507, or a license has not been issued for the drug under section 351 of the Public Health Service Act and if preclinical investigations or investigations under section 505(i) are being conducted with the drug, the manufacturer or sponsor of the drug will notify the Secretary of any decision to discontinue active pursuit of approval of an application under section 505(b), approval of an application for certification under section 507, or approval of a license under section 351 of the Public Health Service Act.

(c) Notice respecting the designation of a drug under subsection (a) shall be made available to the public.

(d) The Secretary shall by regulation promulgate procedures for the implementation of subsection (a).

Protection for Drugs for Rare Diseases or Conditions

SEC. 527 [360cc].

(a) Except as provided in subsection (b), if the Secretary
   (1) approves an application filed pursuant to section 505(b),
   (2) issues a certification under section 507, or
   (3) issues a license under section 351 of the Public Health Service Act for a drug designated under section 526 for a rare disease or condition, the Secretary may not approve another application under section 505(b), issue another certification under section 507, or issue another license under section 351 of the Public Health Service Act for such drug for such disease or condition for a person who is not the holder of such approved application, of such certification, or of such license until the expiration seven years from the date of the approval of the approved application, the issuance of the certification, or the issuance of the license. Section 505(c)(2) does not apply to the refusal to approve an application under the preceding sentence.

(b) If an application filed pursuant to section 505(b) is approved for a drug designated under section 526 for a rare disease or condition, if a certification is issued under section 507 for such a drug, or if a license is issued under section 351 of the Public Health Service Act for such a drug, the Secretary may, during the seven-year period beginning on the date of the application approval, of the issuance of the certification under section 507, or of the issuance of the license, approve another application under section 505(b), issue another certification under section 507, or issue a license under section 351 of the Public Health Service Act, for such drug for such disease or condition for a person who is not the holder of such approved application, of such certification, or of such license if

(1) the Secretary finds, after providing the holder notice and opportunity for the submission of views, that in such period the holder of the approved application, of the certification, or of the license cannot assure the availability of sufficient quantities of the drug to meet the needs of persons with the disease or condition for which the drug was designated; or

(2) such holder provides the Secretary in writing the consent of such holder for the approval of other applications, issuance of other certifications, or the issuance of other licenses before the expiration of such seven-year period.

Open Protocols for Investigations of Drugs for Rare Diseases or Conditions

SEC. 528 [360dd]. If a drug is designated under section 526 as a drug for a rare disease or condition and if notice of a claimed exemption under section 505(i) or regulations issued thereunder is filed for such drug, the Secretary shall encourage the sponsor of such drug to design protocols for clinical investigations of the drug, which may be conducted under the exemption to permit the addition to the investigations of persons with the disease or condition who need the drug to treat the disease or condition and who cannot be satisfactorily treated by available alternative drugs.

Grants and Contracts for Development of Drugs for Rare Diseases and Conditions

SEC. 5. [360ee]

(a) The Secretary may make grants to and enter into contracts with public and private entities and individuals to assist in (1) defraying the costs of qualified clinical testing expenses incurred in connection with the development of drugs for rare diseases and conditions; (2) defraying the costs of developing medical devices for rare diseases or conditions; and (3) defraying the costs of developing medical foods for rare diseases or conditions.

(b) For purposes of subsection (a),

    (1) the term "qualified testing" means

        (A) human clinical testing

            (i) which is carried out under an exemption for a drug for a rare disease or condition under section 505(i) of the Federal Food, Drug, and Cosmetic Act (or regulations issued under such section);

            (ii) which occurs after the date such drug is designated under section 526 of such Act and before the date on which an application with respect to such drug is submitted under section 506(b) or 507 of such Act or under section 351 of the Public Health Service Act; and

(B) preclinical testing involving a drug is designated under section 526 of such Act and before the date on which an application with respect to such drug is submitted under section 505(b) or 507 of such Act or under section 351 of the Public Health Service Act.

(2) The term "rare disease or condition" means

(A) in the case of a drug, any disease, or condition that (A) affects fewer than 200,000 persons in the United States; or (B) affect more than 200,000 in the United States and for which there is no reasonable expectation that the cost of developing and making available in the United States a drug for such disease or condition will be recovered from sales in the United States of such drug;

(B) in the case of a medical device, any disease or condition that occurs so infrequently in the United States that there is no reasonable expectation that a medical device for such disease or condition will be developed without assistance under subsection (a); and

(C) in the case of a medical food, any disease or condition that occurs so infrequently in the United States that there is no reasonable expectation that a medical food for such disease or condition will be developed without assistance under subsection (a). Determinations under the preceding sentence with respect to any drug shall be made on the basis of the facts and circumstances as of the date the request for designation of the drug under section 526 of the Federal Food, Drug, and Cosmetic Act is made;

(D) The term "medical food" means a food that is formulated to be consumed or administered enterally under the supervision of a physician and that is intended for the specific dietary management of a disease or condition for which distinctive nutritional requirements, based on recognized scientific principles, are established by medical evaluation.

(c) For grants and contracts under subsection (a), there are authorized to be appropriated $10,000,000 for fiscal year 1988, $12,000,000 for fiscal year 1989, and $14,000,000 for fiscal year 1990.

(d) STUDY—The Secretary of Health and Human Services shall conduct a study to determine whether the application of subchapter B of chapter V of the Federal Food, Drug, and Cosmetic Act (relating to drugs for rare diseases and conditions) and section 28 of the Internal Revenue Code of 1986 (relating to tax credit) to medical devices or medical foods for rare diseases or conditions or to both is needed to encourage the development of such devices and foods. The Secretary shall report the results of the study to the Committee on Energy and Commerce of the House of

Representatives and the Committee on Labor and Human Resources of the Senate not later than one year after the date of the enactment of this Act. For purposes of this section, the term "rare diseases or conditions" has the meaning prescribed by section 5 of the Orphan-Drug Act (21 US.C. 360ee).

Orphan Products Board

SEC. 227 [236].

(a) There is established in the Department of Health and Human Services a board for the development of drugs (including biologics) and devices (including diagnostic products) for rare diseases or conditions to be known as the Orphan Products Board. The Board shall be composed of the Assistant Secretary for Health of the Department of Health and Human Services and representatives, selected by the Secretary, of the Food and Drug Administration, the National Institutes Health, the Centers for Disease Control, and any other Federal department or agency that the Secretary determines has activities relating to drugs and devices for rare diseases or conditions. The Assistant Secretary for Health shall chair the Board.

(b) The function of the Board shall be to promote the development of drugs and devices for rare diseases or conditions and the coordination among Federal, other public, and private agencies in carrying out their respective functions relating to the development of such articles for such diseases or conditions.

(c) In the case of drugs for rare diseases or conditions, the Board shall
  (1) evaluate
    (A) the effect of subchapter B of the Federal Food, Drug, and Cosmetic Act on the development of such drugs; and
    (B) the implementation of such subchapter;
  (2) evaluate the activities of the National Institutes of Health and the Alcohol, Drug Abuse, and Mental Health Administration for the development of drugs for such diseases or conditions;
  (3) assure appropriate coordination among the Food and Drug Administration, the National Institutes of Health, the Alcohol, Drug Abuse, and Mental Health Administration, and the Centers for Disease Control in the carrying out of their respective functions relating to the development of drugs for such diseases or conditions to assure that the activities of each agency are complementary;
  (4) assure appropriate coordination among all interested Federal agencies, manufacturers, and organizations representing patients, in their activities relating to such drugs;

(5) with the consent of the sponsor of a drug for a rare disease or condition exempt under section 505(i) of the Federal Food, Drug, and Cosmetic Act or regulations issued under such section, inform physicians and the public respecting the availability of such drug for such disease or condition, and inform physicians and the public respecting the availability of drugs approved under section 505(c) of such Act or licensed under section 351 of this Act for rare diseases or conditions;

(6) seek business entities and others to undertake the sponsorship of drugs for rare diseases or conditions, seek investigators to facilitate the development of such drugs, and seek business entities to participate in the distribution of such drugs; and

(7) reorganize the efforts of public and private entities and individuals in seeking the development of drugs for rare diseases or conditions and in developing such drugs.

(d) The Board shall consult with interested persons respecting the activities of the Board under this section and, as part of such consultation, shall provide the opportunity for the submission of oral views.

(e) The Board shall submit to the Committee on Labor and Human Resources of the Senate and the Committee on Energy and Commerce of the House of Representatives an annual report

(1) identifying the drugs that have been designated under section 526 of the Federal Food, Drug, and Cosmetic Act for a rare disease or condition;

(2) describing the activities of the Board; and

(3) containing the results of the evaluations carried out by the Board.

The Director of the National Institutes of Health and the Administrator of the Alcohol, Drug Abuse, and Mental Health Administration shall submit to the Board for inclusion in the annual report a report on the rare disease and condition research activities of the Institutes of the National Institutes of Health and the Alcohol, Drug Abuse, and Mental Health Administration; the Secretary of the Treasury shall submit to the Board for inclusion in the annual report a report on the use of the credit against tax provided by section 44H of the Internal Revenue Code of 1954; and the Secretary of Health and Human Services shall submit to the Board for inclusion in the annual report a report on the program of assistance under section 5 of the ODA for the development of drugs for rare diseases and conditions. Each annual report shall be submitted by June 1 of each year for the preceding calendar year.

CHAPTER 4

Investigational New Drug Applications (INDs)

INDs are among the most complex and critical of regulatory submissions. Most INDs run thousands of pages (often as many as 15 volumes) and may take months of assembly effort.

The IND is the application to allow testing of a new drug (or biological) on human subjects in formal clinical trials. Since the FDA's primary function is to assure the public's health and safety, approval of the IND is contingent on compelling evidence of the relative safety of the drug under consideration and on the safety of the controls built into the proposed clinical studies.

Since the IND is often the first formal communication with the FDA, it often sets the tone for ongoing FDA relations. A reputation for care and diligence, built with a strong IND, can strengthen continuing interactions, while a poorly designed or incomplete IND can sour the same future relationships.

CLASSIFICATION

INDs can be classified on five dimensions: commercial/noncommercial, standard/emergency, paper/electronic, drug/biological, and original/505(b)(2). Additional descriptors can characterize the phase of the proposed study or studies, the medical focus of the drug/biologic, and the design of the proposed study or studies.

Commercial INDs (those intended to lead to eventual production and marketing of a drug) are subject to greater scrutiny and review than INDs submitted by universities, research laboratories, and other not-for-profit organizations. For the noncommercial organizations, IND review tends to focus on the study design and the role of the Institutional Review Board (IRB). Commercial INDs add to these foci more extensive review of the chemistry, manufacturing, and control (CMC), pharmacology, and Investigator's Brochure, as

Guidebook for Drug Regulatory Submissions, by Sandy Weinberg
Copyright © 2009 John Wiley & Sons, Inc.

well as a detailed review of prior human experience and research with the drug.

The result of this different (informal) standard of review is driving initial research into the public not-for-profit sector, with commercial drug companies tending to become involved in later stages (phases 2 and 3) of development. The process effectively provides greater flexibility early in the development process while carefully controlling more extensive and intensive clinical trials.

Emergency INDs (often supplements to or amendments of standard INDs) receive priority review and accelerated consideration. As supplements, emergency INDs are generally abbreviated formats referencing the original IND (with a newly filed 1571 form). Most often, they represent corrections or modifications in the experimental design, chemistry, and/or control of the new drug.

Currently, most INDs are submitted in paper form, often accompanied by an electronic disk with hyperlinks. Purely electronic submissions are still rare, in large part because of a lack of standardization and electronic sophistication on the part of the FDA. There is currently a Clinical Data Interchange Standards Consortium (CDISC) test underway; assuming it proves successful, it is likely that CDISC will emerge as a common electronic submission standard for INDs, New Drug Applications (NDAs), and Abbreviated New Drug Applications (ANDAs) over the next three to five years.

The FDA permits a research organization to rely heavily on referenced studies originating in outside (generally published) sources. This application, termed a 505(b)(2), is described in detail in Chapter 6. However, since an IND can be written in anticipation of a 505(b)(2) NDA, mention here is appropriate.

All INDS include an extensive review of outside (generally published) literature, with particular focus on any administration of the proposed drug to human subjects or on any published toxicology or preclinical studies that may indicate any possible adverse reactions. An eventual 505(b)(2) NDA will rely on some of these studies, in combination with IND-proposed pivotal new clinical studies, to support the application. This plan will be outlined in the IND study proposal and/or discussed at the pre-IND FDA conference.

These five dimensions, along with the FDA Center target of the application (Metabolic, CNS, Oncology, etc.); the proposed study phases 1 (preclinical), 2 (limited clinical), 3 (extensive clinical), and 4 (postmarketing); and the details of the proposed study design are used to classify the IND and its intent.

TEAM EFFORT

Because of its complexity (and resulting extent) the preparation of an IND application is a team effort, involving regulatory (relations, regulatory CMC, submissions, technical writing, and reference research), Quality Assurance (auditing, CMC stability, and analysis results), CMC [active pharmaceutical ingredient (API) and final product manufacture, control, and testing], and clinical research (Investigator's Brochure, study design, scientific analysis, IRB approval). That team is generally headed by the leader of the regulatory unit, who, in the capacity of FDA liaison, signs the 1571 cover form.

There are two kinds of teams, in science, business, and other environments. In some settings, we use the "team" terminology to describe the process of subdividing a task, with each subunit contributing its expertise in turn or simultaneously. Consider, for example, the process of home construction. A framing carpenter puts up the skeleton, a dry-wall unit covers the frame, an electrician installs the wiring, and so forth. Together, the team builds the house, with the contractor or architect integrating the subunits into a cohesive whole.

This kind of subdividing team, while tempting on the surface, is not likely to lead to the most effective and successful IND.

The other meaning of the term "team" involves an integrated unit of individuals representing diverse areas of expertise. On a baseball team, for example, the pitcher, catcher, and fielders all work to integrate their efforts. They plan and practice together to be able to execute a pickoff play or a double out. Each player brings individual expertise to the team, but the success is a result of their cooperative blending of those skills.

The successful IND is most likely a result of cooperative work with an integrated team represented by Regulatory, Quality Assurance, Clinical, CMC, and others. Quality Assurance, for example, is likely to have valuable input into the design of the Investigator's Brochure; Clinical can contribute important direction and focus to the literature review; Regulatory may have CMC input of value; and so forth. The integrated team is more likely to both produce a smoothly integrated document and assure that the content of that document represents a cohesive and systematic assurance of public safety, which is the primary FDA focus.

The integrated IND team brings three important advantages. First, many sections of the IND, while defined in FDA guidance documents as self-standing descriptions, actually represent interactive results of input from different organizational subunits. The connection between CMC stability results and Quality Assurance review of the manufacturing site and procedures is a prime example.

Second, the integrated team can provide immediate and multiperspective feedback on all sections of the IND. The varied experiences of team members can help with questions and issues that extend beyond designated areas of responsibility.

Finally, the integrated team approach mimics and hence best meets the FDA review process. While a variety of FDA groups have input into an IND review, those subunits meet in a committee format to discuss and evaluate the submission. As a result, a number of their questions and concerns represent areas of interaction falling between sections rather than topics isolated within a part of the IND.

The integrated team is most likely to prove efficient, effective, and successful in IND (and other regulatory) submissions.

PROCESS

The process of filing an IND follows a carefully prescribed route, though it may be possible to bypass some of the steps in the case of a clear and non-controversial drug. Generally, there are five steps: meeting request, briefing book, meeting, submission, and remediation.

While a meeting is not mandatory, it does have several advantages. First, it allows the submitting organization to begin building a relationship with the relevant FDA players. Second, it provides advance warning of any key issues likely to be major foci in the IND. Third, it provides an opportunity to obtain "buy-in"—general agreement—on issues that are mutually identified as non-controversial. Finally, the pre-IND meeting provides some insight into the ultimate NDA/IND review.

The process begins with a formal letter to the FDA requesting a pre-IND meeting (see Chapter 1). The letter should identify the drug and intended indication and should list and describe the questions to be raised in the meeting (generally, those areas of potential buy-in, those areas in which clarifying discussion would be useful, and the general approach to be taken in the IND). Questions should be worded in the "Does the Agency agree that ..." format to maximize identification of areas of agreement. In addition, the letter should clearly identify the contact individual, should identify the FDA personnel the company believes should attend (i.e., representatives of Metabolic, Toxicology), and may propose possible meeting dates (generally six to eight weeks in the future).

In rare cases, the FDA will respond by denying the meeting on the ground that there is agreement on all of the questions, and request IND submission. This denial represents acceptance of the proposed positions on all questions.

More often, the FDA will schedule the meeting and request a Briefing Book at a specified time (usually four weeks) prior to the meeting. While the proposed date is open to discussion, FDA calendars are very tight, and alternate meetings should only be proposed in extreme cases.

The Briefing Book provides the rationale evidence behind each questions and abibliography of references (including both the citing and the actual publication). It provides an opportunity to expand on the question and to make a clear case for the submitting organization's position on the issue.

At the meeting, the FDA will focus—often in great detail—on those questions raised in the Briefing Book that are considered controversial. While the meeting is not an inquisition, it may be a detailed cross-examination and represents the submitting organization's best opportunity to explain and justify a key issue.

After the meeting (and a follow-up summary letter from the FDA), the requirements for the specific IND are clearly established. While it is theoretically possible to dispute or appeal that finding letter, it represents the FDA's feedback on what evidence it considers necessary. Unless there has been a misunderstanding or a pressing need for clarification, an appeal is unlikely to change that definition. In effect, the FDA is indicating what relief from the formal requirements or reduction of supporting evidence it is willing to accept; rejection of that position is likely to impose more rather than fewer IND requirements.

As soon as the final IND is completed, it is submitted (see the checklist). The FDA conducts a formal review (response generally issued within 30 days of submission). That response (generally provided in a conference call) may be full approval with permission to conduct the proposed study of studies, approval with some restriction on the proposed study or studies, or a rejection. Each requires a response from the submitter.

If granted, approval of a statement of receipt is appropriate. If restrictions or modifications have been required, a statement accepting or (in rare cases) clarifying those restrictions avoids any future misunderstandings. If the IND is rejected, it can be resubmitted with further evidence, clarification, or modifications.

PROBLEM AREAS

An analysis of successful (and unsuccessful) INDs has identified three key problem areas. These represent major FDA foci and areas often presenting difficult challenges for submitting organizations.

CMC. By far, the greatest challenges come in the CMC area. Questions of stability (of API and product), of impurity profiles, of unknown mechanisms of action, and of packaging/shipping/storage requirements are common stumbling blocks that require careful address in IND submissions. The three key criteria are the three Cs: Careful (accurate, technically correct, supported by documentation), Complete (timely, thorough), and Calculated (accurate formulations and calculations).

Investigator's Brochure. The Investigator's Brochure and accompanying study description will be carefully reviewed to make certain that the design is appropriate, meets standard criteria for blinding and control, and protects the human subjects (in initial screening, disclosure, administration, and followup). Safety of humans is the key element in the review; the Investigator's Brochure should clearly and comprehensively address all relevant safety issues.

Previous human experience. The review of literature should address carefully all published studies (U.S. and international) that have included administration of the drug and any side effects, dropouts, or serious issues that emerged in those studies. Drug licensed (or applied for) in European Medicines Agency (EMEA) or other regulatory environments should be reviewed; any rejections or removal from market must be carefully addressed.

SUMMARY

Since INDs generally mark the first critical step in the drug development process and may well mark the first formal interaction with the FDA on a new drug, the submission assumes a highly significant role in the regulatory process. The document is complex, involving important input from all parts of the researching organization, and often runs to thousand of pages of explanation, data, and published research materials.

INDs are most successful when developed by an integrated team of organizational professions; when focused through the FDA premeeting request (briefing, book, discussion) process; and when careful attention is paid to issues related to CMC, the study and Investigator's Brochure, and the previous (published) human experience with the drug. With these carefully constructed elements and appropriate attention to format requirements, the IND can result not only in permission to launch a program of clinical studies but also in a strong and positive relationship with the FDA.

IND APPLICATION SUBMISSION CHECKLIST

This checklist is intended for use in the preparation and submission of INDs. It is recommended that, prior to transmission to the FDA, a second internal review should be conducted by an individual or department not involved in the preparation of the submission (presumably Quality Assurance).

The checklist was developed through discussions with consultants and Quality Assurance directors and has been field-tested in final form with five successful submissions.

- ☐ Form 1571 completed
- ☐ Cover letter including the following:
    - ☐ Name and address of sponsor
    - ☐ Name, address, title, telephone, and e-mail of contact person
    - ☐ Generic and trade name of drug or drug product
    - ☐ FDA code number (assigned at time of preconference)
- ☐ Three copies of application in indexed binders
- ☐ Pagination: all pages included and properly numbered
- ☐ Headings: section headings confirming to submission subparagraphs, with initial Table of Contents

☐ Integrated references: All referenced articles included in final section, internally referenced in text

☐ Bibliography: complete standard format bibliography listing all referenced articles

☐ Complete CMC information provided, including evidence of purity, stability, toxicology testing, and integrity of API, placebo, and final product

☐ Study design protocol included with sufficient detail to allow evaluation

☐ Investigator's Brochure included with detailed information for investigators and IRB records

☐ Review of literature addresses all available prior instances of human use of drug product, with emphasis on safety, administration, and possible adverse events

☐ Complete pharmacological profile provided for API and final product

☐ Summary of regulatory status and marketing history in the United States and foreign countries

☐ Summary of adverse reactions to proposed drug in any country

☐ IND addresses all issues and questions raised in the pre-IND meeting

FDA IND REVIEW CHECKLIST

This FDA IND review checklist has been designed in consultation with FDA reviewers, industry consultants, and regulatory professionals to serve as a summary tool indicating the evaluative criteria used by the Center for Drug Evaluation and Research (CDER) and the Center for Biologics Evaluation and Research (CBER) to critique and assess applications received. It can be used internally as a part of the Quality Assurance process, as a guideline for regulatory development of an application, and/or as a self-assessment tool to predict likely FDA response to an application.

☐ **Logistics:** Submission conforms to FDA guideline 21 Code of Federal Regulations (CFR) Part 312.23(a)(10), (11), and (b), (c), (d), and (e).

☐ **Receipt:** Application was received in the FDA mail room.

☐ IND jackets: Document is contained in one or more 3-in., three-ring binders.

☐ **Form 1571:** IND is accompanied by completed Form 1571, providing (among other data) contact information including corporate name, contact name, address, telephone number, name and address of drug source, generic and trade name of drug.

☐ **Cover letter:** A cover letter indicates disease and therapy names.

☐ **Three copies:** Photocopies are acceptable.

☐ **Format:** Submission conforms to FDA guideline 21 CFR Part 312.23 (a), (10), (11), and (b), (c), (d), and (e) and to FDA norm standards.

☐ **Pagination:** All pages included and properly numbered

☐ **Headings:** Section headings conforming to submission subparagraphs

☐ **Integrated references:** Copies of all referenced articles, with references integrated into the body of text

☐ **Bibliography:** Complete standard format bibliography as referenced in text

Note: If electronic submission is selected:

☐ Advance notification letter provided.

☐ Format and tables conform to *Guidance for Industry: Providing Regulatory Submissions to CBER in Electronic Format—Investigational New Drug Applications (INDs)*

☐ Electronic submission format conforms to approved list in Docket number 92s-0251 [see 21 CFR 11.1(d) and 11.2].

☐ Electronic signatures conform to emerging guidelines, or a paper copy with appropriate nonelectronic signatures is included.

☐ **CONTENT: Organizational structure**

☐ **Cover sheet:** Form 1571

☐ **Table of contents:** Indicates page and volume of each section

☐ **Introductory statement and general investigational plan:** Two- to three-page summary identifying sponsor needs and general (phase) plans

☐ **Investigator's Brochure:** Conformity with the International Conference on Harmonization *Good Clinical Practice: Guideline for the Investigator's Brochure*

☐ **Protocol:** Copy of the protocol for each proposed clinical study. Note that phase 1 protocols should provide a brief outline including estimation of number of subjects to be included, a description of safety exclusions, and a description of dosing plan (duration, dose, method). All protocols should address monitoring of blood chemistry and vital signs, and toxicity-based modification plans.

☐ **CMC information:** It should contain sufficient detail to assure identification, quality, purity, and strength of the investigational drug. It should include stability data of duration appropriate to the length of the proposed study. FDA concerns to be addressed focus on products made with unknown or impure components, products with chemical structures known to be of likely high toxicity, products known to be chemically unstable, and products with an impurity profile indicative of a health hazard or insufficiently defined to assess potential health hazard, or poorly characterized master or working cell bank.

■ Chemistry and manufacturing introduction

■ Drug substance

  ○ Description: physical, chemical, or biological characteristics

- ○ Name and address of manufacturer
- ○ Method of preparation
- ○ Limits and analytical methods
- ○ Stability information
- ■ Drug product
  - ○ List of components
  - ○ Qualitative composition
  - ○ Name and address of drug product manufacturer
  - ○ Description of manufacturing and packaging procedures
  - ○ Limits and analytical methods: identity, strength, quality, and purity
  - ○ Stability results
- ■ Placebo
- ■ Labels and labeling
- ■ Environmental assessment (or claim for exclusion): 21 CFR 312.23(a)(7)(iv)(e)
- ☐ **Pharmacology and toxicology information [21 CFR 312.23(a)(8)]**
  - ■ Pharmacology and drug distribution [21 CFR 312.23(a)(8)(i)]
    - ○ Description of pharmacological effects and mechanisms of action
    - ○ Description of absorption, distribution, metabolism, and excretion of the drug
  - ■ Toxicology summary [21 CFR 312.23(a)(8)(ii)(a)]: summary of toxicological effects in animals and *in vitro*
    - ○ Description of design of toxicological trials and any deviations from design
    - ○ Systematic presentation of animal toxicology studies and toxicokinetic studies
  - ■ Toxicology full data tabulation [21 CFR 312.23(a)(8)(ii)(b)]: Data points with either
    - ○ brief description of the study or
    - ○ copy of the protocol with amendments
  - ■ Toxicology good laboratory practice (GLP) certification [21 CFR 312.23(a)(8)(iii)]
- ☐ **Previous human experience with the investigational drug:** Summary report of any U.S. or non-U.S. human experience with the drug
- ☐ **References:** Indexed copies of referenced articles with comprehensive bibliography
- ☐ **Support:** Evaluation of the referent support provided
  - ☐ **Key issues:** All key issues appropriately referenced, including
    - ■ Investigator's Brochure
    - ■ Protocols
    - ■ CMC information
    - ■ Pharmacology and toxicology information
    - ■ Previous human experience with the investigational drug

☐ **Credible:** References are from credible scientific journals and/or sources.

☐ **Organized:** References are organized and tied to text.

COMMENTS:
DISPOSITION:
   Receipt date:
   Response due date:
   Disposition:
   Notification date:

IND APPLICATION PROCESS

Introduction

Current Federal law requires that a drug be the subject of an approved marketing application before it is transported or distributed across state lines. Because a sponsor will probably want to ship the investigational drug to clinical investigators in many states, it must seek an exemption from that legal requirement. The IND is the means through which the sponsor technically obtains this exemption from the FDA.

During the early preclinical development of a new drug, the sponsor's primary goal is to determine if the product is reasonably safe for initial use in humans and if the compound exhibits pharmacological activity that justifies commercial development. When a product has been identified as a viable candidate for further development, the sponsor then focuses on collecting the data and information necessary to establish that the product will not expose humans to unreasonable risks when used in limited, early-stage clinical studies.

The FDA's role in the development of a new drug begins when the drug's sponsor (usually the manufacturer or the potential marketer), having screened the new molecule for pharmacological activity and acute toxicity potential in animals, wants to test its diagnostic or therapeutic potential in humans. At that point, the molecule changes in legal status under the Federal Food, Drug, and Cosmetic Act and becomes a new drug subject to specific requirements of the drug regulatory system.

There are three IND types.

- An Investigator IND is submitted by a physician who both initiates and conducts an investigation, and under whose immediate direction the investigational drug is administered or dispensed. A physician might submit a research IND to propose studying an unapproved drug, or an approved product for a new indication or in a new patient population.

- *Emergency Use IND* allows the FDA to authorize use of an experimental drug in an emergency situation that does not allow time for submission of an IND in accordance with 21CFR, Sec. 312.23 or Sec. 312.34. It is also used for patients who do not meet the criteria of an existing study protocol, or if an approved study protocol does not exist.
- *Treatment IND* is submitted for experimental drugs showing promise in clinical testing for serious or immediately life-threatening conditions, while the final clinical work is conducted and the FDA review takes place.

There are two IND categories.

- Commercial
- Research (noncommercial)

The IND application must contain information in three broad areas.

- Animal pharmacology and toxicology studies—preclinical data to permit an assessment as to whether the product is reasonably safe for initial testing in humans. Also included are any previous experience with the drug in humans (often foreign use).
- Manufacturing information—information pertaining to the composition, manufacturer, stability, and controls used for manufacturing the drug substance and the drug product. This information is assessed to ensure that the company can adequately produce and supply consistent batches of the drug.
- Clinical protocols and investigator information—detailed protocols for proposed clinical studies to assess whether the initial-phase trials will expose subjects to unnecessary risks. Also, information on the qualifications of clinical investigators—professionals (generally physicians) who oversee the administration of the experimental compound—to assess whether they are qualified to fulfill their clinical trial duties; finally, commitments to obtain informed consent from the research subjects, to obtain review of the study by an IRB, and to adhere to the IND regulations.

Once the IND is submitted, the sponsor must wait 30 calendar days before initiating any clinical trials. During this time, the FDA has an opportunity to review the IND for safety to ensure that research subjects will not be subjected to unreasonable risks.

The interactive chart at http://www.fda.gov/cder/handbook/ind.htm summarizes the IND process, including how CDER determines if the product is suitable for use in clinical trials.

TheWeb site is designed for individuals from pharmaceutical companies, government agencies, academic institutions, private organizations, or other organizations interested in bringing a new drug to market. Each of the following sections contains information from CDER to assist you in the IND application process. For specific information, click on a link to go directly to a section or a Web page.

Resources for IND Applicationss

The following resources have been gathered to provide you with the legal requirements of an IND application, assistance from CDER to help you meet those requirements, and internal IND review principles, policies, and procedures.

Pre-IND Consultation Program: CDER offers a pre-IND consultation program to foster early communications between sponsors and new drug review divisions in order to provide guidance on the data necessary to warrant IND submission. The review divisions are organized generally along therapeutic class and can each be contacted using the designated Pre-IND Consultation List. (December 5, 2006)

Guidance Documents for INDs. Guidance documents represent the Agency's current thinking on a particular subject. These documents are prepared for FDA review staff and applicants/sponsors to provide guidelines on the processing, content, and evaluation/approval of applications and on the design, production, manufacturing, and testing of regulated products. They also establish policies intended to achieve consistency in the Agency's regulatory approach and establish inspection and enforcement procedures. Because guidances are not regulations or laws, they are not enforceable, either through administrative actions or through the courts. An alternative approach may be used if such approach satisfies the requirements of the applicable statute or regulations or both. For information on a specific guidance document, please contact the originating office.

For the complete list of CDER guidances, please see the Guidance Index. Most of these documents are in Adobe Acrobat format, also known as PDF. The free upgrade to Adobe Acrobat 3.0 or higher is recommended, especially if you have difficulty opening any of the following documents. For information on a specific guidance document, please contact the originating office.

Guidance documents to help prepare INDs include the following:

- *Guidance for Industry: INDs—Approaches to Complying with CGMP's for Phase 1 Drugs* (Draft) (January 12, 2006)
- *Guidance for Industry: Exploratory IND Studies* (January 12, 2006)
- *Content and Format of Investigational New Drug Applications (INDs) for Phase 1 Studies of Drugs Including Well- Characterized, Therapeutic, Biotechnology-Derived Products* provides description of required sections of an application.

- *Q & A—Content and Format of INDs for Phase 1 Studies of Drugs, Including Well-Characterized, Therapeutic, Biotechnology-Derived Products.* Optional Format: PDF. This guidance is intended to clarify when sponsors should submit final, quality-assured toxicology reports and/or update the Agency on any changes in findings since submission of nonquality-assured reports or reports based on nonquality-assured data. (Issued October 2000).

- *Bioavailability and Bioequivalence Studies for Orally Administered Drug Products—General Considerations.* Optional Format: PDF (Issued October 2000, Posted October 27, 2000). This guidance should be useful for applicants planning to conduct bioavailability and bioequivalence (BE) studies during the IND period for an NDA, BE studies intended for submission in an ANDA, and BE studies conducted in the postapproval period for certain changes in both NDAs and ANDAs.

- *IND Exemptions for Studies of Lawfully Marketed Drug or Biological Products for the Treatment of Cancer.* (January 2004)

- Drug Master Files (DMF). DMF is a submission to the FDA that may be used to provide confidential detailed information about facilities, processes, or articles used in the manufacturing, processing, packaging, and storing of one or more human drugs.

- *Required Specifications for the FDA's IND, NDA, and ANDA Drug Master File Binders*

Immunotoxicology Evaluation of IND (PDF) (Issued October 2002, Posted October 31, 2002). This guidance makes recommendations to sponsors of INDs on (1) the parameters that should be routinely assessed in toxicology studies to determine the effects of a drug on immune function; (2) when additional immunotoxicity studies should be conducted; and (3) when additional mechanistic information could help characterize the significance of a given drug's effect on the immune system.

Laws, Regulations, Policies, and Procedures

The mission of the FDA is to enforce laws enacted by the U.S. Congress and regulations established by the Agency to protect the consumers' health, safety, and pocketbook. The Federal Food, Drug, and Cosmetic Act is the basic food and drug law of the United States. With numerous amendments, it is the most extensive law of its kind in the world. The law is intended to assure consumers that foods are pure and wholesome, safe to eat, and produced under sanitary conditions; that drugs and devices are safe and effective for their intended uses; that cosmetics are safe and made from appropriate ingredients; and that all labeling and packaging is truthful, informative, and not deceptive.

CFR. The final regulations published in the Federal Register (daily published record of proposed rules, final rules, meeting notices, etc.) are collected in the CFR. The CFR is divided into 50 titles that represent broad areas subject to Federal regulations. The FDA's portion of the CFR interprets the Federal Food, Drug, and Cosmetic Act and related statutes. Section 21 of the CFR contains most regulations pertaining to food and drugs. The regulations document all actions of all drug sponsors that are required under Federal law.

The following regulations apply to the IND application process.

21CFR Part 312	*Investigational New Drug Application*
21CFR Part 314	*INDA and NDA Applications for FDA Approval to Market a New Drug (New Drug Approval)*
21CFR Part 316	*Orphan Drugs*
21CFR Part 58	*Good Laboratory Practice for Nonclinical Laboratory (Animal) Studies*
21CFR Part 50	*Protection of Human Subjects*
21CFR Part 56	*Institutional Review Boards*
21CFR Part 201	*Drug Labeling*
21CFR Part 54	*Financial Disclosure by Clinical Investigators*

Manual of Policies and Procedures (MaPPs). *CDER's MaPPs* are approved instructions for internal practices and procedures followed by CDER staff to help standardize the new drug review process and other activities. MaPPs define external activities as well. All MAPPs are available for the public to review to get a better understanding of office policies, definitions, staff responsibilities, and procedures. MaPPs of particular interest to IND sponsors include the following:

- 4200.1 Consulting the Controlled Substance Staff on INDs and Protocols That Use Schedule I Controlled Substances and Drugs (Issued May 8, 2003)
- 5210.5 Review of Investigational New Drug Applications (Bio-INDs) by the Office of Generic Drugs
- 6030.1 IND Process and Review Procedures (Including Clinical Holds) includes general IND review principles, policies, and procedures for issuing clinical holds of INDs, and processing and responding to sponsors' complete responses to clinical holds.
- 6030.2 INDs: Review of Informed Consent Documents (Issued November 13, 2002)
- 6030.4 INDs: Screening INDs (Issued May 9, 2001, Posted May 14, 2001). This multiservice provisioning platform (MsPP) describes procedures for the review of multiple active moieties or formulations under the single investigative new drug application (IND) called a screening IND.

- 6030.8 INDs: Exception from Informed Consent Requirements for Emergency Research. (Issued February 4, 2003)

IND Forms and Instructions

Forms for use in submitting INDs include the following:

- FDA 1571 Investigational New Drug Application
- FDA 1572 Statement of Investigator
- Instructions for completing FDA forms 1571 and 1572
- FDA Form Distributions Page includes links to Certification: Financial Interest and Arrangements of Clinical Investigators Disclosure: Financial Interest and Arrangements of Clinical Investigators MedWatch: FDA Medical Product Reporting Program—Voluntary MedWatch: FDA Medical Products Reporting Program—Mandatory
- For electronic form submissions, see Electronic Regulatory and Submission Review (ERSR, at http://www.fda.gov/cder/regulatory/ersr).

Emergency Use of an Investigational Drug or Biologics

- The FDA proposes that rules overhaul to expand the availability of experimental drugs. The Agency also clarifies permissible charges to patients. [FDA News (December 11, 2006)]
- The *Guidance for Institutional Review Boards and Clinical Investigators* contains information on Obtaining an Emergency IND, Emergency Exemption from Prospective IRB, Approval Exception from Informed Consent, and Requirement Planned Emergency Research, Informed Consent Exception.
- For assistance in obtaining unapproved cancer drugs, please go to *Access to Unapproved Drugs* (http://www.fda.gov/cder/cancer/access.htm).
- *Federal Register Notice for Emergency Use of an Investigational New Drug; Technical Amendment*
- *Directions to Sponsors of Emergency Investigational New Drug (EIND) Application.* From the Office of Antimicrobial Products, Division of Antiviral Products (November 29, 2005)

Emergency Use Requests

- For investigational biological products regulated by CBER, call 301-827-2000.
- For all other investigational drugs, call 301-827-4570.
- After working hours, call the FDA's Office of Emergency Operations at 301-443-1240.

Related Topics

- NDA Web page provides resources to assist drug sponsors with submitting applications for approval to market a new drug.
- ANDA Web page provides resources to assist drug sponsors with submitting applications to market a generic drug.
- Biological Therapeutic Products Web page
- Drug Application Regulatory Compliance. The approval process for new drug applications includes a review of the manufacturer's compliance with Current Good Manufacturing Practice. This Web page provides resources to help meet compliance.
- Small Business Assistance Program Web page
- ERSR Web page provides information on electronic drug applications, application reviews, Electronic Document Room, and other ERSR projects.
- Postdrug-approval Activities. The goal of CDER's postdrug-approval activities is to monitor the ongoing safety of marketed drugs. This is accomplished by reassessing drug risks based on new data learned after the drug is marketed and by recommending ways of trying to most appropriately manage that risk.

Information for Sponsor-Investigators Submitting INDs

An IND is a request for FDA authorization to administer an investigational drug to humans. Such authorization must be secured prior to interstate shipment and administration of any new drug that is not the subject of an approved new drug application.

IND regulations are contained in Title 21,CFR, Part 312. Copies of the regulations, further guidance regarding IND procedures, and additional forms are available from the FDA Center for Drug Evaluation and Research, Drug Information Branch (HFD-210), 5600 Fishers Lane, Rockville, MD 20857, Tel: (301) 827-4573 or toll free at 1-888-INFOFDA. In addition, forms, regulations, guidances, and a wide variety of additional information are available online at http://www.fda.gov/cder/. Forms may be accessed directly at http://www.fda.gov/opacom/morechoices/fdaforms/cder.html.

The following instructions address only the administrative aspects of preparing and submitting an IND and are intended primarily to provide assistance to individual Sponsor-Investigator applicants, not pharmaceutical companies.

Where to Send the Application. The initial IND submission and each subsequent submission to the IND should be accompanied by a Form FDA 1571 and must be submitted in triplicate (the original and two photocopies are acceptable). Mailing addresses for initial IND submissions are

For a Drug:
Food and Drug Administration
Center for Drug Evaluation and Research
Central Document Room
5901-B Ammendale Rd.
Beltsville, MD 20705-1266

For a Therapeutic Biological Product:
http://www.fda.gov/cber/transfer/transfer.htm
Food and Drug Administration
Center for Drug Evaluation and Research
Therapeutic Biological Products Document Room
5901-B Ammendale Road
Beltsville, MD 20705-1266

Filling Out the Form FDA 1571. The numbers below correspond to the numbered boxes on the Form FDA 1571.

1. The sponsor is the person who takes responsibility for and initiates a clinical investigation. The sponsor may be a pharmaceutical company, a private or academic organization, or an individual. **A Sponsor-Investigator is an individual who both initiates and conducts a clinical investigation and under whose immediate direction the investigational drug is being administered or dispensed.** For administrative reasons, only one individual should be designated as sponsor.

    If a pharmaceutical company will be supplying the drug but will not itself be submitting the IND, the company is not the sponsor.

2. The date of submission is the date that the application is mailed to the FDA.

3. The address is the address to which written correspondence from the FDA should be directed. If this address is a post office box number, a street address must also be provided.

4. The telephone number is the number where the sponsor is usually available during normal working hours. A telephone number must be provided.

5. For name(s) of drug, list the generic name(s) and trade name, if available. Also, state the dosage form(s).

6. If an emergency IND number was previously assigned by the FDA, or the Form FDA 1571 is being included with an amendment to the original IND, then that IND number should be entered here; otherwise, the space should be left blank.

7. Self-explanatory.

8. This section is to be completed by pharmaceutical firms that are conducting clinical studies in support of a marketing application. Sponsor-Investigators need not complete this section.

9. It is necessary for the sponsor to submit certain information with an IND (such as manufacturing and controls information, pharmacology and toxicology data, or data from prior human studies) unless that information has previously been submitted to the FDA *and* the sponsor of the previously submitted information provides a letter authorizing the FDA to refer to the information. In this case, the letter of authorization including the file identification (IND/DMF/NDA number) must be (1) submitted to the authorizer's application and (2) included in the initial submission of the new sponsor's IND. The sole exception to this requirement is when a marketed drug is used in the study, without modification to its approved packaging, in which case the marketed drug product must be identified by trade name, established name, dosage form, strength, and lot number.

10. Numbering of submissions is primarily intended for pharmaceutical firms. Sponsor-Investigators do not have to complete this section.

11. For an original IND submission, only the "Initial Investigational New Drug Application (IND)" box should be checked. For subsequent submissions, check ALL the boxes that apply since the submission may contain more than one type of information.

    Requests to charge and Treatment Protocols must be submitted separately. Treatment INDs and Treatment Protocols are special cases and are not intended for single patient use. Before checking either of these boxes, the sponsor should be thoroughly familiar with the cited regulations and contact the appropriate FDA reviewing division to discuss the proposed treatment use.

12. For a Sponsor-Investigator IND, items 2, 3, and 4 may be briefly addressed in the cover letter or in a summary.

    Where the investigational drug is obtained from a supplier in a final dosage form, items 5, 7, 8, and 9 may be referenced if authorization is given by the supplier (see explanation in section 9). If the investigational drug is prepared or altered in any way after shipment by the supplier, complete manufacturing (or compounding) and controls information, including information on sterility and pyrogenicity testing for parenteral drugs, must be submitted for that process in Item 7.

    Item 6 requires that the protocol be submitted, along with information on the investigators, facilities, and IRB, copies of the completed Form FDA 1572 with attachments would suffice for 6 b–d.

    Item 7 also requires submission of either a claim of categorical exclusion from the requirement to submit an environmental assessment or an environmental assessment [21 CFR 25.15(a)]. When claiming a categorical exclusion, the sponsor should include the following statements: "I claim categorical exclusion [under 21 CFR 25.31(e)] for the study(ies) under this IND. To my knowledge, no extraordinary circumstances exist."

13. This section does not pertain to a Sponsor-Investigator.

14–15. For a pharmaceutical firm, the name of the person responsible for monitoring the conduct of the clinical investigation and reviewing and evaluating safety information should be entered. For Sponsor-Investigator INDs, the investigator has this responsibility.

Note: Certain important commitments that the IND sponsor makes by signing the form FDA 1571 are listed below box 15.

16–17. For an IND sponsored by a pharmaceutical firm or research organization, the name of the sponsor's authorizing representative would be entered, that individual must sign the form For a Sponsor-Investigator IND, and the Sponsor-Investigator should be named and must sign the form.

18–19. Boxes 18 and 19 need not be completed if they duplicate boxes 3 and 4.

20. The date here is the date the form is signed by the sponsor.

Form FDA 1572. Copies of Form FDA 1572 with its attachments may be sent by the Sponsor-Investigator to the FDA to satisfy Form FDA 1571, box 12, item 6 b–d. Information can be supplied in the form of attachments (such as a curriculum vitae) rather than entering that information directly onto the form, but this should be so noted under the relevant section numbers.

FDA Receipt of the IND. Upon receipt of the IND by the FDA, an IND number will be assigned, and the application will be forwarded to the appropriate reviewing division. The reviewing division will send a letter to the Sponsor-Investigator providing notification of the IND number assigned, date of receipt of the original application, address where future submissions to the IND should be sent, and the name and telephone number of the FDA person to whom questions about the application should be directed. Studies shall not be initiated until 30 days after the date of receipt of the IND by the FDA unless you receive earlier notification by the FDA that studies may begin.

GUIDANCE FOR INDUSTRY: PROVIDING REGULATORY SUBMISSIONS TO CBER IN ELECTRONIC FORMAT—INDS

Additional copies of this guidance document are available from Office of Communication, Training and Manufacturers Assistance (HFM-40), 1401 Rockville Pike, Rockville, MD 20852-1448. Tel: 1-800-835-4709 or 301-827-1800 and online at http//:www.fda.gov/cber/guidelines.htm.

For questions on the content of this document, contact Michael B. Fauntle-roy at 301-827-5132.

This guidance document represents the Agency's current thinking on this topic. It does not create or confer any rights for or on any person and does not operate to bind the FDA or the public. An alternative approach may be used if such approach satisfies the requirements of the applicable statutes and regulations.

Introduction

This is one in a series of guidance documents intended to assist you, sponsors, in making regulatory submissions in electronic format to CBER. We, the FDA, intend to update guidance on electronic submissions regularly to reflect the evolving nature of the technology and the experience of those using this technology. As the FDA develops guidance on electronic IND submissions in the common technical document format, we intend to harmonize this guidance with the common technical document guidance.

In this guidance, we discuss specific issues unique to the electronic submission of INDs and their amendments. We have described general issues such as acceptable file formats, media, and submission procedures that are common to all submissions in the companion guidance, *Providing Regulatory Submissions in Electronic Format—General Considerations*, dated January 1999 (January 28, 1999, 64 FR 4433).

This guidance finalizes the draft guidance entitled *Guidance for Industry: Pilot Program for Electronic Investigational New Drug (eIND) Applications for Biological Products*, dated May 1998, that was announced in the Federal Register on June 1, 1998 (63 FR 104). We have incorporated into this guidance our experiences from the pilot program and comments received from the public, and from our electronic marketing applications guidance entitled *Guidance for Industry: Providing Regulatory Submissions to the Center for Biologics Evaluation and Research (CBER) in Electronic Format-Biologics Marketing Applications [Biologics License Application (BLA), Product License Application (PLA)/Establishment License Application (ELA) and New Drug Application (NDA)]*, dated November 1999 (November 12, 1999; 64 FR 61647).

Purpose

This guidance is intended to facilitate the submission of INDs in electronic format as well as ensure quick and easy information access for the reviewer. The guidance features an IND main folder that is used throughout the life of the application. The IND main folder contains six subfolders, four of which are analogous to the review disciplines within CBER. They are described in section "Folders."

We have employed a table of contents (TOC) and a bookmark-driven navigational construct that is similar to the structure employed in CBER's electronic marketing application. You should include at the top of the bookmark hierarchy the following bookmarks: Roadmap, Main TOC, and Item TOC (i.e., for the item currently under review). When presenting a TOC in your electronic IND submission, analogous bookmarks should reside in the left-hand margin.

Your submission should include individual portable document format (PDF) files that contain numeric prefixes. The numeric prefix should reflect the amendment number in which the file was submitted for review. The numeric prefix will facilitate the loading of new files into a preexisting folder structure that features the IND main folder and its six subfolders (see "Folders"). However, the following PDF files should not contain numeric prefixes: *roadmap.pdf* (see *Appendix A*), *protocolctoc.pdf* [see "Protocol and Protocol Revisions (Amendments)" and *Appendix B*, Figure VI-4], and *adverse_eventstoc.pdf* (see "Adverse Events" and *Appendix B*, Figure VI-5). These files are cumulative and will be replaced in subsequent submissions.

The electronic IND also features the use of the *roadmap.pdf*. This is the recommended entry point for the electronic submission. The *roadmap.pdf* should contain functional hypertext links to the original submissions main TOC and to each subsequent submission's TOC. You should include the submission serial number found in the prefix of each file for that submission (see *Appendix A*). You should update and resubmit this file with each amending submission. As a result, the *roadmap.pdf* always will contain a current comprehensive submission history that will enable a reviewer to easily access the original IND and its subsequent amendments through their main TOCs.

When amending your IND, you should utilize the same IND main folder and subfolder names (that you used) in your original IND submission. The amending submissions' IND main folder should include the appropriate subfolders for the content of that submission (see "Folders"). The files should be identified through the use of the amending submissions serial number in their file name prefix (see "Folders and File Names"). We will load the individual files of the new amendment, which reflect a new submission serial number in their prefix, into the preexisting content subfolders on our server. If the amendment contains a content subfolder not previously submitted to the IND, we will load the entire subfolder into the IND main folder on our server. You should submit an updated overall submission index and an updated subfolder specific index with every amendment to the IND. We will load these indexes into the preexisting folder structure.

General Issues

Regulations in 21 CFR Part 312 provide the general requirements for submitting INDs to CBER. Currently, Form FDA 1571, available at http://www.fda.gov/opacom/morechoices/fdaforms/cber.html, outlines the components required in the submission of an IND.

Harmonization with Guidance for Marketing Applications. We have tried to harmonize the guidance for providing INDs and marketing applications in electronic format whenever possible. You should refer to the *Guidance for Industry: Providing Regulatory Submissions to the Center for Biologics Evaluation and Research (CBER) in Electronic Format—Biologics Marketing Applications [Biologics License Application (BLA), Product License Application (PLA)/Establishment License Application (ELA) and New Drug Application (NDA)]*, November 1999, Revised, as a reference.

Submissions Related to the Initial IND. This guidance applies equally to the original submission of an IND and to the subsequent submissions amending the original application. We have described IND submission types on the Form FDA 1571 under item 11. If you decide to provide an IND in electronic format, you should provide the entire submission in electronic format and all amendments to the original submission in electronic format.

Acceptability of Electronic Submissions. In the Federal Register of March 20, 1997 (62 FR 13467), the Agency announced the establishment of a docket, number 92S-0251, where it will publish the submissions it will accept in electronic format. Once a Center has identified in the docket a submission type as one that can be processed, reviewed, and archived in an electronic-only format, you may provide the submission utilizing electronic media without any paper copies [21 CFR 11.1(d) and 11.2].

Electronic Signatures. We are developing procedures for archiving documents with electronic signatures. Until those procedures are in place, you should include with the electronic document the following:

- Documents for which the regulations require an original signature
- A paper copy that includes the handwritten signature of the sponsor' authorized representative and the IND number to identify the electronic document and attachments.

Cross-References to Other INDs. At times, IND submissions are supported by a cross-reference to another IND [21 CFR 312.23(b)]. The utility of the electronic IND submission will be further increased if all reference materials are supplied with the IND submission. You should handle these files in the same manner as other electronic files submitted to the IND. For example, you should generate the files from electronic source files rather than from scanned paper documents if at all possible. If the electronic source file is not available, we will accept a scanned copy. You should describe the file format and organization of these files as described in this guidance.

If an electronic IND or other form of documentation already exists in CBER and the appropriate letters of authorization are supplied, the IND review team will be granted access to those documents. If the files you choose to reference have been provided in electronic format, you should include the main folder name in which the document resides in place of the volume number required under 21 CFR 312.23(b). You should provide copies of the appropriate letters of authorization in the *admin* folder of the submission.

Folder and File Names. We have provided specific names for the folders (see Table 4.1) and subfolders of the submission as well as the TOC files including the roadmap file. Using these names will minimize confusion among the Center's reviewers.

For file names not specifically described, we ask that you use the following naming conventions.

- Include the submission serial number for the file in the initial four numbers of the file.
- Use a descriptive name for the file up to a total of 28 characters. This is a total of 32 characters including the four-digit serial number.
- Use the appropriate three-character extension for the file (e.g., pdf, xpt).
- Be consistent with the file names. For example, if you use the protocol number as part of the name of the original protocol, you should include the same name for the protocol revision.

For example, protocol 1234 provided in amendment number six could be named *0006_1234.pdf*. The revised protocol submitted as part of amendment 125 would be named *0125_1234.pdf*.

Bookmarks and Hypertext Links. For all documents with a TOC, you should provide bookmarks and hypertext links for each item in the document's TOC including all tables, figures, publications, and appendices even if included in a separate file, to serve as part of the TOC for the submission.

To facilitate the review, you should provide hypertext links to supporting annotations, related sections, references, appendices, tables, or figures that are not located on the same page throughout the body of the document. For a reference list at the end of a document, you should provide a hypertext link from the item listed to the appropriate PDF publication file. In order to provide reviewers maximal flexibility in using electronic documents, please avoid linking items across submission folders. We intend to review the information according to discipline and thus you should present your information in a modular fashion. For example, if you intend to use a reference to support a point in the CMC folder, you should not place the reference in the Clinical folder.

TABLE 4.1 Organization of documents

Folder location	Types of document
Administration (*admin*)	Introductory statement, annual reports, change of address, change of contact, change of sponsor, letters of authorization, meeting minutes, interim reports, final reports request for closure, fast track, inactivation, reactivation, rolling BLA or NDA designation, transfer of obligations, withdrawal, meeting request, responses to a clinical hold or information request correspondence
Chemistry, Manufacturing and Controls (*cmc*)	CMC information [§312.23(a)(7)] and informational amendments related specifically to CMC [§312.31] including product characterization, device information, formulation, labeling, lot release, manufacturing information, shipment of product, source information, specifications, lot release data, stability, sterility, and environmental assessment or claim for exclusion
Nonclinical Pharmacology and Toxicology (*pharmtox*)	Pharmacology and toxicology information [§312.23(a)(8)] and informational amendments related specifically to pharmtox [§312.31] including pharmacology and toxicology data, preclinical information, animal models, in vitro models, pharmacokinetics, preclinical reports and protocols, and toxicology
Clinical (*clinical*)	Protocols [§312.23(a)(6)], protocol amendments [§312.30], previous human experience [§312.23(a)(9)], safety reports [§312.32] and informational amendments related specifically to clinical [§312.31] including adverse reactions, consent forms, investigator information, general investigational plan, Investigator's Brochures, IRB approval, new protocols, revised protocols, site information, investigator data, CVs, and 1572s
Other (*other*)	Cross-referenced files and other information

You should also include a bookmark to the roadmap, the submission's main TOC, and the folder's TOC at the highest level of the bookmark hierarchy for documents that you supplied as part of the submission.

Publications. You should provide each publication as a separate PDF file. Establish a hypertext link between the reference to the publication in the application and the publication. You should include the citation for the publication in the title portion of the Document Information field for each publication file.

Submission Management. Timely communications with the appropriate center and office staff prior to the submission of an electronic document are essential. You should contact us when questions arise.

You should notify us in writing of your intent to submit an electronic IND at least three months prior to the target arrival date for the application. Upon receipt and review of the written notification, our staff will schedule a teleconference to discuss the proposed electronic dossier. You should submit CD-ROM, containing mock-up text and data, conveying your interpretation of the guidance for review by Center staff 45 days before the submission target date. As individual sponsors or product teams gain experience in utilizing this submission type, we may find the CD-ROM demonstration to be unnecessary.

Because the review of an initial IND submission must be completed in 30 days, it is essential that the electronic IND submission function smoothly. The CD-ROM demonstration is a critical part of ensuring that smooth function. The CD-ROM demonstration should facilitate discussions of the planned regulatory submission through the presentations of mock-up text, tables, graphics, and data to CBER from the sponsor. The CD-ROM demonstration will (1) present us with an opportunity to ensure that documents are presented in a standard format across all electronic IND applications; (2) present an opportunity for feedback from the review team on the presentation of regulatory information (e.g. data set structures, hypertext links, bookmarking, and document quality); and (3) present an opportunity for our technical staff to provide feedback on how well the proposed submission structure is consistent with our guidance. Effective use of the demonstration and timely communication with our staff should enhance your understanding of this guidance document and its intent. We have listed the appropriate staff contacts for your submissions in *Appendix C.*

Application Structure. An IND is a compilation of many small submissions collected over an extended period of time. Frequently, during the review of an IND submission, a reviewer will need to refer to earlier submissions. To help reviewers navigate through the entire application, you should provide with each new submission a directory that includes a list of not only the files included in the current submission but all the previously submitted files as well (see *Appendix A*—example *roadmap.pdf* file).

This list should be presented in reverse chronological order, by submission, as part of a PDF file called *roadmap.pdf* (see *Appendix A*). This file is linked to the submission's main TOC, which is in turn linked to the TOC provided in each subfolder. See "IND Table of Contents" for additional details on the TOC's files.

Organizing the Main Folder

You should place in the main folder all electronic documents and data sets that you intend to be part of your electronic IND. The only exception is the application directory (*roadmap.pdf file*). This document should be placed in the root directory (Fig. 4.1).

Naming the Main Folder. The main folder for the original submission should be named IXYZ, where XYZ contains abbreviations for the sponsor name, product, and indication. For this submission, you do not know the IND number nor can you generate it before the arrival of the regulatory submission. All amendments to the application should use the same main folder name as the original submission.

Folders. Inside the main folder, you should provide five folders, Administrative (*admin*), Chemistry, Manufacturing and Controls (*cmc*), Pharmacology and Toxicology (*pharmtox*), Clinical (*clinical*), and Other (*other*) to organize the documents and data sets provided in the original submission and subsequent amendments to your IND (Fig. 4.1). See Table 4.1 for the types of documents that would reside in each folder. In addition, the main folder should contain an *indindex* folder (see "Folder and File Names").

You should name the folders as shown in Fig. 4.1. You should not attach an extension to the submission subfolders. Our intent is to create one set of folders per submission and upload additional supporting information into these folders. This will give our review community one central location as a repository for information germane to their review. Place the types of documents/information listed below into the designated folders.

Cover Letter. You should provide a cover letter as a PDF file named *XXXX_ cover.pdf* inside the main folder, where *XXXX* is the submission serial number. You should include in the cover letter the following.

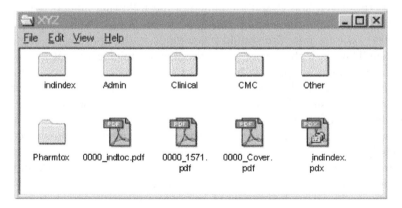

Figure 4.1   IND main folder

- A description of the submission including appropriate regulatory information
- A description of the electronic submission including the type and number of electronic media used (e.g., two CD-ROMs), and the approximate size of the submission (e.g., 1.2 GB)
- A statement that the submission is virus free with a description of the software (name, version, and company) used to check the files for viruses
- Any changes from the recommendations in this guidance document
- The regulatory and information technology points of contact for the application

Form FDA 1571. Inside the main folder, provide a Form FDA 1571, as a PDF file named *XXXX_1571.pdf*, where *XXXX* is the submission serial number. The Agency is developing procedures to allow the submission of electronic signatures. Until procedures are in place, you should attach a paper Form FDA 1571 that is signed by the sponsor's authorized representative to accompany the *1571.pdf* file.

IND TOC. Regulations at 21 CFR 312.23(a)(2) require submission of a TOC.

For the electronic submission, the TOC should contain three levels of detail and the appropriate hypertext links and bookmarks (see *Appendix B*). The first level of detail, the main TOC, will contain a simple listing of the items in section 12 of the Form FDA 1571. You should hypertext link and bookmark these items to the appropriate item TOC for the IND. This single-page PDF file should be named *XXXX_indtoc.pdf*, where *XXXX* is the submission serial number. You should place the main TOC in the main folder.

The second level of detail is the TOC for each folder of the IND. You should provide these TOCs as PDF files named in the following manner, e.g., *0000_admintoc.pdf, 0000_cmctoc.pdf, 0000_pharmtoxtoc.pdf, 0000_clinicaltoc.pdf*, and *0000_othertoc.pdf*. You should place items in the appropriate subfolder. For each TOC, you should list all of the files pertaining to that area in the specific subfolder and provide bookmarks and hypertext links to each document or data set listed in the TOC. In general, these TOCs should consist of a few pages. You should provide bookmarks to the submission's roadmap main TOC and the item's TOC at the highest level of the bookmark hierarchy. This will allow a reviewer to easily navigate throughout the electronic submission.

The third level of detail pertains to reports and protocols. You should fully bookmark and hyperlink the TOC for these documents. For data sets, you should provide a data definition table as a key to the elements being used in the data sets.

Full-Text Index for the Submission. You should provide an index of the full text and the Document Information fields of all items in the submission. The index is generated in PDF by using Acrobat Catalog. Name the index definition file *indindex.pdx.* You should place all associated index files in a folder named *indindex*. Place the *indindex.pdx* definition file and the *indindex* folder in the IND main folder. Associate the *XXXX_indtoc.pdf* file with the index file so that, whenever the TOC file is opened, the associated index is automatically added to the available index list. This will facilitate the use of the search function in Adobe Acrobat. The function enables a reviewer to enter a specific word and search the document for that word's location throughout the documents covered by the indices loaded at the time. The *indindex* folder and file do not have numerical prefixes because they are intended to be cumulative. Index information should be updated each time an amendment is submitted to the IND.

Organizing the Submission

Guidance follows for providing files, in electronic format, for each of the five content folders potentially included in an original submission of an IND and all its subsequent amendments.

Administrative (admin). Table 4.1 lists the types of documents that you should provide in the *admin* folder. You should place all of these files directly into the *admin* subfolder. Do not provide any subfolders within the *admin* folder except for the full text index and publications folders.

Letter of Authorization When referencing information submitted to the Agency by another sponsor, you must provide a written statement that authorizes the reference and that is signed by the person who submitted the information [21 CFR 312.23(b)]. You should provide this letter of authorization as an individual PDF file and place it in the *admin* folder.

Responses to Center Correspondence You should include the actual comments, questions, and requests for additional information communicated in our letter sent to you, as well as your response to these items. You should bookmark each item to facilitate information access and make additional supporting information accessible through a hypertext link contained within your response.

Annual Report Except for the Investigator's Brochure [21 CFR 312.33(d)], you should provide the required information for an annual report as a single PDF file. You will find the items required for the annual report listed in 21 CFR 312.33. As part of the annual report file, you should provide a TOC listing each item detailed in 21 CFR 312.33. You should bookmark and hyperlink each item in the TOC to its referenced information in the document. Information on providing the Investigator's Brochure is provided below.

Other Documents You should provide other documents in this subfolder including those described in Table 4.1 as individual PDF files.

Publications You should provide each publication as a separate PDF file. You should place in alphabetical order and into a single folder named *pubs* all publications that are cited in files contained in the *admin* folder. You should establish a hypertext link between the citation and the publication in the *pubs* folder. Place the *pubs* folder in the *admin* folder. You should include the citation for the publication in the Title portion of the Document Information field for each publication file. You should include the first author's last name, the year of the publication, and the title of the article in the citation.

Full-Text Index You should provide an index of the full text and the Document Information fields of all documents in this folder. You should name the index definition file *admin.pdx*. You should place all associated index files in the *admin* index folder. You should place *admin.pdx* definition file and the *admin* index folder in the *admin* folder. You should associate the *XXXX_ admintoc.pdf* file with the index file so that whenever the TOC file is opened, the associated index is automatically added to the available index list. This will facilitate the use of the search function in Adobe Acrobat. The function enables a reviewer to enter a specific word and search the document for that word's location throughout the documents covered by the indexes loaded at the time. Index files and folders do not have numerical prefixes because they are intended to be cumulative. They should be updated each time an amendment is submitted to the IND.

CMC. Table 4.1 lists the types of documents that you should provide in the *cmc* folder. You should place all files directly into the *cmc* folder. You should not provide any subfolders within the *cmc* folder except for the full-text index and the publications folder.

Documents and Data Sets See *Guidance for Industry: Providing Regulatory Submissions to the Center for Biologics Evaluation and Research (CBER) in Electronic Format—Biologics Marketing Applications [Biologics License Application (BLA), Product License Application (PLA)/Establishment License Application (ELA) and New Drug Application (NDA)]*, November 1999, Revised for guidance on the format of specific documents and data sets files for CMC submissions.

For documents not described in the marketing applications, you should provide documents as individual PDF files and place them in the *cmc* folder.

Publications You should provide each publication as a separate PDF file. You should place in alphabetical order and into a single into a single folder named *pubs* all publications that are cited in files contained in the *cmc* folder. Establish a hyperlink between the citation and the publication in the *pubs* folder. You should place the *pubs* folder in the *cmc* folder. You should include the citation for the publication in the Title portion of the Document Information field for each publication file. The citation should include the first author's last name, the year of the publication, and the title of the article.

Full-Text Index   You should provide an index of the full text and the **Document Information** fields of all documents in this folder. You should name the index definition file *cmc.pdx*. You should place all associated index files in the *cmc* index folder. Place the *cmc.pdx* definition file and the *cmc* index folder in the *cmc* folder. You should associate the *XXXX_cmctoc.pdf* file with the index file so that, whenever the TOC file is opened, the associated index is automatically added to the available index list. This will facilitate the use of the search function in Adobe Acrobat. The function enables a reviewer to enter a specific word and search the document for that word's location throughout the documents covered by the indexes loaded at the time. Index files and folders do not have numerical prefixes because they are intended to be cumulative. They should be updated each time an amendment is submitted to the IND.

Nonclinical Pharmacology and Toxicology (Pharmtox).   Table 4.1 lists the types of documents that you should provide in the *pharmtox* folder. You should place all files directly into the *pharmtox* folder. You should not provide any subfolders within the *pharmtox* folder except for the full-text index and the publications folder.

Documents and Data Sets   See *Guidance for Industry: Providing Regulatory Submissions to the Center for Biologics Evaluation and Research (CBER) in Electronic Format—Biologics Marketing Applications [Biologics License Application (BLA), Product License Application (PLA) / Establishment License Application (ELA) and New Drug Application (NDA)]*, November 1999, Revised, for guidance on the format of specific documents and data sets files for pharmtox submissions.

For documents not described in the marketing applications, you should provide documents as individual PDF files and place them in the *pharmtox* folder.

Publications   You should provide each publication as a separate PDF file. You should place all publications that are cited in files contained in the *pharmtox* folder, in alphabetical order, into a single folder named *pubs*. Establish a hyperlink between the citation and the publication in the *pubs* folder. You should place the *pubs* folder in the *pharmtox* folder. You should include the citation for the publication in the Title portion of the Document Information field for each publication file. You should include the first author's last name, the year of the publication, and the title of the article in the citation.

Full-Text Index   You should provide an index of the full text and the Document Information fields of all documents in this folder. You should name the index definition file *pharmtox.pdx*. You should place all associated index files in the *pharmtox* index folder. Place the *pharmtox.pdx* definition file and the *pharmtox* index folder in the *pharmtox* folder. You should associate the *XXXX_pharmtoc.pdf* file with the index file so that, whenever the TOC file is opened, the associated index is automatically added to the available index list. This will facilitate the use of the search function in Adobe Acrobat. The function enables a reviewer to enter a specific word and search the document for that word's location throughout the documents covered by the indexes loaded at the time. Index files and folders do not have numerical prefixes because they are intended to be cumulative. They should be updated each time an amendment is submitted to the IND.

Clinical. Table 4.1 lists the types of documents that you should provide in the *clinical* folder. You should place all files directly into the clinical folder. You should not provide any subfolders within the *clinical* folder except for the full-text index, publications, protocol, and adverse events folders.

Protocol and Protocol Revisions (amendments)   You should provide each protocol in a separate PDF file in a subfolder labeled Protocols. To help us easily identify the file, use the protocol number as part of the file name. Each protocol should have a TOC. You should hypertext link and bookmark the TOC. For protocol revisions or amendments, you should use the same protocol number that identifies the original protocol. You should submit to the file a complete copy of any revised protocol. This will facilitate the use of the "text compare" function in Adobe Acrobat by our clinical reviewers.

You should create a PDF file named *protocolctoc.pdf* (i.e., protocol cumulative TOC) within the Protocols subfolder. The *protocolctoc.pdf* is a cumulative list of the protocols and revisions with the date of submission presented as a PDF file. The cumulative list should be in inverse chronological order, with the most recent protocol submission at the top of the list. Because this file is cumulative, it does not have a numerical prefix. The *protocolctoc.pdf* should not affect the submission content in any fashion. You should hypertext link the protocols and revisions listed in this file to the documents they reference. You should update this file with the submission of any protocol or protocol revision. The document should function in a manner similar to the *roadmap. pdf* file (see *Appendix A* and *Appendix B*, Figure VI-4).

Adverse Events   You should provide each adverse event report as a separate PDF file in a subfolder labeled "Adverse Events." To aid Center staff in identifying each PDF file, please use a combination of the protocol number, patient number, and event date in each file name (e.g., RIT-02-004_010-023_07132001). Within the Adverse Events subfolder, you should provide a PDF file named *adverse_eventsctoc.pdf* (i.e., adverse events cumulative TOC). The *adverse_ eventsctoc.pdf* is a cumulative list of all adverse events that occurred during the clinical investigation. The cumulative list should be in inverse chronological order with the most recent submission at the top of the list. Because this file is cumulative, it does not have a numerical prefix. The *adverse_eventsctoc. pdf* should not affect the submission content in any fashion. You should hypertext link the adverse event reports listed in this file to the documents they reference. You should update this file with the submission of any adverse event report. The document should function in a manner similar to the *roadmap.pdf* file (see *Appendix A* and *Appendix B*, Figure VI-5).

Investigator's Brochure   You should provide the Investigator's Brochure as a single PDF file. You should include a TOC in the Investigator's Brochure. You should name the file XXXX_*investbrochuretoc.pdf*. You should bookmark and hypertext link the TOC for this file.

General Investigational Plan You should provide the general investigational plan as a single PDF file. You should include a TOC in the general investigational plan. You should name the file *XXXX_geninvestplantoc.pdf*. You should bookmark and hypertext link the TOC for this file.

Clinical Trials Data Bank   We have established a clinical trials data bank to collect information on your clinical trials protocols. Please list your protocols for serious and life-threatening conditions [Food and Drug Administration Modernization Act of 1997 section 113]. When finalized, you should list your protocols in accordance with our *Draft Guidance for Industry—Information Program on Clinical Trials for Serious or Life-Threatening Diseases: Implementation Plan*, June 2001.

Investigator Information   You should provide the investigator information as a single PDF file. If more than one investigator is included in the file, you should provide a bookmark to each investigator.

Previous Human Experience   You should provide previous human experience in a separate PDF file that is reserved for summary information. You should include a TOC in the previous human experience file. You should name the file *XXXX_prevhumexptoc.pdf*. You should bookmark and hypertext link the TOC for this file. If you are providing study reports, you should provide them as described in the appropriate marketing guidance document.

Other Files   See *Guidance for Industry: Providing Regulatory Submissions to the Center for Biologics Evaluation and Research (CBER) in Electronic Format—Biologics Marketing Applications [Biologics License Application (BLA), Product License Application (PLA)/Establishment License Application (ELA) and New Drug Application (NDA)]*, November 1999, Revised, for guidance on the format of specific documents and data sets files for clinical submissions.

For documents not described in the marketing applications, provide documents as individual PDF files and place them in the *clinical* folder.

Publications   You should provide each publication as a separate PDF file. You should place in alphabetical order and into a single folder named *pubs* all publications that are cited in files contained in the *clinical* folder. You should establish a hypertext link between the citation and the publication in the *pubs* folder. You should place the pubs folder in the *clinical* folder. You should include the citation for the publication in the Title portion of the Document Information field for each publication file. You should include in the citation the first author's last name, the year of the publication, and the title of the article.

Full-Text Index   You should provide an index of the full text and the Document Information fields of all documents in this section. You should name the index definition file *clinical.pdx*. You should place all associated index files in the *clinical* folder. Place the *clinical.pdx* definition file and the clinical index folder in the *clinical* folder. You should associate the *XXXX_clinicaltoc.pdf* file with the index file so that, whenever the TOC file is opened, the associated index is automatically added to the available index list. This will facilitate the use of the search function in Adobe Acrobat. The function enables a reviewer to enter a specific word and search the document for that word's location throughout the documents covered by the indexes loaded at the time. Index files and folders do not have numerical prefixes because they are intended to be cumulative. They should be updated each time an amendment is submitted to the IND.

Other.   Table 4.1 lists the types of documents that you should provide in the subfolder. You should place all files directly into the *other* folder. You should not provide any subfolders within the *other* folder except for the full-text index.

Documents   You should provide an individual PDF file for each document.

Full-Text Index   You should provide an index of the full text and the Document Information fields of all documents in the other section. You should name the index definition file *otherindex.pdx*. You should place all associated index files in a folder named *otherindex*. Place the *otherindex.pdx* definition file and the *otherindex* folder in the main *other* folder. You should associate the *XXXX_othertoc.pdf* file with this index so that, whenever the other TOC is opened, the associated index is automatically added to the available index list. This will facilitate the use of the search function in Adobe Acrobat. The function enables a reviewer to enter a specific word and search the document for that word's location throughout the documents covered by the indexes loaded at the time. Index files and folders do not have numerical prefixes because they are intended to be cumulative. They should be updated each time an amendment is submitted to the IND.

APPENDICES

Appendix A: Roadmap File

You should use the *roadmap.pdf* file to establish a hypertext link to the submission's TOC. You should locate the *roadmap.pdf* file in the root directory of the submission. You should update and resubmit the file when you submit amendments to the application. An example of the *roadmap.pdf* file format is shown in Fig. VI-1.

IND submission	Submission date	Submission content	CD-ROM	Hypertext link destination
IND 12345.0003	04-Jul-2001	Cover letter	3.01	amendtoc.pdf
		1571	3.01	
		Protocol 12-345	3.01	
		Investigator information	3.01	
IND 12345.0002	19-Jun-2001	Cover letter	2.01	amendtoc.pdf
		1571	2.01	
		Lot release	2.01	
IND 12345.0001	10-Feb-2001	Cover letter	1.01	amendtoc.pdf
		1571	1.01	
		Revised protocol	1.01	
Sponsor name	15-Jan-2001	Cover letter	0.01	Indtoc.pdf
		1571	0.01	
		Table of contents	0.01	
		Introductory statement	0.01	
		General investigational plan	0.01	
		Investigator's brochure	0.01	
		Protocols	0.01	
		CMC	0.01	
		Pharmacology and toxiology	0.01	
		Previous human experience	0.01	
		Additional information	0.01	

Figure VI-1   Example of a roadmap file electronic roadmap

The *roadmap.pdf* file should not contribute in any way to the content of what is under review. It is a map intended to facilitate navigation through the contents of the submission. You should replace the *roadmap.pdf* file with each new submission of regulatory information.

In addition to providing a navigable guide to the application (i.e., a correspondence history), the *roadmap.pdf* file should include the sponsor's submission date in the DD-MM-YYYY format (e.g., 15-01-2000). You should describe briefly the contents of the original submission and of subsequent amendments in a *roadmap.pdf* table. You should indicate in the *roadmap.pdf* file the location of these files and folders on the submitted CD-ROMs.

Appendix B: IND TOC

The IND TOC should facilitate access to the submission text and data. Examples of the first, second, and third levels for the IND TOC are shown in Figures VI-2 through 7. These examples portray the intent of the IND's multiple TOCs. Protocol is highlighted as a specific example. These files will facilitate a reviewer's ability to navigate throughout an electronic dossier. Bookmarks should mirror the contents of each TOC. At the top of the bookmark hierarchy, three bookmarks (Roadmap, Main TOC, Section/Item TOC) should always reside.

Main IND table of contents		
Section	Description	Electronic folder/file name
	Cover letter	0000_coverletter.pdf
1	Form FDA 1571	0000_1571.pdf
2	Table of contents	0000_indtoc.pdf
3	Introductory statement	0000_intro.pdf
4	General investigational plan	Clinical\0000_clintoc.pdf
5	Investigator's brochure	Clinical\0000_clintoc.pdf
6	Protocols	Clinical\0000_clintoc.pdf
7	Chemistry, manufacturing, and controls	Cmc\0000_cmctoc.pdf
8	Pharmacology and toxicology data	Pharmtox\0000_pharmtoxtoc.pdf
9	Previous human experience	Clinical\0000_clintoc.pdf
10	Additional information/pre-IND information	Admin\0000_admintoc.pdf
11	Other	Other

Figure VI-2 IND main table of contents for original submission 12345. This is the first-level TOC

\multicolumn{3}{c}{Clinical table of contents—items contained within the *clinical* folder}
Item	Description	Folder/file
1	General investigational plan	Clinical\0000_geninvestplantoc.pdf
2	Investigator's brochure	Clinical\0000_investbrochuretoc.pdf
3	Protocol - XOXOXO	Clinical\protocols\protocolcctoc.pdf
4	Sample informed consent	Clinical\0000_consent.pdf
5	Previous human experience	Clinical\0000_prevhumexptoc.pdff
6	Adverse events	Clinical\adverse events\adverse_eventsctoc.pdf

\multicolumn{3}{c}{Pharmtox table of contents—items contained within the *pharmtox* folder}
Item	Description	Folder/file
1	Pharmacology and toxicology summary	Pharmtox\0000_summarytoc.pdf
2	Immunopathology report: cross-reactivity of xxx with normal human tissue	Pharmtox\0000_Immunopath568toc.pdf
3	Immunopathology report: cross-reactivity of XXX with limited normal tissue from rhesus and cynomolgus monkeys	Pharmtox\0000_Immunopath767toc.pdf
4	An MTD/dose range finding intravenous toxicity study in male CD-1 mice	Pharmtoc\0000_Toxicitytoc.pdf
5	A single-intravenous dose pharmacokinetic study in cynomolgus monkeys	Pharmtox\0000_SingleDosetoc.pdf

Figure VI-3 Section-based table of contents. This is the second-level TOC

Submission date	Protocol title	Hyperlink destination
January 15, 2001	The real deal	0005_Pnca101.01.pdf
December 25, 2000	Pure profit	0003_Shazam100.pdf
May 30, 2000	Home cooking	0002_Tcencore50.01.pdf
November 22, 1999	The real deal	0000_Pnca101.pdf
November 22, 1999	Home cooking	0000_TCencore50.pdf

Figure VI-4 Protocol cumulative table of contents

Submission date	Adverse event	Hyperlink destination
13-Jul-2001	Leukocytopenia	0015_RIT-02-004_01023_07132001.pdf
04-Jul-2001	Thrombocytopenia	0012_RIT-02-004_711_07042001.pdf
01-Apr-2000	Alopecia	0007_SUC-01-001_061968_04012000.pdf

Figure VI-5 Adverse event cumulative table of contents

Synopsis
List of abbreviations
1.0 **Overview**
2.0 **Background**
  2.1 Overview
  2.2 Toxicology
  2.3 Pharmacokinetics
  2.4 Human clinical trials
  2.5 Rationale for study design
3.0 **Objectives**
4.0 **Inclusion and exclusion criteria**
  4.1 Inclusion criteria
  4.2 Exclusion criteria
5.0 **Investigational plan**
  5.1 Study design
  5.2 Dose-limiting toxicity and maximum tolerated dose
  5.3 Sample size
  5.4 Treatment
    5.4.1 Clinical trial material
    5.4.2 Drug administration
    5.4.3 Dosage modification
    5.4.4 Criteria for continuation of treatment beyond cycle 1
    5.4.5 Retreatment eligibility criteria
    5.4.6 Concomitant therapy
  5.5 Outcome measures
    5.5.1 Safety outcome measures

Figure VI-6 Part of a protocol table of contents—pure profit. This is the third-level TOC

List of abbreviations

1.0 **Chemistry**

    1.1 Development of the expression construct

        1.1.1 Construction of genes encoding the light and heavy chain variable regions

        1.1.2 Construction of the light and heavy chain plasmids, pp. 1933, 1937

        1.1.3 Construction of the expression plasmid, p. 1937

        1.1.4 Cloning and expression of soluble

            1.1.4.1 Expression plasmid for soluble

            1.1.4.2 Cloning of the cDNA encoding and development of expression plasmid

            1.1.4.3 Development of cell line for production of

            1.1.4.4 Production and purification of

    1.2 Development of the production cell line for

        1.2.1 History of cell line

        1.2.2 Development of the producing cell line

        1.2.3 Preparation and characterization of the clone master cell bank
            and working cell bank

        1.2.4 Preparation and storage of MCB

        1.2.5 Preparation and storage of MWCB

        1.2.6 Characterization of MCB and MWCB

            1.2.6.1 Growth and ING-1 productivity of MCB and MWCB

            1.2.6.2 Sterility testing

            1.2.6.3 Mycoplasma testing

            1.2.6.4 Isoenzyme analysis

            1.2.6.5 Karyotyping

            1.2.6.6 Hamster antibody production (HAP) assay

            1.2.6.7 *In vitro* assay for the presence of viral contaminants

            1.2.6.8 Detection of inapparent viruses by *in vitro* inoculation

            1.2.6.9 Detection of viral particles by thin section electron microscopy

            1.2.6.10 Assay for murine xenotropic viruses by extended S+ L– focus assay

            1.2.6.11 Assay for bovine adventitious agents

            1.2.6.12 Reverse transcriptase testing

            1.2.6.13 Summary of characterization of MCB abd MWCB

Figure VI-7 Part of a CMC table of contents. This is the third-level TOC

Appendix C: CBER Electronic Submission Coordinators

Office of the Director	Mr. Michael B. Fauntleroy Director, Electronic Submissions	(301) 827-5132
Office of Therapeutic Research and Review, Division of Application Review and Policy	Dr. Bradley Glasscock, Pharm.D Ms. Lori Tull	(301) 827-5101
Office of Vaccines Research and Review, Division of Vaccines and Related Product Applications	Dr. Rakesh Pandey, PhD Ms. Gale Heavner, RN Dr. Joseph Temenak, PhD	(301) 827-307
Office of Blood Research and Review, Division of Blood Applications	Ms. Daria Reed	(301) 827-3524

CHAPTER 5

New Drug Applications (NDAs)

THE PINNACLE

The pinnacle goal of most preapproval regulatory submissions is the NDA. The NDA approval grants a practical license to manufacture and sell the product in the United States, significantly increases the equity value of the applying organization, and represents the culmination of the scientific process of discovery, testing, and development.

Just as a pinnacle peak is built upon the structure of surrounding and underlying foundations, the NDA incorporates, references, and contextually includes the preceding Investigational New Drug Application (IND), annual IND reports, and other submissions that together make up the complete filing package. All related filings are identified by a common project number, and will be reviewed as a part of the NDA review even if not referenced in the NDA.

Partly because the NDA is such an important filing and partly because it is the culmination step before market approval, the filing logistical requirements and review requirements are much more stringent than with any other submission. A noncompliant index page, an out-of-specification binder, or an error in pagination can delay a drug approval for months or years. While all FDA submissions require careful review and proofing prior to submission, the NDA has much higher stakes and requires an even higher primary, secondary, and tertiary review.

Those high stakes have led the FDA into a very detailed review process, focusing on both the trivia of the application logistics and the fundamental and critically important questions of drug safety and efficacy. In effect, pressures to respond relatively rapidly, pressures related to the tremendous financial stakes represented by a NDA, and altruistic concerns related to dangers of approving a drug with undesirable side effects or hidden problems have led to tendency to default toward rejection on grounds related to less than critical—some say trivial—matters.

Guidebook for Drug Regulatory Submissions, by Sandy Weinberg
Copyright © 2009 John Wiley & Sons, Inc.

Years ago, as corporate America was racing to replace limited-access mainframe computers with personal computers on every employee's desk, a market survey was conducted to see why so many companies were purchasing IBM PCs when comparable computers, often manufactured (accept for the outer casing) by the same overseas Asian companies, were selling for half the price. The answer they heard from purchasing manager after purchasing manager was that "nobody ever got fired for buying IBM." The same sort of mentality has entered the NDA review process: No reviewer was ever criticized or internally disciplined for rejecting an NDA, particularly if that reviewer could point to some unambiguous (if unimportant) rationale.

That attitude is, of course, self-defeating. At the same time that it may alleviate immediate pressures on an individual reviewer, the resultant delays and increased costs result in more general criticism of the process and of the FDA. As those costs increase—a result of the increasingly stringent regulatory requirements and of the lost market share and decreasing patent duration and value as regulatory reviews and appeals drag on—the pressures on the agency to efficiently and rapidly rule on NDAs increases. Political, media, and public demands for lower drug prices are met with (accurate) industry finger pointing at the agency: every year, delay in drug approval results in a 1/20th loss of patent protection to recover drug costs (compare the six- to eight-year average patent loss during the FDA review to the European method of freezing patent duration during the review process and you can account for most of the cost differential between U.S. and international prices). When headlines about drug recalls due to unexpected side effects are coupled with widespread (if questionable) beliefs that many Americans are rationing their health care because of drug costs, the pressure to rapidly review—and to avoid approval—is immense. If you were the FDA commissioner, facing congressional hearings or an irate public, your optimum strategy would be to very rapidly reject as many NDAs as possible, decreasing you review time statistics while minimizing the potential negative publicity of a recall. Yet, while that strategy would work short term, you would quickly be overwhelmed by public and pressure group demands to allow new products on the market. Perhaps the best advice for an FDA commissioner: either grow very thick skin or find an alternate career.

In short, the public praises the industry when new drugs are introduced, curses the agency when drug approvals are delayed, and criticizes both when drugs are recalled.

DETAILED SUBMISSION REQUIREMENTS

The specific and detailed submission requirements for a NDA are found in "Required Specifications for FDAs IND, NDA, ANDA, Drug Master File Binders," and Title 21 Chapter I Part 314 "Applications for FDA Approval to Market a New Drug or an Antibiotic Drug." Three copies are required: an archival copy, a review copy, and a field copy. Each generally contains an application form, an index, a summary, the appropriate technical sections (CMC, drug analysis, etc.), case report tabulations of patient data, case report forms, drug samples, and labeling (some variations in the technical sections may be appropriate if the drug is not a new drug entity). See Chapter 6 on 505(b)2 NDAs for further appropriate variations.

With the exception of these minor variations as noted, all guidelines and requirements for the format and content should be very closely followed. If any deviations or modifications are anticipated, they should be raised and discussed at the pre-NDA meeting (see below). Note that this creates somewhat of a "chicken and egg" dilemma: It is, of course, desirable to await final drafting of the NDA until after the pre-NDA meeting, yet that meeting may be only opportunity to explain and gain acceptance of any variations in the final NDA draft. The solution, of course, is to prepare a penultimate NDA before the meeting and use the meeting results to tweak that draft into the final submission.

PRE-NDA MEETING

With the exceptions of duration, detail, and perhaps importance, the pre-NDA meeting does not differ significantly from the pre-IND meeting. Again, a meeting request letter initiates the process and raises the specific issues to be addressed—worded to arrive at an agreement of the agency with the stated opinion of the submitter (or to determine the specific areas of disagreement for subsequent discussion).

Again, a Briefing Book should be submitted (usually two weeks prior to the meeting) to allow the FDA team to rapidly come up to speed on the issues raised and to provide appropriate context for the questions under discussion. There is sometimes a regrettable tendency to bury or attempt to disguise controversial questions or problems. The better strategy in almost all cases is to identify these issues clearly, analyze their implications, propose remediation of response, and clearly defend that response. Consider the statement:

> a disproportionate number of subjects voluntarily withdrew from the study, stating that the number of administrations caused hardship. The problem was shared with the Advisory Panel (names appended). Noting that in actual distribution once the product is approved administration will take place at more conveniently located decentralized locations, the panel conducted a statistic power analysis and determined that the dropouts did not adversely affect the study results (report appended).

Such an inclusion would likely generate some FDA discussion and possible eventual concurrence. On the other hand, an FDA investigator discovering the same dropout rate independently, without the context of the advisory panel review, would be likely to increase skepticism about all other aspects of the submission while rejecting the results of the particular study.

INDEPENDENT REVIEW

All regulatory documents presumably are subject to a tripartite review process. The submission is reviewed by the corporate Regulatory group, which proofs, considers issues of conformity to internal policy and to FDA guidance; and checks the factual statements. A Quality Assurance review then rechecks all the previous items and independently confirms all facts and statements. Finally, a corporate review (at or near the top of the organization) precedes the final signatures and confirms conclusions and plans.

In the case of the NDA, a fourth review is recommended. This is an appropriate occasion to bring in one or more outside independent consultants to act as a "mock FDA" review panel. The panel should be thoroughly familiar with all FDA guidelines, style requirements, and policies. The panel should review the NDA in great deal, using the same two-tier review process as is employed at the FDA (first: review for conformity to logistical requirements; second: review of content).

Then, preferably at an off-site location (to avoid any interruptions) the panel should meet with the corporate regulatory NDA team [presumably Regulatory Director, Medical Director, Chemistry, Manufacturing, and Control (CMC) Director, and others as appropriate] with a detailed grilling and discussion. The idea is to dissect the entire document and to closely question the corporate team on all aspects.

This process serves three important purposes. First, it provides a fourth detailed review of the document. Second, it serves as practice for the FDA presentation meeting. And third, it provides an opportunity to discuss strategy and tactics. While this independent review is certainly not mandatory (it does not appear as even a suggestion in any FDA guidance document), it is a common practice and highly recommended.

SUGGESTIONS

Based upon an analysis of NDAs that were rejected as well as those approved over a five-year period (2002–2006), here are 11 suggestions to maximize the probability of success.

1. Conform exactly to the paper or electronic logistical/formatting requirements. The initial review of logistical conformity can slow ultimate approval by months. Make certain that all components are present and clearly labeled as required.

2. In the CMC section, make certain that stability data clearly support the submitted data and the requested label. Avoid reliance on accelerated stability tests whenever possible.

3. Again, in the CMC section, account for all significant impurities, with particular attention to any that has been tied to carcinogens or serious side effects in the past.

4. Complete Patient Records (case forms) should be included, with any gaps clearly indicated and discussed. The natural FDA assumption is that any missing case record form represents either (a) an adverse reaction, (b) sloppy procedures, or (c) an attempt at fraud. Clearly document the reason for any missing case form, including the results of a Quality Assurance follow-up investigation.

5. Analyses should be complete ("show your work"), replicable, and clearly explained. Most FDA complaints about analyses related to overly complex procedures without a sound explanation for the design.

6. Formulations should be consistent, particularly when multiple active pharmaceutical ingredient (API) vendors or multiple manufacturers are utilized. Any differences in the drug profiles should be clearly discussed and analyzed. If different batches or manufacturers are used in a study, a statistical analysis comparing formulations is appropriate.

7. Label details are highly negotiable and can be used to provide a rational response to product limitations revealed in the study. An NDA that shows some food effects may be rejected; the same NDA, with a requested label that says "not to be taken with food" may be acceptable. Propose the strongest label the data support but do not push beyond that logical limit.

8. The basic safety studies, including the International Conference on Harmonization (ICH) standard series of preclinical tests, receive close attention in the NDA review. Even if specific ICH studies were never discussed in the pre-IND meeting, the IND review, and the pre-NSDA meeting, they should be addressed in the NDA.

9. There is no requirement that a new drug represent a unique treatment or therapy or even that it represent an improvement over existing therapies (the new drug may be recommended, for example, only for people with certain sensitivities or for use in settings where one delivery system is not appropriate). An application may be delayed or rejected; however, if there is an alternate therapy that lacks significant side effects or potential dangers inherent in the new drug. It is important, therefore, that alternate therapies and their comparative risk/benefit analyses be addressed.

10. Some NDAs are rejected for failure to appropriately analyze Non-U.S. experiences with the drug. European and other recalls, warnings, and

adverse studies should be carefully reviewed—perhaps with input from the panel of experts' advisory board—and a determination should be made concerning their importance and significance.

11. The extensive IND literature review, evaluating all relevant international publications concerning the drug, should be carefully updated and reanalyzed for trends and emerging problems. This requires more than just an addition to the first IND literature review to reflect the years that have passed; the reanalysis of the composite body of literature may reveal hidden problems that should be addressed.

While these 11 suggestions may seem basic, they cover the vast majority of (nondrug-specific) reasons why NDAs are delayed or rejected.

SUMMARY: THE KEY QUESTIONS

The apparently trivial requirements surrounding an NDA may seem so overwhelmingly complex that they may blot out the real key questions that drive the review process. For best results with an NDA, pay attention to the minutiae but also keep uppermost in mind the two real issues underlying everything else:

- Is the drug safe? If used in the manner prescribed in the proposed label, is there clear and compelling evidence that the drug will do no harm or that any side effects are insignificant when compared with the potential benefits? Note that the question is not composite and asked across all patients: A drug that cures 70% of the population but kills the remaining 30% to whom it is administered is not acceptable. For any and every individual patient, is there a strong reason to believe that the drug is fundamentally safe?
- Is the drug effective? The relative safety is balanced in a cost/benefit analysis: Unless there is a demonstrable, clear benefit, no drug is sufficiently desirable to deserve approval. The FDA does not approve placebos whose only benefit is subconscious. Compelling evidence of effectiveness, ideally tied to sound theory, is required.

If there is sound evidence of safety, well-designed and well-conducted studies of effectiveness, and conformity to the logistical requirements, the NDA should be approved with a minimum of difficulty.

NDA SUBMISSION CHECKLIST

This checklist is intended for use in the preparation and submission of NDAs. It is recommended that, prior to transmission to the FDA, a second internal review be conducted by an individual or department not involved in the preparation of the submission (presumably Quality Assurance).

The checklist was developed through discussions with consultants and Quality Assurance directors and has been field-tested in final form with three successful submissions.

- ☐ Form 1571 completed
- ☐ Cover letter
    - ☐ Name and address of sponsor
    - ☐ Name, address, title, telephone, and e-mail of contact person
    - ☐ Generic and trade name of drug or drug product
    - ☐ FDA Code Number (assigned at time of preconference)
- ☐ Form 3674 "Certification of Compliance with Requirements of Clinical-Trails.gov Data Bank" completed
- ☐ Three copies of application in indexed binders
- ☐ Pagination: All pages included and properly numbered
- ☐ Headings: Section headings confirming to submission subparagraphs, with initial Table of Contents
- ☐ Integrated references: All referenced articles included in final section, internally referenced in text
- ☐ Bibliography: Complete standard format bibliography listing all referenced articles
- ☐ Container closure and packaging system information provided
- ☐ Microbiological analysis provided
- ☐ Human Pharmacokinetics and Bioavailability information provided
- ☐ Complete CMC Information provided, including evidence of purity, stability, toxicology testing, and integrity of API, placebo, and final product.
- ☐ Analysis of all cited published studies and of all cited FDA findings, summarizing relevance and results
- ☐ Complete study protocol of BE/BA study and for any additional studies conducted by applicant
- ☐ Raw data for all applicant-conducted studies
- ☐ Drug Master File (DMF) completed, including information on facilities, processes, and articles used in manufacturing, processing, packaging, and storage
- ☐ Analysis of all applicant-conducted studies
- ☐ Investigators Brochure for all applicant-conducted studies included with detailed information for investigators and Institutional Review Board records

☐ Review of literature addresses all available prior instances of human use of drug product with emphasis on safety, administration, and possible adverse events

☐ Complete pharmacological profile provided for API and final product

☐ Summary of regulatory status and marketing history in United States and foreign countries

☐ Summary of adverse reactions to proposed drug in any country

☐ NDA addresses all issues and questions raised in the pre-NDA meeting

☐ Prescription Drug user Fee information provided

If NDA is submitted electronically:

☐ Form FDA-356h, Application to Market, is included.

☐ Form FDA-3397, User Fees, is included.

☐ Form FDA-3331, NDA Field Report, is included.

[For more details concerning electronic submissions, see Electronic Regulatory Submission and Review (ERSR) guidelines.]

FDA NDA REVIEW CHECKLIST

This FDA NDA Review checklist has been designed in consultation with FDA reviewers, industry consultants, and regulatory professionals to serve as a summary tool indicating the evaluative criteria used by the Center for Drug Evaluation and Research (CDER) and the Center for Biologics Evaluation and Research (CBER) to critique and assess applications received. It can be used internally as a part of the Quality Assurance process, as a guideline for regulatory development of an application, and/or as a self-assessment tool to predict likely FDA response to an application.

☐ **Logistics:** Submission conforms to FDA guideline "New Drug Application (NDA) Review Process Chart."

   ☐ **Receipt:** Application was received in the FDA mail room.

   ☐ **NDA jackets:** Document is contained in one or more 3-inch, two-ring binders.

   ☐ **Form 1571:** NDA is accompanied by completed Form 1571, providing (among other data) contact information including corporate name, contact name, address, telephone number, name and address of drug source, and generic and trade name of drug.

   ☐ **Cover letter:** A cover letter indicates disease and therapy names.

☐ **Three copies:** Photocopies are acceptable.

☐ Form 3674 "Certification of Compliance with Requirements of Clinical-Trails.gov Data Bank" completed.

☐ **Format:** Submission conforms to FDA guideline 21 Code of Federal Regulations (CFR) Part 312.23(a)(10), (11), and (b), (c), (d), and (e) and to FDA norm standards

 ☐ **Pagination:** All pages included and properly numbered

 ☐ **Headings:** Section headings conforming to submission subparagraphs

 ☐ **Integrated references:** Copies of all referenced articles, with references integrated into the body of text

 ☐ **Bibliography:** Complete standard format bibliography as referenced in text

If NDA is submitted electronically:

☐ Form FDA-356h, Application to Market, is included.

☐ Form FDA-3397, User Fees, is included.

☐ Form FDA-3331, NDA Field Report, is included.

☐ Advance notification letter is provided.

☐ Format and tables conform to *Guidance for Industry: Providing Regulatory Submissions to CBER in Electronic Format.*

☐ Electronic submission format conforms to approved list in Docket number 92s-0251 [see 21 CFR 11.1(d) and 11.2].

☐ Electronic Signatures conform to emerging guidelines, or a paper copy with appropriate nonelectronic signatures is included.

(For more details concerning Electronic Submissions, see ERSR guidelines)

☐ Drug Master File completed, including information on facilities, processes, and articles used in manufacturing, processing, packaging, and storage

☐ **CONTENT: Overview**

☐ NDA provides sufficient information to permit determination of whether the drug is safe and effective in its proposed use(s) and whether the benefits of the drug outweigh the risks.

☐ NDA provides sufficient information to permit determination of whether the drug's proposed labeling (package insert) is appropriate and what it should contain.

☐ NDA provides sufficient information to permit determination of whether the methods used in manufacturing the drug and the controls used to maintain the drug's quality are adequate to preserve the drug's identity, strength, quality, and purity.

☐ **CONTENT: Organizational structure**

  ☐ **Cover sheet:** Form 1571

  ☐ **Table of contents:** Indicates page and volume of each section

  ☐ **Summary of published studies/industry actions:** Complete with summary, analysis, and evaluation.

  ☐ **Investigator's Brochure:** Conformity with ICH *Good Clinical Practice: Guideline for the Investigator's Brochure*

  ☐ **Protocol:** Copy of the protocol for each conducted clinical study. Note that Phase 1 protocols should provide a brief outline, including estimation of number of subjects to be included, description of safety exclusions, and description of dosing plan (duration, dose, method). All protocols should address monitoring of blood chemistry and vital signs, and toxicity-based modification plans.

  ☐ **CMC information** should contain sufficient detail to assure identification, quality, purity, and strength of the investigational drug and should include stability data of duration appropriate to the length of the proposed study. FDA concerns to be addressed focus on products made with unknown or impure components; products with chemical structures known to be of high likely toxicity, products known to be chemically unstable, products with an impurity profile indicative of a health hazard or insufficiently defined to assess potential health hazard, or poorly characterized master or working cell bank.

    ■ Chemistry and manufacturing introduction

    ■ Drug substance

      ○ Description: physical, chemical, or biological characteristics

      ○ Name and address of manufacturer

      ○ Method of preparation

      ○ Limits and analytical methods

      ○ Stability information

    ■ Drug product

      ○ List of components

      ○ Qualitative composition

      ○ Name and address of drug product manufacturer

      ○ Description of manufacturing and packaging procedures

      ○ Limits and analytical methods: identity, strength, quality, and purity

      ○ Stability results

    ■ Placebo

    ■ Labels and labeling

    ■ Environmental assessment (or claim for exclusion): 21 CFR 312.23(a)(7)(iv)(e)

□ **Pharmacology and toxicology information [21 CFR 312.23(a)(8)]**

- Pharmacology and drug distribution [21 CFR 312.23(a)(8)(i)]
  - ○ Description of pharmacological effects and mechanisms of action
  - ○ Description of absorption, distribution, metabolism, and excretion of the drug
- Toxicology summary [21 CFR 312.23(a)(8)(ii)(a)]: Summary of toxicological effects in animals and *in vitro*
  - ○ Description of design of toxicological trials and any deviations from design
  - ○ Systematic presentation of animal toxicology studies and toxicokinetic studies
- Toxicology full data tabulation [21 CFR 312.23(a)(8)(ii)(b)]: data points with either:
  - brief description of the study or
  - copy of the protocol with amendments
- Toxicology GLP certification [21 CFR 312.23(a)(8)(iii)]

□ **Previous human experience with the investigational drug:** Summary report of any U.S. or non-U.S. human experience with the drug

□ **References:** Indexed copies of referenced articles with comprehensive bibliography

□ **Support:** Evaluation of the referent support provided

□ **Key issues:** All key issues appropriately referenced, including

- □ Investigator's Brochure
- □ Protocols
- □ CMC information
- □ Pharmacology and toxicology information
- □ Previous human experience with the investigational drug
- □ **Credible:** References are from credible scientific journals and/or sources.
- □ **Organized:** References are organized and tied to text.

COMMENTS:
DISPOSITION:
   Receipt date:
   Response due date:
   Disposition:
   Notification date:

GUIDANCE FOR INDUSTRY[1]: BIOAVAILABILITY AND BIOEQUIVALENCE STUDIES FOR ORALLY ADMINISTERED DRUG PRODUCTS—GENERAL CONSIDERATIONS (DRAFT GUIDANCE)[2]

Comments and suggestions regarding this draft document should be submitted within 30 days of publication in the Federal Register of the notice announcing the availability of the draft guidance. Submit comments to Dockets Management Branch (HFA-305), Food and Drug Administration, 5630 Fishers Lane, Rm. 1061, Rockville, MD 20852. All comments should be identified with the docket number listed in the notice of availability that publishes in the Federal Register.

For questions regarding this draft document, contact (CDER) Aida Sanchez at 301-827-5847.

U.S. Department of Health and Human Services
Food and Drug Administration
Center for Drug Evaluation and Research (CDER)
July 2002

Additional copies are available from:
Office of Training and Communication
Division of Drug Information, HFD-240
Center for Drug Evaluation and Research
Food and Drug Administration
5600 Fishers Lane
Rockville, MD 20857
Tel: 301-827-4573
http://www.fda.gov/cder/guidance/index.htm

This draft guidance represents the FDA's current thinking on this topic. It does not create or confer any rights for or on any person and does not operate to bind the FDA or the public. An alternative approach may be used if such approach satisfies the requirements of the applicable statutes and regulations.

Introduction

This guidance is intended to provide recommendations to sponsors and/or applicants planning to include bioavailability (BA) and bioequivalence (BE) information for orally administered drug products in INDs, NDAs, abbrevi-

---

[1] This guidance was prepared by the Biopharmaceutics Coordinating Committee in CDER at the FDA.

[2] This guidance document is being distributed for comment purposes only.

ated new drug applications (ANDAs), and their supplements. This guidance is a revision of the October 2000 guidance. This revised guidance changes recommendations regarding (1) study design and dissolution methods development, (2) comparisons of BA measures, (3) the definition of proportionality, and (4) waivers for BE studies. The guidance also makes other revisions for clarification. The revisions should provide better guidance to sponsors conducting BA and BE studies for orally administered drug products. This guidance contains advice on how to meet the BA and BE requirements set forth in part 320 (21 CFR Part 320) as they apply to dosage forms intended for oral administration.[3] The guidance is also generally applicable to nonorally administered drug products where reliance on systemic exposure measures is suitable to document BA and BE (e.g., transdermal delivery systems and certain rectal and nasal drug products). The guidance should be useful for applicants planning to conduct BA and BE studies during the IND period for an NDA, BE studies intended for submission in an ANDA, and BE studies conducted in the postapproval period for certain changes in both NDAs and ANDAs.[4]

Background

General. Studies to measure BA and/or establish BE of a product are important elements in support of INDs, NDAs, ANDAs, and their supplements. As part of INDs and NDAs for orally administered drug products, BA studies focus on determining the process by which a drug is released from the oral dosage form and moves to the site of action. BA data provide an estimate of the fraction of the drug absorbed, as well as its subsequent distribution and elimination. BA can be generally documented by a systemic exposure profile obtained by measuring drug and/or metabolite concentration in the systemic circulation over time. The systemic exposure profile determined during clinical trials in the IND period can serve as a benchmark for subsequent BE studies.

Studies to establish BE between two products are important for certain changes before approval for a pioneer product in NDA and ANDA submissions and in the presence of certain postapproval changes in NDAs and ANDAs. In BE studies, an applicant compares the systemic exposure profile of a test drug product with that of a reference drug product. For two orally administered drug products to be bioequivalent, the active drug ingredient or active moiety in the test product should exhibit the same rate and extent of absorption as the reference drug product.

---

[3]These dosage forms include tablets, capsules, solutions, suspensions, conventional/immediate release, and modified (extended, delayed) release drug products.
[4]Other Agency guidances are available that consider specific scale-up and postapproval changes (SUPAC) for different types of drug products to help satisfy regulatory requirements in Part 320 and § 314.70 (21 CFR 314.70).

Both BA and BE studies are required by regulations, depending on the type of application being submitted. Under § 314.94, BE information is required to ensure therapeutic equivalence between a pharmaceutically equivalent test drug product and a reference-listed drug. Regulatory requirements for documentation of BA and BE are provided in part 320, which contains two subparts. Subpart A covers general provisions, while subpart B contains 18 sections delineating the following general BA/BE requirements:

- Requirements for submission of BA and BE data (§ 320.21)
- Criteria for waiver of an *in vivo* BA or BE study (§ 320.22)
- Basis for demonstrating *in vivo* BA or BE (§ 320.23)
- Types of evidence to establish BA or BE (§ 320.24)
- Guidelines for conduct of *in vivo* BA studies (§ 320.25)
- Guidelines on design of single-dose BA studies (§ 320.26)
- Guidelines on design of multiple-dose *in vivo* BA studies (§ 320.27)
- Correlations of BA with an acute pharmacological effect or clinical evidence (§ 320.28)
- Analytical methods for an *in vivo* BA study (§ 320.29)
- Inquiries regarding BA and BE requirements and review of protocols by the FDA (§ 320.30)
- Applicability of requirements regarding an IND application (§ 320.31)
- Procedures for establishing and amending a BE requirement (§ 320.32)
- Criteria and evidence to assess actual or potential BE problems (§ 320.33)
- Requirements for batch testing and certification by the FDA (§ 320.34)
- Requirements for *in vitro* batch testing of each batch (§ 320.35)
- Requirements for maintenance of records of BE testing (§ 320.36)
- Retention of BA samples (§ 320.38)
- Retention of BE samples (§ 320.63)

Bioavailability. Bioavailability is defined in § 320.1 as

> the rate and extent to which the active ingredient or active moiety is absorbed from a drug product and becomes available at the site of action. For drug products that are not intended to be absorbed into the bloodstream, bioavailability may be assessed by measurements intended to reflect the rate and extent to which the active ingredient or active moiety becomes available at the site of action.

This definition focuses on the processes by which the active ingredients or moieties are released from an oral dosage form and move to the site of action.

From a pharmacokinetic perspective, BA data for a given formulation provide an estimate of the relative fraction of the orally administered dose that is absorbed into the systemic circulation when compared with the BA data for a solution, suspension, or intravenous dosage form [21 CFR 320.25(d)(2) and (3)]. In addition, BA studies provide other useful pharmacokinetic information related to distribution, elimination, the effects of nutrients on absorption of the drug, dose proportionality, linearity in pharmacokinetics of the active moieties, and, where appropriate, inactive moieties. BA data may also provide information indirectly about the properties of a drug substance before entry into the systemic circulation, such as permeability and the influence of presystemic enzymes and/or transporters (e.g., p-glycoprotein).

BA for orally administered drug products can be documented by developing a systemic exposure profile obtained from measuring the concentration of active ingredients and/or active moieties and, when appropriate, its active metabolites over time in samples collected from the systemic circulation. Systemic exposure patterns reflect both release of the drug substance from the drug product and a series of possible presystemic/systemic actions on the drug substance after its release from the drug product. Additional comparative studies should be performed to understand the relative contribution of these processes to the systemic exposure pattern.

One regulatory objective is to assess, through appropriately designed BA studies, the performance of the formulations used in the clinical trials that provide evidence of safety and efficacy [21 CFR 320.25(d)(1)]. The performance of the clinical trial dosage form may be optimized, in the context of demonstrating safety and efficacy, before marketing a drug product. The systemic exposure profiles of clinical trial material can be used as a benchmark for subsequent formulation changes and may be useful as a reference for future BE studies.

Although BA studies have many pharmacokinetic objectives beyond formulation performance as described above, it should be noted that subsequent sections of this guidance focus on using relative BA (referred to as product quality BA) and, in particular, BE studies as a means to document product quality. *In vivo* performance, in terms of BA/BE, may be considered to be one aspect of product quality that provides a link to the performance of the drug product used in clinical trials and to the database containing evidence of safety and efficacy.

Bioequivalence. Bioequivalence is defined in § 320.1 as

> the absence of a significant difference in the rate and extent to which the active ingredient or active moiety in pharmaceutical equivalents or pharmaceutical alternatives becomes available at the site of drug action when administered at the same molar dose under similar conditions in an appropriately designed study.

As noted in the statutory definitions, both BE and product quality BA focus on the release of a drug substance from a drug product and subsequent absorption into the systemic circulation. For this reason, similar approaches to measuring BA in an NDA should generally be followed in demonstrating BE for an NDA or an ANDA. Establishing product quality BA is a benchmarking effort with comparisons to an oral solution, oral suspension, or an intravenous formulation. In contrast, demonstrating BE is usually a more formal comparative test that uses specified criteria for comparisons and predetermined BE limits for such criteria.

1. *IND/NDAs*   BE documentation may be useful during the IND or NDA period to establish links between (1) early and late clinical trial formulations; (2) formulations used in clinical trial and stability studies, if different; (3) clinical trial formulations and to-be-marketed drug product; and (4) other comparisons, as appropriate. In each comparison, the new formulation or new method of manufacture is the test product, and the prior formulation or method of manufacture is the reference product. The determination to redocument BE during the IND period is generally left to the judgment of the sponsor, who may wish to use the principles of relevant guidances (in this guidance, see "Postapproval Changes" and "*In Vitro* Studies") to determine when changes in components, composition, and/or method of manufacture suggest further *in vitro* and/or *in vivo* studies should be performed.

   A test product may fail to meet BE limits because the test product has higher or lower measures of rate and extent of absorption compared with the reference product or because the performance of the test or reference product is more variable. In some cases, nondocumentation of BE may arise because of inadequate numbers of subjects in the study relative to the magnitude of intrasubject variability, not because of either high or low relative BA of the test product. Adequate design and execution of a BE study will facilitate understanding of the causes of nondocumentation of BE.

   Where the test product generates plasma levels that are substantially above those of the reference product, the regulatory concern is not therapeutic failure but the adequacy of the safety database from the test product. Where the test product has levels that are substantially below those of the reference product, the regulatory concern becomes therapeutic efficacy. When the variability of the test product rises, the regulatory concern relates to both safety and efficacy because it may suggest that the test product does not perform as well as the reference product, and the test product may be too variable to be clinically useful.

   Proper mapping of individual dose-response or concentration-response curves is useful in situations where the drug product has plasma levels that are either higher or lower than those of the reference product and are outside usual BE limits. In the absence of individual data, population dose-response or concentration-response data acquired over a range of doses, including doses above the recommended therapeutic doses, may be sufficient to demonstrate that the increase in plasma levels would not be accompanied by additional risk. Similarly, population dose- or concentration-response relationships observed over a lower range of doses, including doses below the recommended therapeutic doses, may be able to demonstrate that reduced levels of the test product compared with the reference product are associated with adequate efficacy. In either event, the burden is on the sponsor to demonstrate the adequacy of the clinical trial dose-response or concentration-response data to provide evidence of therapeutic equivalence. In the absence of this evidence, a failure to document BE may suggest that the product should be reformulated, the method of manufacture for the test product should be changed, and/or the BE study should be repeated.

2. *ANDAs* BE studies are a critical component of ANDA submissions. The purpose of these studies is to demonstrate BE between a pharmaceutically equivalent generic drug product and the corresponding reference listed drug [21 CFR 314.94 (a)(7)]. Together with the determination of pharmaceutical equivalence, establishing BE allows a regulatory conclusion of therapeutic equivalence.

3. *Postapproval Changes* Information on the types of *in vitro* dissolution and *in vivo* BE studies that should be conducted for immediate-release and modified-release drug products approved as either NDAs or ANDAs in the presence of specified postapproval changes is provided in the FDA guidances for industry entitled *SUPAC-IR: Immediate Release Solid Oral Dosage Forms: Scale-Up and Post-Approval Changes: Chemistry, Manufacturing, and Controls*, In Vitro *Dissolution Testing, and* In Vivo *Bioequivalence Documentation* (November 1995); and *SUPAC-MR: Modified Release Solid Oral Dosage Forms: Scale-Up and Post-Approval Changes: Chemistry, Manufacturing, and Controls*, In Vitro *Dissolution Testing, and* In Vivo *Bioequivalence Documentation* (September 1997). In the presence of certain major changes in components, composition, and/or method of manufacture after approval, *in vivo* BE should be redemonstrated. For approved NDAs, the drug product after the change should be compared with the drug product before the change. For approved ANDAs, the drug product after the change should be compared with the reference-listed drug. Under section 506A(c)(2)(B) of the Federal Food, Drug, and Cosmetic Act (the Act) [21 U.S.C. 356a(c)(2)(B)], postapproval changes requiring completion of studies in accordance with part 320 must be submitted in a supplement and approved by the FDA before distributing a drug product made with the change.

Methods to Document BA and BE

As noted in § 320.24, several *in vivo* and *in vitro* methods can be used to measure product quality BA and establish BE. In descending order of preference, these include pharmacokinetic, pharmacodynamic, clinical, and *in vitro* studies. These general approaches are discussed in the following sections of this guidance. Product qualities BA and BE frequently rely on pharmacokinetic measures such as area under the curve (AUC) and maximum plasma concentration (Cmax) that are reflective of systemic exposure.

Pharmacokinetic Studies

1. *General Considerations*   The statutory definitions of BA and BE, expressed in terms of rate and extent of absorption of the active ingredient or moiety to the site of action, emphasize the use of pharmacokinetic measures in an accessible biological matrix such as blood, plasma, and/or serum to indicate release of the drug substance from the drug product into the systemic circulation.[5] This approach rests on an understanding that measuring the active moiety or ingredient at the site of action is generally not possible and, furthermore, that some relationship exists between the efficacy/safety and concentration of active moiety and/or its important metabolite or metabolites in the systemic circulation. To measure product quality BA and establish BE, reliance on pharmacokinetic measurements may be viewed as a bioassay that assesses release of the drug substance from the drug product into the systemic circulation. A typical study is conducted as a crossover study. In this type of study, clearance, volume of distribution, and absorption, as determined by physiological variables (e.g. gastric emptying, motility, pH), are assumed to have less interoccasion variability compared with the variability arising from formulation performance. Therefore, differences between two products because of formulation factors can be determined.

2. *Pilot Study*   If the sponsor chooses, a pilot study in a small number of subjects can be carried out before proceeding with a full BE study. The study can be used to validate analytical methodology, assess variability, optimize sample-collection time intervals, and provide other information. For example, for conventional immediate-release products, careful timing of initial samples may avoid a subsequent finding in a full-scale study that the first sample collection occurs after the plasma concentration peak. For modified-release products, a pilot study can help determine the sampling schedule to assess lag time and dose dumping. A pilot study that documents BE may be appropriate, provided its design and execution are suitable and a sufficient number of subjects (e.g., 12) have completed the study.

---

[5] If serial measurements of the drug or its metabolites in plasma, serum, or blood cannot be accomplished, measurement of urinary excretion may be used to document BE.

3. *Pivotal Bioequivalence Studies*   General recommendations for a standard BE study based on pharmacokinetic measurements are provided in Attachment A.

4. *Study Designs*   Nonreplicate study designs are recommended for BE studies of immediate-release and modified-release dosage forms. However, sponsors and/or applicants have the option of using replicate designs for BE studies for these drug products. Replicate study designs offer several scientific advantages compared with nonreplicate designs. The advantages of replicate study designs are that they (1) allow comparisons of within-subject variances for the test and reference products, (2) indicate whether a test product exhibits higher or lower within-subject variability in the bioavailability measures when compared to the reference product, (3) provide more information about the intrinsic factors underlying formulation performance, and (4) reduce the number of subjects needed in the BE study. The recommended method of analysis of nonreplicate or replicate studies to establish BE is average BE, as discussed in section IV. General recommendations for nonreplicate study designs are provided in Attachment A. Recommendations for replicate study designs can be found in the Guidance for Industry *Statistical Approaches to Establishing Bioequivalence* (January 2001).

5. *Study Population*   Unless otherwise indicated by a specific guidance, subjects recruited for *in vivo* BE studies should be 18 years old or older and capable of giving informed consent. This guidance recommends that *in vivo* BE studies be conducted in individuals representative of the general population, taking into account age, sex, and race. If the drug product is intended for use in both sexes, the sponsor should attempt to include similar proportions of males and females in the study. If the drug product is to be used predominantly in the elderly, the sponsor should attempt to include as many subjects of 60 years old or older as possible. The total number of subjects in the study should provide adequate power for BE demonstration, but it is not expected that there will be sufficient power to draw conclusions for each subgroup. Statistical analysis of subgroups is not recommended. Restrictions on admission into the study should generally be based solely on safety considerations. In some instances, it may be useful to admit patients into BE studies for whom a drug product is intended. In this situation, sponsors and/or applicants should attempt to enter patients whose disease process is stable for the duration of the BE study. In accordance with § 320.31, for some products that will be submitted in ANDAs, an IND may be required for BE studies to ensure patient safety.

6. *Single-Dose/Multiple-Dose Studies*   Instances where multiple-dose studies may be useful are defined under § 320.27(a)(3). However, this guidance generally recommends single-dose pharmacokinetic studies for both immediate- and modified-release drug products to demonstrate BE

because they are *generally* more sensitive in assessing release of the drug substance from the drug product into the systemic circulation (see "Documentation of BA and BE"). If a multiple-dose study design is important, appropriate dosage administration and sampling should be carried out to document attainment of steady state.

7. *Bioanalytical Methodology* Bioanalytical methods for BA and BE studies should be accurate, precise, selective, sensitive, and reproducible. A separate FDA guidance entitled *Bioanalytical Method Validation* (May 2001) is available to assist sponsors in validating bioanalytical methods.

8. *Pharmacokinetic Measures of Systemic Exposure* Both direct (e.g., rate constant, rate profile) and indirect (e.g., Cmax, Tmax, mean absorption time, mean residence time, Cmax normalized to AUC) pharmacokinetic measures are limited in their ability to assess rate of absorption. This guidance, therefore, recommends a change in focus from these direct or indirect measures of absorption rate to measures of systemic exposure. Cmax and AUC can continue to be used as measures for product quality BA and BE, but more in terms of their capacity to assess exposure than their capacity to reflect rate and extent of absorption. Reliance on systemic exposure measures should reflect comparable rate and extent of absorption, which in turn should achieve the underlying statutory and regulatory objective of ensuring comparable therapeutic effects. Exposure measures are defined relative to early, peak, and total portions of the plasma, serum, or blood concentration-time profile, as follows:

   a. Early Exposure For orally administered immediate-release drug products, BE may generally be demonstrated by measurements of peak and total exposure. An early exposure measure may be informative on the basis of appropriate clinical efficacy/safety trials and/or pharmacokinetic/pharmacodynamic studies that call for better control of drug absorption into the systemic circulation (e.g., to ensure rapid onset of an analgesic effect or to avoid an excessive hypotensive action of an antihypertensive). In this setting, the guidance recommends use of partial AUC as an early exposure measure. The partial area should be truncated at the population median of Tmax values for the reference formulation. At least two quantifiable samples should be collected before the expected peak time to allow adequate estimation of the partial area.

   b. Peak Exposure Peak exposure should be assessed by measuring the peak drug concentration (Cmax) obtained directly from the data without interpolation.

   c. Total Exposure For single-dose studies, the measurement of total exposure should be
      - area under the plasma/serum/blood concentration-time curve from time zero to time t (AUC_{0-t}), where t is the last time point with measurable concentration for individual formulation.

• area under the plasma/serum/blood concentration-time curve from time 0 to time infinity (AUC_{0-}), where $AUC_{0-} = AUC_{0-t} + C_t/_{-z}$, Ct is the last measurable drug concentration and $_{-z}$ is the terminal or elimination rate constant calculated according to an appropriate method. The terminal half-life ($t_{1/2}$) of the drug should also be reported.

For steady-state studies, the measurement of total exposure should be the area under the plasma, serum, or blood concentration-time curve from time 0 to time _ over a dosing interval at steady state (AUC_{0-}), where _ is the length of the dosing interval.

Pharmacodynamic Studies. Pharmacodynamic studies are not recommended for orally administered drug products when the drug is absorbed into the systemic circulation and a pharmacokinetic approach can be used to assess systemic exposure and establish BE. However, in those instances where a pharmacokinetic approach is not possible, suitably validated pharmacodynamic methods can be used to demonstrate BE.

Comparative Clinical Studies. Where there are no other means, well-controlled clinical trials in humans may be useful to provide supportive evidence of BA or BE. However, the use of comparative clinical trials as an approach to demonstrate BE is generally considered insensitive and should be avoided where possible (21 CFR 320.24). The use of BE studies with clinical trial end points may be appropriate to demonstrate BE for orally administered drug products when measurement of the active ingredients or active moieties in an accessible biological fluid (pharmacokinetic approach) or pharmacodynamic approach is infeasible.

In Vitro Studies. Under certain circumstances, product quality BA and BE can be documented using *in vitro* approaches [21 CFR 320.24(b)(5) and 21 CFR 320.22(d)(3)]. For highly soluble, highly permeable, rapidly dissolving, orally administered drug products, documentation of BE using an *in vitro* approach (dissolution studies) is appropriate based on the biopharmaceutics classification system.[6] This approach may also be suitable under some circumstances in assessing BE during the IND period, for NDA and ANDA submissions, and in the presence of certain postapproval changes to approved NDAs and ANDAs. In addition, *in vitro* approaches to document BE for *nonbioproblem* drugs approved before 1962 remain acceptable (21 CFR 320.33).

Dissolution testing is also used to assess batch-to-batch quality, where the dissolution tests, with defined procedures and acceptance criteria, are used to allow batch release. Dissolution testing is also used to (1) provide process

---

[6] See the FDA guidance for industry on Waiver of *In Vivo* Bioavailability and Bioequivalence Studies for Immediate Release Solid Oral Dosage Forms Based on a Biopharmaceutics Classification System (August 2000) at http://www.fda.gov/cvm/guidance/guide171.pdf. This document provides complementary information on the Biopharmaceutics Classification System.

control and quality assurance, and (2) assess whether further BE studies relative to minor postapproval changes should be conducted, where dissolution can function as a signal of bioinequivalence. *In vitro* dissolution characterization is encouraged for all product formulations investigated (including prototype formulations), particularly if *in vivo* absorption characteristics are being defined for the different product formulations. Such efforts may enable the establishment of an *in vitro–in vivo* correlation. When an *in vitro–in vivo* correlation or association is available [21 CFR 320.24(b)(1)(ii)], the *in vitro* test can serve not only as a quality control specification for the manufacturing process but also as an indicator of how the product will perform *in vivo*. The following guidances provide recommendations on the development of dissolution methodology, setting specifications, and the regulatory applications of dissolution testing: (1) *Dissolution Testing of Immediate Release Solid Oral Dosage Forms* (August 1997) and (2) *Extended Release Oral Dosage Forms: Development, Evaluation, and Application of* In Vitro/In Vivo *Correlations* (September 1997).

The following information should generally be included in the dissolution method development report for solid oral dosage forms:

For NDAs:

- The pH solubility profile of the drug substance
- Dissolution profiles generated at different agitation speeds [e.g., 100–150 rpm for U.S. Pharmacopeia (USP) Apparatus I (basket), and 50–100 rpm for USP Apparatus II (paddle)]
- Dissolution profiles generated on all strengths in at least three dissolution media (pH 1.2, 4.5, and 6.8 buffer). Water can be used as an additional medium. If the drug being considered is poorly soluble, appropriate concentrations of surfactants should be used.

The agitation speed and medium that provide the best discriminating ability, taking into account all the available *in vitro* and *in vivo* data, will be selected.

For ANDAs:

- USP method
- If a USP method is not available, the FDA method for the reference listed drug should be used.
- If USP and/or FDA methods are not available, the dissolution method development report described above should be submitted.

This guidance recommends that dissolution data from three batches for both NDAs and ANDAs be used to set dissolution specifications for modified-release dosage forms, including extended-release dosage forms.

Comparison of BA Measures in BE Studies

An equivalence approach has been and continues to be recommended for BE comparisons. The recommended approach relies on (1) a criterion to allow the comparison, (2) a confidence interval (CI) for the criterion, and (3) a BE limit. Log-transformation of exposure measures before statistical analysis is recommended. BE studies are performed as single-dose, crossover studies. To compare measures in these studies, data have been analyzed using an average BE criterion. This guidance recommends continued use of an average BE criterion to compare BA measures for replicate and nonreplicate BE studies of both immediate- and modified-release products.

Documentation of BA and BE

An *in vivo* study is generally recommended for all solid oral dosage forms approved after 1962 and for *bioproblem* drug products approved before 1962. Waiver of *in vivo* studies for different strengths of a drug product may be granted under § 320.22(d)(2) when (1) the drug product is in the same dosage form, but in a different strength; (2) this different strength is *proportionally similar* in its active and inactive ingredients to the strength of the product for which the same manufacturer has conducted an acceptable *in vivo* study; and (3) the new strength meets an appropriate *in vitro* dissolution test. This guidance defines *proportionally similar* in the following ways:

- All active and inactive ingredients are in exactly the same proportion between different strengths (e.g., a tablet of 50-mg strength has all the inactive ingredients, exactly half that of a tablet of 100-mg strength, and twice that of a tablet of 25-mg strength).
- Active and inactive ingredients are not in exactly the same proportion between different strengths as stated above, but the ratios of inactive ingredients to total weight of the dosage form are within the limits defined by the SUPAC-IR and SUPAC-MR guidances (up to Level II).
- For high potency drug substances, where the amount of the active drug substance in the dosage form is relatively low, the total weight of the dosage form remains nearly the same for all strengths (within ±10% of the total weight of the strength on which a biostudy was performed), the same inactive ingredients are used for all strengths, and the change in any strength is obtained by altering the amount of the active ingredients and one or more of the inactive ingredients. The changes in the inactive ingredients are within the limits defined by the SUPAC-IR and SUPAC-MR guidances (up to Level II).

Exceptions to the above definitions may be possible, if adequate justification is provided.

Solutions. For oral solutions, elixirs, syrups, tinctures, or other solubilized forms, *in vivo* BA and/or BE can be waived [21 CFR 320.22(b)(3)(i)]. Generally, *in vivo* BE studies are waived for solutions on the assumptions that release of the drug substance from the drug product is self-evident and that the solutions do not contain any excipient that significantly affects drug absorption [21 CFR 320.22(b)(3)(iii)]. However, there are certain excipients, such as sorbitol or mannitol, that can reduce the BA of drugs with low intestinal permeability in amounts sometimes used in oral liquid dosage forms.

Suspensions. BA and BE for a suspension should generally be established as for immediate-release solid oral dosage forms, and both *in vivo* and *in vitro* studies are recommended.

Immediate-Release Products: Capsules and Tablets

1. *General Recommendations*

   For product qualities BA and BE studies, where the focus is on release of the drug substance from the drug product into the systemic circulation, a single-dose, fasting study should be performed. *In vivo* BE studies should be accompanied by *in vitro* dissolution profiles on all strengths of each product. For ANDAs, the BE study should be conducted between the test product and reference listed drug using the strength(s) specified in *Approved Drug Products with Therapeutic Equivalence Evaluations (Orange Book)*.

2. *Waivers of* In Vivo *BE Studies (Biowaivers)*

   a. INDs, NDAs, and ANDAs: Preapproval

   When the drug product is in the same dosage form but in a different strength and is proportionally similar in its active and inactive ingredients to the reference-listed drug, an *in vivo* BE demonstration of one or more lower strengths can be waived to the reference-listed drug based on dissolution tests and an in vivo study on the highest strength.[7]

   For an NDA, biowaivers of a higher strength will be determined to be appropriate based on (1) clinical safety and/or efficacy studies including data on the dose and the desirability of the higher strength, (2) linear elimination kinetics over the therapeutic dose range, (3) the higher strength being proportionally similar to the lower strength, and (4) the same dissolution procedures being used for both strengths and similar dissolution results obtained. A dissolution profile should be generated for all strengths.

   If an appropriate dissolution method has been established (see "*In Vitro* Studies"), and the dissolution results indicate that the dissolu-

---

[7]This recommendation modifies a prior policy of allowing biowaivers for only three lower strengths on ANDAs.

tion characteristics of the product are not dependent on the product strength, then dissolution profiles in one medium are usually sufficient to support waivers of *in vivo* testing. Otherwise, dissolution data in three media (pH 1.2, 4.5, and 6.8) are recommended.

The f_2 test should be used to compare profiles from the different strengths of the product. An f_2 value of ≥50 indicates a sufficiently similar dissolution profile such that further *in vivo* studies are not necessary. For an f_2 value of <50, further discussions with CDER review staff may help to determine whether an *in vivo* study is necessary [21 CFR 320.22(d)(2)(ii)]. The f_2 approach is not suitable for rapidly dissolving drug products (e.g., ≥85% dissolved in 15 min or less).

For an ANDA, conducting an *in vivo* study on a strength that is not the highest may be appropriate for reasons of safety, subject to approval by the Division of Bioequivalence, Office of Generic Drugs, and provided that the following conditions are met.

- Linear elimination kinetics has been shown over the therapeutic dose range.
- The higher strengths of the test and reference products are proportionally similar to their corresponding lower strength.
- Comparative dissolution testing on the higher strength of the test and reference products is submitted and found to be appropriate.

b. NDAs and ANDAs: Postapproval

Information on the types of *in vitro* dissolution and *in vivo* BE studies for immediate-release drug products approved as either NDAs or ANDAs in the presence of specified postapproval changes are provided in an FDA guidance for industry entitled *SUPAC-IR: Immediate Release Solid Oral Dosage Forms: Scale-Up and Post-Approval Changes: Chemistry, Manufacturing, and Controls, In Vitro Dissolution Testing, and In Vivo Bioequivalence Documentation* (November 1995). For postapproval changes, the *in vitro* comparison should be made between the prechange and postchange products. In instances where dissolution profile comparisons are recommended, an f_2 test should be used. An f_2 value of ≥50 suggests a sufficiently similar dissolution profile, and no further *in vivo* studies are needed. When *in vivo* BE studies are recommended, the comparison should be made for NDAs between the prechange and postchange products, and for ANDAs between the postchange and reference-listed drug products.

Modified-Release Products. Modified-release products include delayed-release products and extended (controlled)-release products.

As defined in the USP, delayed-release drug products are dosage forms that release the drugs at a time later than immediately after administration (i.e., these drug products exhibit a lag time in quantifiable plasma concentrations).

Typically, coatings (e.g., enteric coatings) are intended to delay the release of medication until the dosage form has passed through the acidic medium of the stomach. *In vivo* tests for delayed-release drug products are similar to those for extended-release drug products. *In vitro* dissolution tests for these products should document that they are stable under acidic conditions and that they release the drug only in a neutral medium (e.g., pH 6.8).

Extended-release drug products are dosage forms that allow a reduction in dosing frequency as compared with when the drug is present in an immediate-release dosage form. These drug products can also be developed to reduce fluctuations in plasma concentrations. Extended-release products can be capsules, tablets, granules, pellets, and suspensions. If any part of a drug product includes an extended-release component, the following recommendations apply.

1. *NDAs: BA and BE Studies*

   An NDA can be submitted for a previously unapproved new molecular entity, or for a new salt, new ester, prodrug, or other noncovalent derivative of a previously approved new molecular entity, formulated as a modified-release drug product. The first modified-release drug product for a previously approved immediate-release drug product should be submitted as an NDA. Subsequent modified-release products that are pharmaceutically equivalent and bioequivalent to the listed drug product should be submitted as ANDAs. BA requirements for the NDA of an extended-release product are listed in § 320.25(f). The purpose of an *in vivo* BA study for which a controlled-release claim is made is to determine if all of the following conditions are met.

   • The drug product meets the controlled release claims made for it.

   • The BA profile established for the drug product rules out the occurrence of any dose dumping.

   • The drug product's steady-state performance is equivalent to a currently marketed, noncontrolled release or controlled-release drug product that contains the same active drug ingredient or therapeutic moiety and that is subject to an approved full NDA.

   • The drug product's formulation provides consistent pharmacokinetic performance between individual dosage units.

   As noted in § 320.25(f)(2), "the reference material(s) for such a bioavailability study shall be chosen to permit an appropriate scientific evaluation of the controlled release claims made for the drug product," such as

   • a solution or suspension of the active drug ingredient or therapeutic moiety;

   • a currently marketed noncontrolled-release drug product containing the same active drug ingredient or therapeutic moiety and administered according to the dosage recommendations in the labeling; and

• a currently marketed controlled-release drug product subject to an approved full NDA containing the same active drug ingredient or therapeutic moiety and administered according to the dosage recommendations in the labeling.

This guidance recommends that the following BA studies be conducted for an extended-release drug product submitted as an NDA:

• A single-dose, fasting study on all strengths of tablets and capsules and highest strength of beaded capsules
• A single-dose, food-effect study on the highest strength
• A steady-state study on the highest strength

BE studies are recommended when substantial changes in the components or composition and/or method of manufacture for an extended-release drug product occur between the to-be-marketed NDA dosage form and the clinical trial material.

2. *ANDAs: BE Studies*

For modified-release products submitted as ANDAs, the following studies are recommended: (1) a single-dose, nonreplicate, fasting study comparing the highest strength of the test and reference-listed drug product, unless the drug or drug product is highly variable in which case a replicate design study is recommended; and (2) a food-effect, nonreplicate study comparing the highest strength of the test and reference product (see "Solutions"). Because single-dose studies are considered more sensitive in addressing the primary question of BE (i.e., release of the drug substance from the drug product into the systemic circulation), multiple-dose studies are generally not recommended, even in instances where nonlinear kinetics are present.

3. *Waivers of In Vivo BE Studies (Biowaivers): NDAs and ANDAs*

   a. Beaded Capsules—Lower Strength

   For modified-release beaded capsules where the strength differs only in the number of beads containing the active moiety, a single-dose, fasting BE study should be carried out only on the highest strength, with waiver of in vivo studies for lower strengths based on dissolution profiles. A dissolution profile should be generated for each strength using the recommended dissolution method. The f_2 test should be used to compare profiles from the different strengths of the product. An f_2 value of ≥ 50 can be used to confirm that further in vivo studies are not needed.

   b. Tablets—Lower Strength

   For modified-release tablets, when the drug product is in the same dosage form but in a different strength, is proportionally similar in its active and inactive ingredients, and has the same drug release mechanism, an *in vivo* BE determination of one or more lower strengths can be waived based on dissolution profile comparisons, with an *in vivo* study only on the highest strength. The drug products should exhibit similar dissolution profiles between the highest strength and the lower strengths based on the f_2 test in at least three dissolution media (e.g., pH 1.2, 4.5, and 6.8). The dissolution profile should be generated on the test and reference products of all strengths.

4. *Postapproval Changes*

Information on the types of *in vitro* dissolution and *in vivo* BE studies for extended-release drug products approved as either NDAs or ANDAs in the presence of specified postapproval changes are provided in an FDA guidance for industry entitled *SUPAC-MR: Modified Release Solid Oral Dosage Forms: Scale-Up and Post-Approval Changes: Chemistry, Manufacturing, and Controls,* In Vitro *Dissolution Testing, and* In Vivo *Bioequivalence Documentation* (September 1997). For postapproval changes, the *in vitro* comparison should be made between the prechange and postchange products. In instances where dissolution profile comparisons are recommended, an f_2 test should be used. An f_2 value of ≥ 50 suggests a similar dissolution profile. A failure to demonstrate similar dissolution profiles may indicate that an *in vivo* BE study should be performed. When *in vivo* BE studies are conducted, the comparison should be made for NDAs between the prechange and postchange products, and for ANDAs between the postchange product and reference-listed drug.

Miscellaneous Dosage Forms. Rapidly dissolving drug products, such as buccal and sublingual dosage forms, should be tested for *in vitro* dissolution and *in vivo* BA and/or BE. Chewable tablets should also be evaluated for *in vivo* BA and/or BE. Chewable tablets (as a whole) should be subject to *in vitro* dissolution because they might be swallowed by a patient without proper chewing. In general, *in vitro* dissolution test conditions for chewable tablets should be the same as for nonchewable tablets of the same active ingredient or moiety. Infrequently, different test conditions or acceptance criteria may be indicated for chewable and nonchewable tablets, but these differences, if they exist, should be resolved with the appropriate review division.

Special Topics

Food-Effect Studies. Coadministration of food with oral drug products may influence drug BA and/or BE. Food-effect BA studies focus on the effects of food on the release of the drug substance from the drug product as well as the absorption of the drug substance. BE studies with food focus on demonstrating comparable BA between test and reference products when coadministered with meals. Usually, a single-dose, two-period, two-treatment, two-sequence crossover study is recommended for both food-effect BA and BE studies.

Moieties to Be Measured

1. *Parent Drug Versus Metabolites*

   The moieties to be measured in biological fluids collected in BA and BE studies are either the active drug ingredient or its active moiety in the administered dosage form (parent drug) and, when appropriate, its active metabolites [21 CFR 320.24(b)(1)(i)].[8] This guidance recommends the following approaches for BA and BE studies.

   For BA studies (see "Bioavailability"), determination of moieties to be measured in biological fluids should take into account both concentration and activity. *Concentration* refers to the relative quantity of the parent drug or one or more metabolites in a given volume of an accessible biological fluid such as blood or plasma. *Activity* refers to the relative contribution of the parent drug and its metabolite(s) in the biological fluids to the clinical safety and/or efficacy of the drug. For BA studies, both the parent drug and its major active metabolites should be measured, if analytically feasible.

   For BE studies, measurement of only the parent drug released from the dosage form, rather than the metabolite, is generally recommended. The rationale for this recommendation is that the concentration-time profile of the parent drug is more sensitive to changes in formulation performance than a metabolite, which is more reflective of metabolite formation, distribution, and elimination. The following are exceptions to this general approach.

   - Measurement of a metabolite may be preferred when parent drug levels are too low to allow reliable analytical measurement in blood, plasma, or serum for an adequate length of time. The metabolite data obtained from these studies should be subject to a CI approach for BE demonstration. If there is a clinical concern related to efficacy or safety for the parent drug, sponsors and/or applicants should contact the appropriate review division to determine whether the parent drug should be measured and analyzed statistically.
   - A metabolite may be formed as a result of gut wall or other presystemic metabolism. If the metabolite contributes meaningfully to safety and/or efficacy, the metabolite and the parent drug should be measured. When the relative activity of the metabolite is low and does not contribute meaningfully to safety and/or efficacy, it does not need to be measured. The parent drug measured in these BE studies should be analyzed using a CI approach. The metabolite data can be used to provide supportive evidence of comparable therapeutic outcome.

[8] A dosage form contains active and, usually, inactive ingredients. The active ingredient may be a prodrug that requires further transformation *in vivo* to become active. An active moiety is the molecule or ion, excluding those appended portions of the molecule that cause the drug to be an ester, salt, or other noncovalent derivative of the molecule, responsible for the physiological or pharmacological action of the drug substance.

2. *Enantiomers Versus Racemates*

For BA studies, measurement of individual enantiomers may be important. For BE studies, this guidance recommends measurement of the racemate using an achiral assay. Measurement of individual enantiomers in BE studies is recommended only when all of the following conditions are met: (1) The enantiomers exhibit different pharmacodynamic characteristics. (2) The enantiomers exhibit different pharmacokinetic characteristics. (3) Primary efficacy and safety activity resides with the minor enantiomer. (4) Nonlinear absorption is present (as expressed by a change in the enantiomer concentration ratio with change in the input rate of the drug) for at least one of the enantiomers. In such cases, BE criteria should be applied to the enantiomers separately.

3. *Drug Products with Complex Mixtures as the Active Ingredients*

Certain drug products may contain complex drug substances (i.e., active moieties or active ingredients that are mixtures of multiple synthetic and/or natural source components). Some or all of the components of these complex drug substances cannot be characterized with regard to chemical structure and/or biological activity. Quantification of all active or potentially active components in pharmacokinetic studies to document BA and BE is neither necessary nor desirable. Rather, BA and BE studies should be based on a small number of markers of rate and extent of absorption. Although necessarily a case-by-case determination, criteria for marker selection include amount of the moiety in the dosage form, plasma or blood levels of the moiety and biological activity of the moiety relative to other moieties in the complex mixture. Where pharmacokinetic approaches are not feasible to assess rate and extent of absorption of a drug substance from a drug product, *in vitro* approaches may be preferred. Pharmacodynamic or clinical approaches may be called for if no quantifiable moieties are available for *in vivo* pharmacokinetic or *in vitro* studies.

Long Half-Life Drugs. In a BA or pharmacokinetic study involving an oral product with a long half-life drug, adequate characterization of the half-life calls for blood sampling over a long period of time. For a BE determination of an oral product with a long half-life drug, a nonreplicate, single-dose, crossover study can be conducted, provided an adequate washout period is used. If the crossover study is problematic, a BE study with a parallel design can be used. For either a crossover or parallel study, sample collection time should be adequate to ensure completion of gastrointestinal transit (approximately two to three days) of the drug product and absorption of the drug substance. Cmax and a suitably truncated AUC can be used to characterize peak and total drug exposure, respectively. For drugs that demonstrate low intrasubject variability in distribution and clearance, an AUC truncated at 72h (AUC_{0-72h}) can be used in place of AUC_{0-t} or $AUC_{0-\infty}$. For drugs demonstrating high intrasubject variability in distribution and clearance, AUC truncation warrants caution. In such cases, sponsors and/or applicants should consult the appropriate review staff.

First-Point Cmax. The first point of a concentration-time curve in a BE study based on blood and/or plasma measurements is sometimes the highest point, which raises a question about the measurement of true Cmax because of insufficient early sampling times. A carefully conducted pilot study may avoid this problem. Collection of an early time point between 5 and 15 min after dosing followed by additional sample collections (e.g., two to five) in the first hour after dosing may be sufficient to assess early peak concentrations. If this sampling approach is followed, data sets should be considered adequate, even when the highest observed concentration occurs at the first time point.

Orally Administered Drugs Intended for Local Action. Documentation of product quality BA for NDAs where the drug substance produces its effects by local action in the gastrointestinal tract can be achieved using clinical efficacy and safety studies and/or suitably designed and validated *in vitro* studies. Similarly, documentation of BE for ANDAs and for both NDAs and ANDAs in the presence of certain postapproval changes can be achieved using BE studies with clinical efficacy and safety end points and/or suitably designed and validated *in vitro* studies if the latter studies are either reflective of important clinical effects or are more sensitive to changes in product performance compared to a clinical study. To ensure comparable safety, additional studies with and without food may help to understand the degree of systemic exposure that occurs following administration of a drug product intended for local action in the gastrointestinal tract.

Narrow Therapeutic Range Drugs. This guidance defines *narrow therapeutic range*[9] drug products as those containing certain drug substances that are subject to therapeutic drug concentration or pharmacodynamic monitoring, and/or where product labeling indicates a narrow therapeutic range designation. Examples include digoxin, lithium, phenytoin, theophylline, and warfarin. Because not all drugs subject to therapeutic drug concentration or pharmacodynamic monitoring are narrow therapeutic range drugs, sponsors and/or applicants should contact the appropriate review division at CDER to determine whether a drug should or should not be considered to have a narrow therapeutic range.

This guidance recommends that sponsors consider additional testing and/or controls to ensure the quality of drug products containing narrow therapeutic range drugs. The approach is designed to provide increased assurance of interchangeability for drug products containing specified narrow therapeutic range drugs. It is not designed to influence the practice of medicine or pharmacy.

---

[9]This guidance uses the term "narrow therapeutic range" instead of "narrow therapeutic index" drug, although the latter is more commonly used.

Unless otherwise indicated by a specific guidance, this guidance recommends that the traditional BE limit of 80% to 125% for nonnarrow therapeutic range drugs remain unchanged for the BA measures (AUC and Cmax) of narrow therapeutic range drugs.

Attachment A

General Pharmacokinetic Study Design and Data Handling. For both
replicate and nonreplicate *in vivo* pharmacokinetic BE studies, the following general approaches are recommended, recognizing that the elements may be adjusted for certain drug substances and drug products.

Study Conduct

- The test or reference products should be administered with about 8 oz (240 mL) of water to an appropriate number of subjects under fasting conditions, unless the study is a food-effect BA and BE study.
- Generally, the highest marketed strength should be administered as a single unit. If warranted for analytical reasons, multiple units of the highest strength can be administered, providing the total single-dose remains within the labeled dose range.
- An adequate washout period (e.g., more than five half-lives of the moieties to be measured) should separate each treatment.
- The lot numbers of both test and reference listed products and the expiration date for the reference product should be stated. The drug content of the test product should not differ from that of the reference listed product by more than 5%. The sponsor should include a statement of the composition of the test product and, if possible, a side-by-side comparison of the compositions of test and reference-listed products. In accordance with § 320.38, samples of the test and reference-listed product must be retained for five years.
- Before and during each study phase, subjects should (1) be allowed water as desired except for 1 h before and after drug administration, (2) be provided standard meals no less than 4 h after drug administration, and (3) abstain from alcohol for 24 h before each study period and until after the last sample from each period is collected.

Sample Collection and Sampling Times

- Under normal circumstances, blood, rather than urine or tissue, should be used. In most cases, drug or metabolites are measured in serum or plasma. However, in certain cases, whole blood may be more appropriate for analysis. Blood samples should be drawn at appropriate times to describe the absorption, distribution, and elimination phases of the drug. For most drugs, 12 to 18 samples, including a predose sample, should be collected per subject per dose. This sampling should continue for at least three or more terminal half-lives of the drug. The exact timing for sample collection depends on the nature of the drug and the input from the administered dosage form. The sample collection should be spaced in such a way that the maximum concentration of the drug in the blood (Cmax) and terminal elimination rate constant ($\_z$) can be estimated accurately. At least three to four samples should be obtained during the terminal log-linear phase to obtain an accurate estimate of $\_z$ from linear regression. The actual clock time when samples are drawn, as well as the elapsed time related to drug administration, should be recorded.

Subjects with Predose Plasma Concentrations

- If the predose concentration is less than or equal to 5% of Cmax value in that subject, the subject's data without any adjustments can be included in all pharmacokinetic measurements and calculations. If the predose value is greater than 5% of Cmax, the subject should be dropped from all BE study evaluations.

Data Deletion Due to Vomiting

- Data from subjects who experience emesis during the course of a BE study for immediate-release products should be deleted from statistical analysis if vomiting occurs at or before two times median Tmax. In the case of modified-release products, the data from subjects who experience emesis any time during the labeled dosing interval should be deleted.

   The following pharmacokinetic information is recommended for submission.
- Plasma concentrations and time points
- Subject, period, sequence, treatment
- AUC_{0-t}, $AUC_{0-\infty}$, Cmax, Tmax, $\_z$, and $t_{1/2}$
- Intersubject, intrasubject, and/or total variability, if available
- Cmin (concentration at the end of a dosing interval), Cav (average concentration during a dosing interval), degree of fluctuation [(Cmax − Cmin)/Cav], and swing [(Cmax − Cmin)/Cmin] if steady-state studies are employed
- Partial AUC, requested only as discussed in "Early Exposure"

In addition, the following statistical information should be provided for AUC_{0-t}, $AUC_{0-\infty}$, and Cmax:

geometric mean
arithmetic mean
ratio of means
CIs

Logarithmic transformation should be provided for measures used for BE demonstration.

Rounding Off of CI Values

- CI values should not be rounded off; therefore, to pass a CI limit of 80 to 125, the value should be at least 80.00 and not more than 125.00.

GUIDANCE FOR INDUSTRY[9]—NDAS: IMPURITIES IN DRUG SUBSTANCES

U.S. Department of Health and Human Services
Food and Drug Administration
Center for Drug Evaluation and Research
February 2000
CMC

Additional copies are available from:
Drug Information Branch, HFD-210
Center for Drug Evaluation and Research
5600 Fishers Lane, Rockville, MD 20857
Tel: 301-827-4573
http://www.fda.gov/cder/guidance/index.htm

This guidance recommends that applicants refer to *Q&A Impurities in New Drug Substances* (January 4, 1996, 61 FR 371) when seeking guidance on identification, qualification and reporting of impurities in drug substances that are not considered new drug substances. Although Q3A was developed by the ICH to provide guidance on the information that should be provided in an NDA in support of impurities in *new* drug substances that are produced by chemical syntheses, the Agency believes that the guidance provided there on identification, qualification, and reporting of impurities should also be considered when evaluating impurities in drug substances produced by chemical syntheses that are *not* considered new drug substances.[10]

This recommendation applies to applicants planning to submit NDAs and supplements for changes in drug substance synthesis or process. It also applies to holders of Type II DMFs that support such applications. Applicants should note that this recommendation would not apply to DMFs cited in an NDA or

[9]This guidance was prepared by the Drug Substance Technical Committee of the CMC Coordinating Committee in CDER at the FDA. This guidance represents the Agency's current thinking on reporting impurities in drug substances for certain NDAs and DMFs. It does not create or confer any rights for or on any person and does not operate to bind FDA or the public. An alternative approach may be used if such approach satisfies the requirements of the applicable statutes, regulations, or both.

[10]ICH Q3A defines a *new drug substance* (also referred to as a new molecular entity or new chemical entity) as a designated therapeutic moiety that has not been previously registered in a region or member state. The definition also states that a *new drug substance* may be a complex, a simple ester, or a salt of a previously approved drug substance.

supplement if the DMF information has been deemed acceptable for that dosage form, route of administration, and daily intake prior to the publication of the final version of this guidance. Examples of NDAs affected by the recommendation include those submitted for new dosage forms of already approved drug products, or drug products containing two or more active moieties that are individually used in already approved drug products but have not previously been approved or marketed together in a drug product.

This guidance does not apply to applications for biological, biotechnological, peptide, oligonucleotide, radiopharmaceutical, fermentation and semisynthetic products derived therefrom, herbal products, or crude products of animal or plant origin, nor does it apply to ANDAs. Guidance on drug substances used for ANDA products is available in the FDA's guidance on *ANDAs: Impurities in Drug Substances* (November 1999).

FDA IND, NDA, ANDA, OR DMF BINDERS

Effective, Wednesday, April 1, 1998, all interested parties can call the following number to order FDA IND, NDA, ANDA and Drug Master File binders:

U.S. Government Printing Office (GPO)
Washington, DC 20404-0001
202) 512-1800
Program #B511-S

Quantity of binders that can be order at any one time is to be determined by GPO.

Required Specifications for the FDA's IND, NDA, ANDA, DMF Binders

As of June 10, 1997, the FDA no longer provides IND, NDA, ANDA or DMF application binders to outside firms. Firms are required to have their own binders made and printed according to the following specifications. If you have any questions or need additional information, please contact Mia Prather at 301-796-0618.

Polyethylene Binders

Front (flat size): 248 × 292 mm (9¾ × 11½")
Back (flat size): 248 × 305 mm (9¾ × 12") [size includes 13 mm (½") lip at top]

Must be high-impact linear plastic (matte finish or similar). Must be able to withstand temperatures up to 150 degrees. Material should have a surface smooth enough to allow printing with a complete bonding of ink to the surface after a minimum of 1-h drying time. Should be free from streaks, blisters, scratches, and mottling.

Binder weight **must** be 0.023–0.025 gauge. Ink color **must** be **black**.

Polyethylene binders include

- FDA Form 2626–Blue–NDA archival binder
- FDA Form 2675–Red–IND archival binder
- FDA Form 3316–Red–DMF archival binder
- FDA Form 3316a–Blue–DMF binder

Paper Binders

Front (flat size): 267 × 292 mm (10½ × 11½″)
Back (flat size): 267 × 305 mm (10½ × 12″) [size includes 13 mm (½″) lip at top

Binder MUST be of 11-point plate rope stock of extra heavy weight. Ink color **must** be **black**. Maroon binder ink color **must** be **white**.

Paper binders include

- FDA Form 2626a–Red–NDA chemistry binder
- FDA Form 2626b–Yellow–NDA pharmacology binder
- FDA Form 2626c–Orange–NDA Pharmacokinetic binder
- FDA Form 2626d–White–NDA microbiology binder
- FDA Form 2626e–Tan–NDA clinical data binder
- FDA Form 2626f–Green –NDA statistics binder
- FDA Form 2626h–Maroon–NDA field Submission chemistry binder
- FDA Form 2675a–Green–IND chemistry binder
- FDA Form 2675b–Orange–IND microbiology binder

Printing

Required on front folder in a clear, sharp, permanent-type print in **black** ink. Permanent adhesive labels may be used in a clear, sharp print. Printing must withstand a "Scotch Tape Test," which consists of pressing a strip of "Scotch" tape firmly on the printed area and removing it. There should be **no** transfer of the printed area on the tape.

Binding. Polyethylene binders (front and back) **must** contain an internal (hidden) hinge formed in the material by heat and pressure. Hinge should extend along the entire left-hand binding edge of the binder and be of a depth to provide a clean, straight fold free from wrinkle when created or folded on the hinge. Hinge holes should be reinforced with metal eyelets and suitable for accommodating an ACCO-type fastener allowing for expansion. Outside binder surfaces MUST be smooth with NO exposed hinges or fastener.

Paper binders (front and back) **must** have two hinge holes scored along the entire left-hand binding edge and must be of a depth to provide a clean, straight fold free from wrinkle when creased or folded on the score. Hinge holes should be reinforced and suitable for accommodating an ACCO-type fastener allowing for expansion.

Round corner the inside edge of tab on back folder and outside edges of the front and back folders on polyethylene and paper binders.

Finished margins **must** conform to binder sizes indicated above

Below are cover samples for FDA Form 2626, 2626a thru h—NDA Applications, FDA Form 2675, 2675a and b—IND Applications, and FDA Form 3316, 3316a—DMFs.

Sample Cover—Form FDA 2626 (series a–h)
NOTE: Sample is **smaller** in print (font) size than actual cover. Printing **must** match layout of previously submitted section binders.

VOLUME _____
NEW DRUG APPLICATION
NDA No. _____
NAME OF APPLICANT
NAME OF NEW DRUG
SECTION NAME (*see below)
This submission: VOL._____OF_____VOLS.

Listed below are FDA NDA/ANDA binders identical to sample above. Section cover name is **only** difference.

*Form #	Color	Ink	Section cover name
2626	Blue	Black	Archival Copy
2626a	Red	Black	NDA chemistry
2626b	Yellow	Black	NDA pharmacology
2626c	Orange	Black	NDA pharmacokinetic
2626d	White	Black	NDA microbiology
2626e	Tan	Black	NDA clinical data
2626f	Green	Black	NDA statistics
2626h	Maroon	White	NDA Field submission chemistry

Sample Cover—Form FDA 2675 (series a–b)
NOTE: Sample is smaller in print (font) size than actual cover. Printing MUST match layout of previously submitted section binders.

VOLUME _____
NOTICE OF CLAIMED
INVESTIGATIONAL
EXEMPTION FOR A
NEW DRUG
IND. NO._____
SPONSOR
NAME OF DRUG (*see below)
This submission: VOL.____OF_____VOLS.

Listed below are FDA IND binders identical to sample above. Section cover name is **only** difference.

*Form #	Color	Ink	Cover drug name
2675	Red	Black	IND name of drug
2675a	Green	Black	IND name of drug
2675b	Orange	Black	IND name of drug

Sample Cover—FDA Form 3316
NOTE: Sample is **smaller** in p.rint (font) size than actual cover. Printing **must** match layout of previously submitted section binders.

VOLUME _____
DRUG MASTER FILE
NO. _____
NAME OF APPLICANT
(*see below)
TYPE:
This submission: VOL._____OF_____VOLS.

Listed below are DMF binders identical to sample above. File # and Type will be **only** difference.

*Form #	Color	Ink	Cover name
3316	Red	Black	Drug Master File
3316a	Blue	Black	Drug Master File

Most federal laws administered through the FDA are codified into the Food, Drug and Cosmetic Act, Other significant laws enforced by the FDA include the Public Health Service Act, Controlled Substrances Act, and Federal Anti-Tampering Act.

Title 21—Food and Drugs

CHAPTER I—FOOD AND DRUG ADMINISTRATION, DEPARTMENT OF
HEALTH AND HUMAN SERVICES
PART 314: APPLICATIONS FOR FDA APPROVAL TO MARKET A NEW
DRUG OR AN ANTIBIOTIC DRUG

(Code of Federal Regulations)
(Title 21, Volume 5, Parts 300 to 499)
(Revised as of April 1, 1998)
From the U.S. Government Printing Office via GPO Access
(CITE: 21 CFR 314.50)
(Pages 102–112)
Title 21: Food and Drugs
Chapter I: Food and Drug Administration, Department of Health and Human
    Services—Continued
Part 314: Applications for FDA Approval to MARKET A NEW DRUG OR
    AN ANTIBIOTIC DRUG—Table of Contents
Subpart B: Applications
Sec. 314.50: Content and Format of an Application

Applications and supplements to approved applications are required to be submitted in the form and contain the information, as appropriate for the particular submission, required under this section. Three copies of the application are required: An archival copy, a review copy, and a field copy. An application for a new chemical entity will generally contain an application form, an index, a summary, five or six technical sections, case report tabulations of patient data, case report forms, drug samples, and labeling. Other applications will generally contain only some of those items, and information will be limited to that needed to support the particular submission. These include an application of the type described in section 505(b)(2) of the act, an amendment, and a supplement. The application is required to contain reports of all investigations of the drug product sponsored by the applicant, and all other information about the drug pertinent to an evaluation of the application that is received or otherwise obtained by the applicant from any source. The FDA will maintain guidelines on the format and content of applications to assist applicants in their preparation.

(a) Application form. The applicant shall submit a completed and signed application form that contains the following:

    (1) The name and address of the applicant; the date of the application; the application number if previously issued (for example, if the application is a resubmission, an amendment, or a supplement); the name of the drug product, including its established, proprietary, code, and chemical names; the dosage form and strength; the route of administration; the identification numbers of all investigational new drug applications that are referenced in the application; the identification numbers of all drug master files and other applications under this part that are referenced in the application; and the drug product's proposed indications for use.

(2) A statement whether the submission is an original submission, a 505(b)(2) application, a resubmission, or a supplement to an application under Sec. 314.70.

(3) A statement whether the applicant proposes to market the drug product as a prescription or an over-the-counter product.

(4) A checklist identifying what enclosures required under this section the applicant is submitting.

(5) The applicant, or the applicant's attorney, agent, or other authorized official shall sign the application. If the person signing the application does not reside or have a place of business within the United States, the application is required to contain the name and address of, and be countersigned by, an attorney, agent, or other authorized official who resides or maintains a place of business within the United States.

(b) Index. The archival copy of the application is required to contain a comprehensive index by volume number and page number to the summary under paragraph (c) of this section, the technical sections under paragraph (d) [[Page 103]] of this section, and the supporting information under paragraph (f) of this section.

(c) Summary

(1) An application is required to contain a summary of the application in enough detail that the reader may gain a good general understanding of the data and information in the application, including an understanding of the quantitative aspects of the data. The summary is not required for supplements under Sec. 314.70. Resubmissions of an application should contain an updated summary, as appropriate. The summary should discuss all aspects of the application, and synthesize the information into a well-structured and unified document. The summary should be written at approximately the level of detail required for publication in, and meet the editorial standards generally applied by, refereed scientific and medical journals. In addition to the agency personnel reviewing the summary in the context of their review of the application, the FDA may furnish the summary to FDA advisory committee members and agency officials whose duties require an understanding of the application. To the extent possible, data in the summary should be presented in tabular and graphic forms. The FDA has prepared a guideline under Sec. 10.90(b) that provides information about how to prepare a summary. The summary required under this paragraph may be used by the FDA or the applicant to prepare the Summary Basis of Approval document for public disclosure [under Sec. 314.430(e)(2)(ii)] when the application is approved.

(2) The summary is required to contain the following information:

   (i) The proposed text of the labeling for the drug, with annotations to the information in the summary and technical sections of the application that support the inclusion of each statement in the labeling, and, if the application is for a prescription drug, statements describing the reasons for omitting a section or subsection of the labeling format in Sec. 201.57.

   (ii) A statement identifying the pharmacologic class of the drug and a discussion of the scientific rationale for the drug, its intended use, and the potential clinical benefits of the drug product.

   (iii) A brief description of the marketing history, if any, of the drug outside the United States, including a list of the countries in which the drug has been marketed, a list of any countries in which the drug has been withdrawn from marketing for any reason related to safety or effectiveness, and a list of countries in which applications for marketing are pending. The description is required to describe both marketing by the applicant and, if known, the marketing history of other persons.

   (iv) A summary of the chemistry, manufacturing, and controls section of the application.

   (v) A summary of the nonclinical pharmacology and toxicology section of the application.

   (vi) A summary of the human pharmacokinetics and bioavailability section of the application.

   (vii) A summary of the microbiology section of the application (for anti-infective drugs only).

   (viii) A summary of the clinical data section of the application, including the results of statistical analyses of the clinical trials.

   (ix) A concluding discussion that presents the benefit and risk considerations related to the drug, including a discussion of any proposed additional studies or surveillance the applicant intends to conduct postmarketing.

(d) Technical sections. The application is required to contain the technical sections described below. Each technical section is required to contain data and information in sufficient detail to permit the agency to make a knowledgeable judgment about whether to approve the application or whether grounds exist under section 505(d) or 507 of the act to refuse to approve the application. The required technical sections are as follows:

   (1) Chemistry, manufacturing, and controls section. A section describing the composition, manufacture, and specification of the drug substance and the drug product, including the following:

      (i) Drug substance. A full description of the drug substance including its physical and chemical characteristics and stability; the name and address of [[Page 104]] its manufacturer; the method of synthesis (or isolation) and purification of the drug substance; the process controls used during manufacture and packaging; and such specifications and analytical methods as are necessary to assure the identity, strength, quality, and purity of the drug substance and the bioavailability of the drug products made from the substance, including, for example, specifications relating to stability, sterility, particle size, and crystalline form. The application may provide additionally for the use of alternatives to meet any of these requirements, including alternative sources, process controls, methods, and specifications. Reference to the current edition of the U.S. Pharmacopeia and the National Formulary may satisfy relevant requirements in this paragraph.

(ii)

(a) Drug product. A list of all components used in the manufacture of the drug product (regardless of whether they appear in the drug product); and a statement of the composition of the drug product; a statement of the specifications and analytical methods for each component; the name and address of each manufacturer the drug product; a description of the manufacturing and packaging procedures and in-process controls for the drug product; such specifications and analytical methods as are necessary to assure the identity, strength, quality, purity, and bioavailability of the drug product, including, for example, specifications relating to sterility, dissolution rate, containers and closure systems; and stability data with proposed expiration dating. The application may provide additionally for the use of alternatives to meet any of these requirements, including alternative components, manufacturing and packaging procedures, in-process controls, methods, and specifications. Reference to the current edition of the U.S. Pharmacopeia and the National Formulary may satisfy relevant requirements in this paragraph.

(b) Unless provided by paragraph (d)(1)(ii)(a) of this section, for each batch of the drug product used to conduct a bioavailability or bioequivalence study described in Sec. 320.38 or Sec. 320.63 of this chapter or used to conduct a primary stability study: The batch production record; the specifications and test procedures for each component and for the drug product; the names and addresses of the sources of the active and noncompendial inactive components and of the container and closure system for the drug product; the name and address of each contract facility involved in the manufacture, processing, packaging, or testing of the drug product and identification of the operation performed by each contract facility; and the results of any test performed on the components used in the manufacture of the drug product as required by Sec. 211.84(d) of this chapter and on the drug product as required by Sec. 211.165 of this chapter.

(c) The proposed or actual master production record, including a description of the equipment, to be used for the manufacture of a commercial lot of the drug product or a comparably detailed description of the production process for a representative batch of the drug product.

(iii) Environmental impact. The application is required to contain either a claim for categorical exclusion under Sec. 25.30 or 25.31 of this chapter or an environmental assessment under Sec. 25.40 of this chapter.

(iv) The applicant may, at its option, submit a complete chemistry, manufacturing, and controls section 90 to 120 days before the anticipated submission of the remainder of the application. The FDA will review such early submissions as resources permit.

(v) Except for a foreign applicant, the applicant shall include a statement certifying that the field copy of the application has been provided to the applicant's home FDA district office.

(2) Nonclinical pharmacology and toxicology section. A section describing, with the aid of graphs and tables, animal and *in vitro* studies with drug, including the following:

(i) Studies of the pharmacological actions of the drug in relation to its proposed therapeutic indication and studies that otherwise define the pharmacologic properties of the drug or are pertinent to possible adverse effects.

(ii) Studies of the toxicological effects of the drug as they relate to the [[Page 105]] drug's intended clinical uses, including, as appropriate, studies assessing the drug's acute, subacute, and chronic toxicity; carcinogenicity; and studies of toxicities related to the drug's particular mode of administration or conditions of use.

(iii) Studies, as appropriate, of the effects of the drug on reproduction and on the developing fetus.

(iv) Any studies of the absorption, distribution, metabolism, and excretion of the drug in animals.

(v) For each nonclinical laboratory study subject to the good laboratory practice regulations under part 58 a statement that it was conducted in compliance with the good laboratory practice regulations in part 58, or, if the study was not conducted in compliance with those regulations, a brief statement of the reason for the noncompliance.

(3) Human pharmacokinetics and bioavailability section. A section describing the human pharmacokinetic data and human bioavailability data, or information supporting a waiver of the submission of *in vivo* bioavailability data under subpart B of part 320, including the following:

   (i) A description of each of the bioavailability and pharmacokinetic studies of the drug in humans performed by or on behalf of the applicant that includes a description of the analytical and statistical methods used in each study and a statement with respect to each study that it either was conducted in compliance with the institutional review board regulations in part 56, or was not subject to the regulations under Sec. 56.104 or Sec. 56.105, and that it was conducted in compliance with the informed consent regulations in part 50.

   (ii) If the application describes in the chemistry, manufacturing, and controls section specifications or analytical methods needed to assure the bioavailability of the drug product or drug substance, or both, a statement in this section of the rationale for establishing the specification or analytical methods, including data and information supporting the rationale.

   (iii) A summarizing discussion and analysis of the pharmacokinetics and metabolism of the active ingredients and the bioavailability or bioequivalence, or both, of the drug product.

(4) Microbiology section. If the drug is an anti-infective drug, a section describing the microbiology data, including the following:

   (i) A description of the biochemical basis of the drug's action on microbial physiology.

   (ii) A description of the antimicrobial spectra of the drug, including results of *in vitro* preclinical studies to demonstrate concentrations of the drug required for effective use.

   (iii) A description of any known mechanisms of resistance to the drug, including results of any known epidemiologic studies to demonstrate prevalence of resistance factors.

   (iv) A description of clinical microbiology laboratory methods (for example, *in vitro* sensitivity discs) needed for effective use of the drug.

(5) Clinical data section. A section describing the clinical investigations of the drug, including the following:

   (i) A description and analysis of each clinical pharmacology study of the drug, including a brief comparison of the results of the human studies with the animal pharmacology and toxicology data.

(ii) A description and analysis of each controlled clinical study pertinent to a proposed use of the drug, including the protocol and a description of the statistical analyses used to evaluate the study. If the study report is an interim analysis, this is to be noted and a projected completion date provided. Controlled clinical studies that have not been analyzed in detail for any reason (e.g., because they have been discontinued or are incomplete) are to be included in this section, including a copy of the protocol and a brief description of the results and status of the study.

(iii) A description of each uncontrolled clinical study, a summary of the results, and a brief statement explaining why the study is classified as uncontrolled.

(iv) A description and analysis of any other data or information relevant to an evaluation of the safety and effectiveness of the drug product obtained or otherwise received by the applicant from any source, foreign or domestic, including information derived from [[Page 106]] clinical investigations, including controlled and uncontrolled studies of uses of the drug other than those proposed in the application, commercial marketing experience, reports in the scientific literature, and unpublished scientific papers.

(v) An integrated summary of the data demonstrating substantial evidence of effectiveness for the claimed indications. Evidence is also required to support the dosage and administration section of the labeling, including support for the dosage and dose interval recommended. The effectiveness data shall be presented by gender, age, and racial subgroups and shall identify any modifications of dose or dose interval needed for specific subgroups. Effectiveness data from other subgroups of the population of patients treated, when appropriate, such as patients with renal failure or patients with different levels of severity of the disease, also shall be presented.

(vi) A summary and updates of safety information, as follows:

    (a) The applicant shall submit an integrated summary of all available information about the safety of the drug product, including pertinent animal data, demonstrated or potential adverse effects of the drug, clinically significant drug/drug interactions, and other safety considerations, such as data from epidemiological studies of related drugs. The safety data shall be presented by gender, age, and racial subgroups. When appropriate, safety data from other subgroups of the population of patients treated also shall be presented, such as for patients with renal failure or patients with different levels of severity of the disease. A description of any statistical analyses performed in analyzing safety data should also be included, unless already included under paragraph (d)(5)(ii) of this section.

(b) The applicant shall, under section 505(i) of the act, update periodically its pending application with new safety information learned about the drug that may reasonably affect the statement of contraindications, warnings, precautions, and adverse reactions in the draft labeling. These "safety update reports" are required to include the same kinds of information (from clinical studies, animal studies, and other sources) and are required to be submitted in the same format as the integrated summary in paragraph (d)(5)(vi)(a) of this section. In addition, the reports are required to include the case report forms for each patient who died during a clinical study or who did not complete the study because of an adverse event (unless this requirement is waived). The applicant shall submit these reports

    (1) 4 months after the initial submission;

    (2) following receipt of an approvable letter; and

    (3) at other times as requested by the FDA. Prior to the submission of the first such report, applicants are encouraged to consult with the FDA regarding further details on its form and content.

(vii) If the drug has a potential for abuse, a description and analysis of studies or information related to abuse of the drug, including a proposal for scheduling under the Controlled Substances Act. A description of any studies related to overdosage is also required, including information on dialysis, antidotes, or other treatments, if known.

(viii) An integrated summary of the benefits and risks of the drug, including a discussion of why the benefits exceed the risks under the conditions stated in the labeling.

(ix) A statement with respect to each clinical study involving human subjects that it either was conducted in compliance with the institutional review board regulations in part 56, or was not subject to the regulations under Sec. 56.104 or Sec. 56.105, and that it was conducted in compliance with the informed consent regulations in part **50**.

(x) If a sponsor has transferred any obligations for the conduct of any clinical study to a contract research organization, a statement containing the name and address of the contract research organization, identification of the clinical study, and a listing of the obligations transferred. If all obligations governing the conduct of the study have been transferred, a general statement of this transfer—in lieu of a listing of the specific obligations transferred—may be submitted.

(xi) If original subject records were audited or reviewed by the sponsor in the course of monitoring any clinical [[Page 107]] study to verify the accuracy of the case reports submitted to the sponsor, a list identifying each clinical study so audited or reviewed.

(6) Statistical section. A section describing the statistical evaluation of clinical data, including the following:

(i) A copy of the information submitted under paragraph (d)(5)(ii) of this section concerning the description and analysis of each controlled clinical study, and the documentation and supporting statistical analyses used in evaluating the controlled clinical studies.

(ii) A copy of the information submitted under paragraph (d)(5)(vi)(a) of this section concerning a summary of information about the safety of the drug product, and the documentation and supporting statistical analyses used in evaluating the safety information.

(e) Samples and labeling.

(1) Upon request from the FDA, the applicant shall submit the samples described below to the places identified in the agency's request. The FDA will generally ask applicants to submit samples directly to two or more agency laboratories that will perform all necessary tests on the samples and validate the applicant's analytical methods.

(i) Four representative samples of the following, each sample in sufficient quantity to permit the FDA to perform three times each test described in the application to determine whether the drug substance and the drug product meet the specifications given in the application:

(a) The drug product proposed for marketing;

(b) The drug substance used in the drug product from which the samples of the drug product were taken; and

(c) Reference standards and blanks (except that reference standards recognized in an official compendium need not be submitted).

(ii) Samples of the finished market package, if requested by the FDA.

(2) The applicant shall submit the following in the archival copy of the application:

(i) Three copies of the analytical methods and related descriptive information contained in the chemistry, manufacturing, and controls section under paragraph (d)(1) of this section for the drug substance and the drug product that are necessary for the FDA's laboratories to perform all necessary tests on the samples and to validate the applicant's analytical methods. The related descriptive information includes a description of each sample; the proposed regulatory specifications for the drug; a detailed description of the methods of analysis; supporting data for accuracy, specificity, precision and ruggedness; and complete results of the applicant's tests on each sample.

    (ii) Copies of the label and all labeling for the drug product (4 copies of draft labeling or 12 copies of final printed labeling).

(f) Case report forms and tabulations. The archival copy of the application is required to contain the following case report tabulations and case report forms:

    (1) Case report tabulations. The application is required to contain tabulations of the data from each adequate and well-controlled study under Sec. 314.126 (Phase 2 and Phase 3 studies as described in Secs. 312.21 (b) and (c) of this chapter), tabulations of the data from the earliest clinical pharmacology studies (Phase 1 studies as described in Sec. 312.21(a) of this chapter), and tabulations of the safety data from other clinical studies. Routine submission of other patient data from uncontrolled studies is not required. The tabulations are required to include the data on each patient in each study, except that the applicant may delete those tabulations which the agency agrees, in advance, are not pertinent to a review of the drug's safety or effectiveness. Upon request, the FDA will discuss with the applicant in a "pre-NDA" conference those tabulations that may be appropriate for such deletion. Barring unforeseen circumstances, tabulations agreed to be deleted at such a conference will not be requested during the conduct of the FDA's review of the application. If such unforeseen circumstances do occur, any request for deleted tabulations will be made by the director of the FDA division responsible for reviewing the application, in accordance with paragraph (f)(3) of this section.[[Page 108]]

    (2) Case report forms. The application is required to contain copies of individual case report forms for each patient who died during a clinical study or who did not complete the study because of an adverse event, whether believed to be drug related or not, including patients receiving reference drugs or placebo. This requirement may be waived by the FDA for specific studies if the case report forms are unnecessary for a proper review of the study.

    (3) Additional data. The applicant shall submit to FDA additional case report forms and tabulations needed to conduct a proper review of the application, as requested by the director of the FDA division responsible for reviewing the application. The applicant's failure to submit information requested by the FDA within 30 days after receipt

of the request may result in the agency viewing any eventual submission as a major amendment under Sec. 314.60 and extending the review period as necessary. If desired by the applicant, the FDA division director will verify in writing any request for additional data that was made orally.

(4) Applicants are invited to meet with the FDA before submitting an application to discuss the presentation and format of supporting information. If the applicant and the FDA agree, the applicant may submit tabulations of patient data and case report forms in a form other than hard copy, for example, on microfiche or computer tapes.

(g) Other. The following general requirements apply to the submission of information within the summary under paragraph (c) of this section and within the technical sections under paragraph (d) of this section.

(1) The applicant ordinarily is not required to resubmit information previously submitted, but may incorporate the information by reference. A reference to information submitted previously is required to identify the file by name, reference number, volume, and page number in the agency's records where the information can be found. A reference to information submitted to the agency by a person other than the applicant is required to contain a written statement that authorizes the reference and that is signed by the person who submitted the information.

(2) The applicant shall submit an accurate and complete English translation of each part of the application that is not in English. The applicant shall submit a copy of each original literature publication for which an English translation is submitted.

(3) If an applicant who submits a new drug application under section 505(b) of the act obtains a "right of reference or use," as defined under Sec. 314.3(b), to an investigation described in clause (A) of section 505(b)(1) of the act, the applicant shall include in its application a written statement signed by the owner of the data from each such investigation that the applicant may rely on in support of the approval of its application, and provide the FDA access to, the underlying raw data that provide the basis for the report of the investigation submitted in its application.

(h) Patent information. The application is required to contain the patent information described under Sec. 314.53.

(i) Patent certification—

(1) Contents. A 505(b)(2) application is required to contain the following:

(i) Patents claiming drug, drug product, or method of use.

(A) Except as provided in paragraph (i)(2) of this section, a certification with respect to each patent issued by the

United States Patent and Trademark Office that, in the opinion of the applicant and to the best of its knowledge, claims a drug (the drug product or drug substance that is a component of the drug product) on which investigations that are relied upon by the applicant for approval of its application were conducted or that claims an approved use for such drug and for which information is required to be filed under section 505(b) and (c) of the act and Sec. 314.53. For each such patent, the applicant shall provide the patent number and certify, in its opinion and to the best of its knowledge, one of the following circumstances:

(1) That the patent information has not been submitted to the FDA. The applicant shall entitle such a certification "Paragraph I Certification";

(2) That the patent has expired. The applicant shall entitle such a certification "Paragraph II Certification"; [[Page 109]]

(3) The date on which the patent will expire. The applicant shall entitle such a certification "Paragraph III Certification"; or

(4) That the patent is invalid, unenforceable, or will not be infringed by the manufacture, use, or sale of the drug product for which the application is submitted. The applicant shall entitle such a certification "Paragraph IV Certification." This certification shall be submitted in the following form:

I, (name of applicant), certify that Patent No. _____ _____ (is invalid, unenforceable, or will not be infringed by the manufacture, use, or sale of) (name of proposed drug product) for which this application is submitted.

The certification shall be accompanied by a statement that the applicant will comply with the requirements under Sec. 314.52(a) with respect to providing a notice to each owner of the patent or their representatives and to the holder of the approved application for the drug product which is claimed by the patent or a use of which is claimed by the patent and with the requirements under Sec. 314.52(c) with respect to the content of the notice.

(B) If the drug on which investigations that are relied upon by the applicant were conducted is itself a licensed generic drug of a patented drug first approved under section 505(b) of the act, the appropriate patent certification under this section with respect to each patent that claims the first-approved patented drug or that claims an approved use for such a drug.

(ii) No relevant patents. If, in the opinion of the applicant and to the best of its knowledge, there are no patents described in paragraph (i)(1)(i) of this section, a certification in the following form:

In the opinion and to the best knowledge of (name of applicant), there are no patents that claim the drug or drugs on which investigations that are relied upon in this application were conducted or that claim a use of such drug or drugs.

(iii) Method of use patent.

(A) If information that is submitted under section 505(b) or (c) of the act and Sec. 314.53 is for a method of use patent, and the labeling for the drug product for which the applicant is seeking approval does not include any indications that are covered by the use patent, a statement explaining that the method of use patent does not claim any of the proposed indications.

(B) If the labeling of the drug product for which the applicant is seeking approval includes an indication that, according to the patent information submitted under section 505(b) or (c) of the act and Sec. 314.53 or in the opinion of the applicant, is claimed by a use patent, the applicant shall submit an applicable certification under paragraph (i)(1)(i) of this section.

(2) Method of manufacturing patent. An applicant is not required to make a certification with respect to any patent that claims only a method of manufacturing the drug product for which the applicant is seeking approval.

(3) Licensing agreements. If a 505(b)(2) application is for a drug or method of using a drug claimed by a patent and the applicant has a licensing agreement with the patent owner, the applicant shall submit a certification under paragraph (i)(1)(i)(A)(4) of this section ("Paragraph IV Certification") as to that patent and a statement that it has been granted a patent license. If the patent owner consents to an immediate effective date upon approval of the 505(b)(2) application, the application shall contain a written statement from the patent owner that it has a licensing agreement with the applicant and that it consents to an immediate effective date.

(4) Late submission of patent information. If a patent described in paragraph (i)(1)(i)(A) of this section is issued and the holder of the

approved application for the patented drug does not submit the required information on the patent within 30 days of issuance of the patent, an applicant who submitted a 505(b)(2) application that, before the submission of the patent information, contained an appropriate patent certification is not required to submit an amended certification. An applicant whose 505(b)(2) application is filed after a late submission of patent information or whose 505(b)(2) application was previously filed but did not contain an appropriate patent certification at the time of the patent submission shall submit a certification under paragraph (i)(1)(i) or (i)(1)(ii) of this section or a [[Page 110]] statement under paragraph (i)(1)(iii) of this section as to that patent.

(5) Disputed patent information. If an applicant disputes the accuracy or relevance of patent information submitted to the FDA, the applicant may seek a confirmation of the correctness of the patent information in accordance with the procedures under Sec. 314.53(f). Unless the patent information is withdrawn or changed, the applicant must submit an appropriate certification for each relevant patent.

(6) Amended certifications. A certification submitted under paragraphs (i)(1)(i) through (i)(1)(iii) of this section may be amended at any time before the effective date of the approval of the application. An applicant shall submit an amended certification as an amendment to a pending application or by letter to an approved application. If an applicant with a pending application voluntarily makes a patent certification for an untimely filed patent, the applicant may withdraw the patent certification for the untimely filed patent. Once an amendment or letter for the change in certification has been submitted, the application will no longer be considered to be one containing the prior certification.

(i) After finding of infringement. An applicant who has submitted a certification under paragraph (i)(1)(i)(A)(4) of this section and is sued for patent infringement within 45 days of the receipt of notice sent under Sec. 314.52 shall amend the certification if a final judgment in the action is entered finding the patent to be infringed unless the final judgment also finds the patent to be invalid. In the amended certification, the applicant shall certify under paragraph (i)(1)(i)(A)(3) of this section that the patent will expire on a specific date.

(ii) After removal of a patent from the list. If a patent is removed from the list, any applicant with a pending application (including a tentatively approved application with a delayed effective date) who has made a certification with respect to such patent shall amend its certification. The applicant shall certify under paragraph (i)(1)(ii) of this section that no patents described in paragraph (i)(1)(i) of this section claim the drug or, if other relevant patents claim the drug, shall amend the certification to refer only to those relevant patents. In the amendment, the applicant shall state the reason for the change in certification (that the patent is or has been removed from the list). A patent that is the subject of a lawsuit under Sec. 314.107(c) shall not be removed from the list until the FDA determines either that no delay in effective dates of approval is required under that section as a result of the lawsuit, that the patent has expired, or that any such period of delay in effective dates of approval is ended. An applicant shall submit an amended certification as an amendment to a pending application. Once an amendment for the change has been submitted, the application will no longer be considered to be one containing a certification under paragraph (i)(1)(i)(A)(4) of this section.

(iii) Other amendments.

   (A) Except as provided in paragraphs (i)(4) and (i)(6)(iii)(B) of this section, an applicant shall amend a submitted certification if, at any time before the effective date of the approval of the application, the applicant learns that the submitted certification is no longer accurate.

   (B) An applicant is not required to amend a submitted certification when information on an otherwise applicable patent is submitted after the effective date of approval for the 505(b)(2) application.

(j) *Claimed exclusivity.* A new drug product, upon approval, may be entitled to a period of marketing exclusivity under the provisions of Sec. 314.108. If an applicant believes its drug product is entitled to a period of exclusivity, it shall submit with the new drug application prior to approval the following information:

(1) A statement that the applicant is claiming exclusivity.

(2) A reference to the appropriate paragraph under Sec. 314.108 that supports its claim.

(3) If the applicant claims exclusivity under Sec. 314.108(b)(2), information to show that, to the best of its knowledge or belief, a drug has not previously been approved under section 505(b) of the act containing any active moiety [[Page 111]] in the drug for which the applicant is seeking approval.

(4) If the applicant claims exclusivity under Sec. 314.108(b)(4) or (b)(5), the following information to show that the application contains "new clinical investigations" that are "essential to approval of the application or supplement" and were "conducted or sponsored by the applicant":

(i) "New clinical investigations." A certification that to the best of the applicant's knowledge each of the clinical investigations included in the application meets the definition of "new clinical investigation" set forth in Sec. 314.108(a).

(ii) "Essential to approval." A list of all published studies or publicly available reports of clinical investigations known to the applicant through a literature search that are relevant to the conditions for which the applicant is seeking approval, a certification that the applicant has thoroughly searched the scientific literature and, to the best of the applicant's knowledge, the list is complete and accurate and, in the applicant's opinion, such published studies or publicly available reports do not provide a sufficient basis for the approval of the conditions for which the applicant is seeking approval without reference to the new clinical investigation(s) in the application, and an explanation as to why the studies or reports are insufficient.

(iii) "Conducted or sponsored by." If the applicant was the sponsor named in the Form FDA-1571 for an investigational new drug application (IND) under which the new clinical investigation(s) that is essential to the approval of its application was conducted, identification of the IND by number. If the applicant was not the sponsor of the IND under which the clinical investigation(s) was conducted, a certification that the applicant or its predecessor in interest provided substantial support for the clinical investigation(s) that is essential to the approval of its application, and information supporting the certification. To demonstrate "substantial support," an applicant must either provide a certified statement from a certified public accountant that the applicant provided **50** percent or more of the cost of conducting the study or provide an explanation of why the FDA should consider the applicant to have conducted or sponsored the study if the applicant's financial contribution to the study is less than **50** percent or the applicant did not sponsor the investigational new drug. A predecessor in interest is an entity, e.g., a corporation, that the applicant has taken over, merged with, or purchased, or from which the applicant has purchased all rights to the drug. Purchase of nonexclusive rights to a clinical investigation after it is completed is not sufficient to satisfy this definition.

(k) *Financial certification or disclosure statement.* The application shall contain a financial certification or disclosure statement or both as required by part 54 of this chapter.

(l) Format of an original application. (1) The applicant shall submit a complete archival copy of the application that contains the information required under paragraphs (a) through (f) of this section. The FDA will maintain the archival copy during the review of the application to permit individual reviewers to refer to information that is not contained in their particular technical sections of the application, to give other agency personnel access to the application for official business, and to maintain in one place a complete copy of the application. An applicant may submit on microfiche the portions of the archival copy of the application described in paragraphs (b) through (d) of this section. Information relating to samples and labeling, described in paragraph (e) of this section, is required to be submitted in hard copy. Tabulations of patient data and case report forms, described in paragraph (f) of this section, may be submitted on microfiche only if the applicant and the FDA agree. If the FDA agrees, the applicant may use another suitable microform system.

(2) The applicant shall submit a review copy of the application. Each of the technical sections, described in paragraphs (d)(1) through (d)(6) of this section, in the review copy is required to be separately bound with a copy of the application form required under paragraph (a) of this section and a copy of the summary required under paragraph (c) of this section. [[Page 112]]

(3) The applicant shall submit a field copy of the application that contains the technical section described in paragraph (d)(1) of this section, a copy of the application form required under paragraph (a) of this section, a copy of the summary required under paragraph (c) of this section, and a certification that the field copy is a true copy of the technical section described in paragraph (d)(1) of this section contained in the archival and review copies of the application.

(4) The applicant may obtain from the FDA sufficient folders to bind the archival, the review, and the field copies of the application. (Collection of information requirements approved by the Office of Management and Budget under control number 0910-0001)

[50 FR 7493, Feb. 22, 1985; 50 FR 14212, Apr. 11, 1985, as amended at 50 FR 16668, Apr. 26, 1985; 50 FR 21238, May 23, 1985; 52 FR 88\47, Mar. 19, 1987; 55 FR 11580, Mar. 29, 1990; 57 FR 17982, Apr. 28, 1992; 58 FR 47351, Sept. 8, 1993; 59 FR 13200, Mar. 21, 1994; 59 FR 50361, Oct. 3, 1994; 59 FR 60051, Nov. 21, 1994; 62 FR 40599, July 29, 1997; 63 FR 5252, Feb. 2, 1998; 63 FR 6862, Feb. 11, 1998]

Effective Date Note:

1. At 63 FR 5252, Feb. 2, 1998, Sec. 314.50 was amended by redesignating paragraph (k) as paragraph (l) and by adding a new paragraph (k), effective Feb. 2, 1999.

2. At 63 FR 6862, Feb. 11, 1998, Sec. 314.50 was amended by revising the second sentence and adding two new sentences after the second sentence in paragraph (d)(5)(v), and by adding two new sentences after the first sentence in paragraph (d)(5)(vi)(a), effective Aug. 10, 1998. For the convenience of the user, the superseded text is set forth as follows:

Sec. 314.50: Content and format of an application.

(d)

(5)

(v) Evidence is also required to support the dosage and administration section of the labeling, including support for the dosage and dose interval recommended, and modifications for specific subgroups (for example, pediatrics, geriatrics, patients with renal failure).

(Code of Federal Regulations)

(Title 21, Volume 5, Parts 300 to 499)

(Revised as of April 1, 1998)

From the U.S. Government Printing Office via GPO Access

(Cite: 21 CFR 314.126)

(Pages 153–155)

Title 21: Food and Drugs

Chapter I: Food and Drug Administration, Department of Health and Human Services—Continued

Part 314: Applications for FDA Approval to Market a New Drug or an Antibiotic Drug—Table of Contents

Subpart D: FDA Action on Applications and Abbreviated Applications

Sec. 314.126: Adequate and Well-Controlled Studies

(a) The purpose of conducting clinical investigations of a drug is to distinguish the effect of a drug from other influences, such as spontaneous change in the course of the disease, placebo effect, or biased observation. The characteristics described in paragraph (b) of this section have been developed over a period of years and are recognized by the scientific community as the essentials of an adequate and well-controlled clinical investigation. The Food and Drug Administration considers these characteristics in determining whether an investigation is adequate and well-controlled for purposes of sections 505 and 507 of the act. Reports of adequate and well-controlled investigations provide the primary basis for determining whether there is "substantial evidence" to support the claims of effectiveness for new drugs and antibiotics. Therefore, the study report should provide sufficient details of study design, conduct, and analysis to allow critical evaluation and a determination of whether the characteristics of an adequate and well-controlled study are present.

(b) An adequate and well-controlled study has the following characteristics:

(1) There is a clear statement of the objectives of the investigation and a summary of the proposed or actual methods of analysis in the protocol for the study and in the report of its results. In addition, the protocol should contain a description of the proposed methods of analysis, and the study report should contain a description of the methods of analysis ultimately used. If [[Page 154]] the protocol does not contain a description of the proposed methods of analysis, the study report should describe how the methods used were selected.

(2) The study uses a design that permits a valid comparison with a control to provide a quantitative assessment of drug effect. The protocol for the study and report of results should describe the study design precisely; for example, duration of treatment periods, whether treatments are parallel, sequential, or crossover, and whether the sample size is predetermined or based upon some interim analysis. Generally, the following types of control are recognized:

(i) Placebo concurrent control. The test drug is compared with an inactive preparation designed to resemble the test drug as far as possible. A placebo-controlled study may include additional treatment groups, such as an active treatment control or a dose-comparison control, and usually includes randomization and blinding of patients or investigators, or both.

(ii) Dose-comparison concurrent control. At least two doses of the drug are compared. A dose-comparison study may include additional treatment groups, such as placebo control or active control. Dose-comparison trials usually include randomization and blinding of patients or investigators, or both.

(iii) No treatment concurrent control. Where objective measurements of effectiveness are available and placebo effect is negligible, the test drug is compared with no treatment. No treatment concurrent control trials usually include randomization.

(iv) Active treatment concurrent control. The test drug is compared with known effective therapy; for example, where the condition treated is such that administration of placebo or no treatment would be contrary to the interest of the patient. An active treatment study may include additional treatment groups, however, such as a placebo control or a dose-comparison control. Active treatment trials usually include randomization and blinding of patients or investigators, or both. If the intent of the trial is to show similarity of the test and control drugs, the report of the study should assess the ability of the study to have detected a difference between treatments. Similarity of test drug and active control can mean either that both drugs were effective or that neither was effective. The analysis of the study should explain why the drugs should be considered effective in the study, for example, by reference to results in previous placebo-controlled studies of the active control drug.

(v) Historical control. The results of treatment with the test drug are compared with experience historically derived from the adequately documented natural history of the disease or condition, or from the results of active treatment, in comparable patients or populations. Because historical control populations usually cannot be as well assessed with respect to pertinent variables as can concurrent control populations, historical control designs are usually reserved for special circumstances. Examples include studies of diseases with high and predictable mortality (for example, certain malignancies) and studies in which the effect of the drug is self-evident (general anesthetics, drug metabolism).

(3) The method of selection of subjects provides adequate assurance that they have the disease or condition being studied, or evidence of susceptibility and exposure to the condition against which prophylaxis is directed.

(4) The method of assigning patients to treatment and control groups minimizes bias and is intended to assure comparability of the groups with respect to pertinent variables such as age, sex, severity of disease, duration of disease, and use of drugs or therapy other than the test drug. The protocol for the study and the report of its results should describe how subjects were assigned to groups. Ordinarily, in a concurrently controlled study, assignment is by randomization, with or without stratification.

(5) Adequate measures are taken to minimize bias on the part of the subjects, observers, and analysts of the data. The protocol and report of the study should describe the procedures used to accomplish this, such as blinding.

(6) The methods of assessment of subjects' response are well-defined and reliable. The protocol for the study and [[Page 155]] the report of results should explain the variables measured, the methods of observation, and criteria used to assess response.

(7) There is an analysis of the results of the study adequate to assess the effects of the drug. The report of the study should describe the results and the analytic methods used to evaluate them, including any appropriate statistical methods. The analysis should assess, among other things, the comparability of test and control groups with respect to pertinent variables, and the effects of any interim data analyses performed.

(c) The Director of the Center for Drug Evaluation and Research may, on the Director's own initiative or on the petition of an interested person, waive in whole or in part any of the criteria in paragraph (b) of this section with respect to a specific clinical investigation, either prior to the investigation or in the evaluation of a completed study. A petition for a waiver is required to set forth clearly and concisely the specific criteria from which waiver is sought, why the criteria are not reasonably applicable to the particular clinical investigation, what alternative procedures, if any, are to be, or have been employed, and what results have been obtained. The petition is also required to state why the clinical investigations so conducted will yield, or have yielded, substantial evidence of effectiveness, notwithstanding non-conformance with the criteria for which waiver is requested.

(d) For an investigation to be considered adequate for approval of a new drug, it is required that the test drug be standardized as to identity, strength, quality, purity, and dosage form to give significance to the results of the investigation.

(e) Uncontrolled studies or partially controlled studies are not acceptable as the sole basis for the approval of claims of effectiveness. Such studies carefully conducted and documented, may provide corroborative support of well-controlled studies regarding efficacy and may yield valuable data regarding safety of the test drug. Such studies will be considered on their merits in the light of the principles listed here, with the exception of the requirement for the comparison of the treated subjects with controls. Isolated case reports, random experience, and reports lacking the details which permit scientific evaluation will not be considered.

(Collection of information requirements approved by the Office of Management and Budget under control number 0910-0001)

(50 FR 7493, Feb. 22, 1985, as amended at 50 FR 21238, May 23, 1985; 55 FR 11580, Mar. 29, 1990)

(Code of Federal Regulations)
(Title 21, Volume 5, Parts 300 to 499)
(Revised as of April 1, 1998)
From the U.S. Government Printing Office via GPO Access
(Cite: 21 CFR 314.420)
(Pages 173–174)

Title 21: Food and Drugs
Chapter I: Food and Drug Administration, Department of Health and Human Services—Continued
Part 314: Applications for FDA Approval to Market a New Drug or an Antibiotic Drug—Table of Contents

Subpart G: Miscellaneous Provisions
Sec. 314.420: Drug Master Files

(a) A drug master file is a submission of information to the Food and Drug Administration by a person (the drug master file holder) who intends it to be used for one of the following purposes: To permit the holder to incorporate the information by reference when the holder submits an investigational new drug application under part 312 or submits an application or an abbreviated application or an amendment or supplement to them under this part, or to permit the holder to authorize other persons to rely on the information to support a submission to the FDA without the holder having to disclose the information to the person. The FDA ordinarily neither independently reviews drug master files nor approves or disapproves submissions to a drug master file. Instead, the agency customarily reviews the information only in the context of an application under part 312 or this part. A drug master file may contain information of the kind required for any submission to the agency, including information about the following:

  (1) Manufacturing site, facilities, operating procedures, and personnel (because an FDA on-site inspection of a foreign drug manufacturing facility presents unique problems of planning and travel not presented by an inspection of a domestic manufacturing facility, this information is only recommended for foreign manufacturing establishments);

  (2) Drug substance, drug substance intermediate, and materials used in their preparation, or drug product;

  (3) Packaging materials;

  (4) Excipient, colorant, flavor, essence, or materials used in their preparation; [[Page 174]]

  (5) FDA-accepted reference information. (A person wishing to submit information and supporting data in a drug master file (DMF) that is not covered by Types I through IV DMF's must first submit a letter of intent to the Drug Master File Staff, Food and Drug Administration, 12420 Parklawn Dr., Rm. 2-14, Rockville, MD 20852. The FDA will then contact the person to discuss the proposed submission.)

(b) An investigational new drug application or an application, abbreviated application, amendment, or supplement may incorporate by reference all or part of the contents of any drug master file in support of the submission if the holder authorizes the incorporation in writing. Each incorporation by reference is required to describe the incorporated material by name, reference number, volume, and page number of the drug master file.

(c) A drug master file is required to be submitted in two copies. The agency has prepared under Sec. 10.90(b) a guideline that provides information about how to prepare a well-organized drug master file. If the drug master file holder adds, changes, or deletes any information in the file, the holder shall notify in writing, each person authorized to reference that information. Any addition, change, or deletion of information in a drug master file (except the list required under paragraph (d) of this section) is required to be submitted in two copies and to describe by name, reference number, volume, and page number the information affected in the drug master file.

(d) The drug master file is required to contain a complete list of each person currently authorized to incorporate by reference any information in the file, identifying by name, reference number, volume, and page number the information that each person is authorized to incorporate. If the holder restricts the authorization to particular drug products, the list is required to include the name of each drug product and the application number, if known, to which the authorization applies.

(e) The public availability of data and information in a drug master file, including the availability of data and information in the file to a person authorized to reference the file, is determined under part 20 and Sec. 314.430.

(Collection of information requirements approved by the Office of Management and Budget under control number 0910-0001)

[50 FR 7493, Feb. 22, 1985, as amended at 50 FR 21238, May 23, 1985; 53 FR 33122, Aug. 30, 1988; 55 FR 28380, July 11, 1990]

CHAPTER 6

505(b)2 New Drug Applications (NDAs)

THE CONTROVERSY

The 505(b)2 application process is mired in controversy. Many reviewers in the Agency seem obstructionist, apparently viewing the process as an attempt to skirt important regulatory controls. Many in the industry are (as a result) skeptical of the value of the approach, fearing it enters the process with a "red flag" mark against it. Yet the intent and value of the 505(b)2 provision are clear and positive.

For years, the industry, the public, and congressional oversight committees have railed against the high cost and long delays involved in FDA regulation. In a time when many Americans fear rationing of health care based upon a patient's financial and insurance resources, any added cost not directly contributing to product safety is viewed skeptically. And horror stories about unnecessary regulation—often distorted in the multiple retelling—seem to be adding costs to the development of new drugs without proportionately assuring a safety value.

The 505(b)2 provision is a response. It permits the submission of an NDA [and, working backward, the design of an investigational new drug application (IND)] based at least in part on other studies not conducted (or with right of reference) by the applicant. In effect, 505(b)2 recognizes the use of supporting studies published in the public literature or FDA decisions and findings of safety and effectiveness, in support of a new drug application. The data requirement is not lowered: 505(b)2 simply permits the use of supporting data generated outside of the applying organization.

Despite this relatively mild loss of control, skeptics are concerned that published articles for which the applicant (and Agency) lacks a right of reference, and hence access to raw data and audit controls, represent a lower level of scrutiny than that which is present in traditional submissions. Intended to speed the approval of changes to existing drugs (dosage adjustments, route of administration changes, formulation modifications, etc.), the use of 505(b)2 applications for new drug entities, while permitted, may seem to be an attempt

Guidebook for Drug Regulatory Submissions, by Sandy Weinberg
Copyright © 2009 John Wiley & Sons, Inc.

to minimize regulatory review. The dynamic tension between pressures to speed the approval process and to maintain standards of review is being fought out unofficially with the 505(b)2 applications.

505(b)2 DEFINED

The 505(b)2 provision allows the submission of a NDA and supporting submissions (such as an IND application) in situations in which some or all of the supporting data come from a source or sources outside of the applicant organization. If all supporting data come from studies conducted by the applicant (or the applicant's agents) or from studies to which the applicant has right of reference (and access to raw data and analyses), the 505(b)2 process is not appropriate.

Outside sources are generally of two types.

- **Published literature**, generally peer reviewed, in which public access to the conclusions, results of analysis, and summary of data are included but for which the applicant does not have a right of reference including access to the raw data and the ability to replicate or supplement the analyses.
- **Agency findings** reporting the FDA's analytical conclusions of drug safety and/or effectiveness. These findings are usually the result of prior review of supporting data related to the drug in question.

Covered under the 505(b)2 provision are new chemical entities—though note the internal skepticism described above—as well as changes to previously approved drugs, including changes in dosage, route of administration, formulation, active ingredients, and strength. The 505(b)2 application is not appropriate for drugs that are simply duplications of existing drugs, that represent changes only in the projects absorption pattern, or that report only changes in the unintentional absorption pattern.

Patent Issues

The 505(b)2 application raises some patent issues beyond the scope of this book but that need to be considered if the option is under review. Generally, the 505(b)2 provides a patent exclusivity if (and only if) the applicant conducts one or more critical studies in support of the application. If all support studies are referenced from published literature of Agency findings, the patent exclusivity will not apply. While the definition of "critical studies" is subject to some interpretation, in this context, it most commonly refers to studies that demonstrate the link between the applicant drug and other formulations used in outside studies or previously approved by the Agency. These studies fall under the headings of Bioequivalence (BE) or Bioavailability (BA). While some exceptions are possible, in practicality, the three-year patent exclusivity is dependent upon the successful completion of a BE/BA study.

In addition, the formal granting of the three-year patent exclusivity requires the formal notification of the original patent holder of the approval of a 505(b)2 NDA.

The 505(b)2 Process

A 505(b)2 NDA does not differ significantly from a traditional NDA and follows the same general format. Of course, the traditional NDA contains the details of the actual collected study data and the analyses conducted, while the 505(b)2 simply references the results summarized and published in outside sources.

Because of the Agency skepticism described above and because of the relative weakness of not having automatic and immediate access to the data as would be the case in a traditional study, there are four recommendations that can strengthen the 505(b)2 application and, to a large degree, offset the perceived weaknesses.

First, 505(b)2 applications are encouraged to communicate directly with the researchers of any referenced studies, requesting access to data, discussing analyses, and generally exploring the details of the study process. The depth of these interactions adds credibility to the published studies and further supports the application. For example, obtaining and including an analytical profile of the drug administered in the published study (or obtaining a sample and conducting a profile) can help establish the purity (or impurity profile) and bolster the applicability of the study to the actual drug under application.

Second, 505(b)2 applicants (and other applicants, generally) should establish an outside and independent board of scientific advisors that can conduct a further peer review of the published studies included in the application. The analysis of this board, particularly focusing on study weaknesses or product dissimilarities, can again increase the credibility of the application.

Third, referenced FDA findings included in the application are most useful when they meet the three tests of recency, expertise, and relevance. Citations should carefully deal with any agency and industry evolutionary changes in requirement or research sophistication between the finding date and the submission: the more recent the finding, the more credibility it will seem. The issuer of the finding—specifically, the FDA group or team—will also affect the credibility of the reference. A finding from the same group to which the application is directed is ideal; a finding from a rival feuding group is of considerably lesser value. Finally, the more exact the match between the finding and application drug product, the stronger the credibility. Minor variations are more likely to fall under the previous finding umbrella than are major reformulations or significant modifications.

Finally, and perhaps most subjectively, a 505(b)2 application is likely to be positively received in direct proportion to the quantity and quality of perceived effort expended by the applying organization. The inclusion of a BE/BA study and of even a limited dosing study establishes the familiarity of the applicant with the drug product. 505(b)2 applications relying entirely on outside studies, without any research conducted by the applicant, seem to start the process with several strikes against them.

These four suggestions—build a relationship with the authors of published studies; have a scientific review board add a second peer review; establish the credibility of any FDA referenced findings; and add at least minimal applicant-conducted studies to the mix—while not mandatory, formal, or official, are likely to enhance perception of the application:.

Summary

Despite a perception of FDA skepticism and a resulting hesitation by some industry leaders, the 505(b)2 NDA can be a valuable tool for efficiently and effectively gaining approval of a product in outside clinical research use or closely related to an approved drug entity. The same principles of any NDA apply, with the advantage of substituting some clinical research with published results and/or previous Agency findings.

While the FDA is under intense congressional and public pressure to shorten the approval process, however, more profound responsibilities and pressures assure that an abbreviated process does not compromise safety and quality. Therefore, there is an inverse relationship between the amount of outside referral in a 505(b)2 and the skepticism it engenders. Subjectively viewing the process, a 505(b)2 that relies entirely on published studies and Agency findings would face maximum opposition (and, without at least a BE/BA study, no real patent projection). A 505(b)2 that represents a combination of outside published studies and/or FDA findings with applicant-conducted studies can reduce costs, shorten the research process, and stand an excellent chance in the NDA review.

505(b)2 NDA SUBMISSION CHECKLIST

This checklist is intended for use in the preparation and submission of 505(b)2 NDAs. It is recommended that, prior to transmission to the FDA, a second internal review should be conducted by an individual or department not involved in the preparation of the submission (presumably Quality Assurance).

The checklist was developed through discussions with consultants and Quality Assurance directors and has been field-tested in final form with three successful submissions.

- ☐ Form 1571 completed
- ☐ Cover letter
    - ☐ Name and address of sponsor
    - ☐ Name, address, title, telephone, and e-mail of contact person
    - ☐ Generic and trade name of drug or drug product
    - ☐ FDA code number (assigned at time of preconference)
- ☐ Form 3674 "Certification of Compliance with Requirements of Clinical-Trails.gov Data Bank" completed
- ☐ Three copies of application in indexed binders
- ☐ Pagination: All pages included and properly numbered
- ☐ Headings: Section headings confirming to submission subparagraphs, with initial Table of Contents
- ☐ Integrated references: All referenced articles included in final section, internally referenced in text
- ☐ Bibliography: Complete standard format bibliography listing all referenced articles
- ☐ Container closure and packaging system information provided
- ☐ Microbiological analysis provided
- ☐ Human pharmacokinetics and BA information provided
- ☐ Complete Chemistry, Manufacturing, and Control (CMC) information provided, including evidence of purity, stability, toxicology testing, and integrity of active pharmaceutical ingredient (API), placebo, and final product.
- ☐ Analysis of all cited published studies, and of all cited FDA findings, summarizing relevance and results
- ☐ Complete study protocol of BE/BA study and for any additional studies conducted by applicant
- ☐ Raw data for all applicant-conducted studies
- ☐ Drug Master File completed, including information on facilities, processes, and articles used in manufacturing, processing, packaging, and storage
- ☐ Analysis of all applicant-conducted studies
- ☐ Investigator's Brochure for all applicant-conducted studies included with detailed information for investigators and Institutional Review Board records
- ☐ Review of literature addresses all available prior instances of human use of drug product with emphasis on safety, administration, and possible adverse events
- ☐ Complete pharmacological profile provided for API and final product
- ☐ Summary of regulatory status and marketing history in the United States and foreign countries

☐ Summary of adverse reactions to proposed drug in any country
☐ NDA addresses all issues and questions raised in the pre-NDA meeting
☐ Prescription Drug User Fee Act information provided

If 505(b)2 NDA is submitted electronically:

☐ Form FDA-356h, Application to Market, is included.
☐ Form FDA-3397, User Fees, is included.
☐ Form FDA-3331, NDA Field Report, is included.

(For more details concerning electronic submissions, see Electronic Regulatory Submission and Review guidelines at http://www.fda.gov/cder/regulatory/ersr.)

FDA 505(b)2 NDA REVIEW CHECKLIST

This FDA 505(b)2 NDA Review checklist has been designed in consultation with FDA reviewers, industry consultants, and regulatory professionals to serve as a summary tool indicating the evaluative criteria used by the Center for Drug Evaluation and Research (CDER) and the Center for Biologics Evaluation and Research (CBER) to critique and assess applications received. It can be used internally as a part of the Quality Assurance process, as a guideline for regulatory development of an application, and/or as a self-assessment tool to predict likely FDA response to an application.

☐ **Logistics:** Submission conforms to FDA guideline "NDA Review Process Chart."

   ☐ **Receipt:** Application was received in the FDA mail room.
   ☐ **NDA jackets:** Document is contained in one or more 3-in., three-ring binders.
   ☐ **Form 1571:** NDA is accompanied by completed Form 1571, providing (among other data) contact information including corporate name, contact name, address, telephone number, name and address of drug source, generic and trade name of drug.
   ☐ **Cover letter:** A cover letter indicates disease and therapy names.
   ☐ **Three copies:** Photocopies acceptable.
   ☐ Form 3674 "Certification of Compliance with Requirements of Clinical Trails.gov Data Bank" completed
   ☐ **Format:** Submission conforms to FDA guideline 21 Code of Federal Regulations (CFR) Part 312.23(a)(10), (11), and (b), (c), (d), and (e) and to FDA norm standards.
   ☐ **Pagination:** All pages included and properly numbered
   ☐ **Headings:** Section headings conforming to submission subparagraphs
   ☐ **Integrated references:** Copies of all referenced articles, with references integrated into the body of text

☐ **Bibliography:** Complete standard format bibliography as referenced in text

If 505(b)2 NDA is submitted electronically:

☐ Form FDA-356h, Application to Market, is included.

☐ Form FDA-3397, User Fees, is included.

☐ Form FDA-3331, New Drug Application Field Report, is included.

☐ Advance notification letter provided

☐ Format and tables conform to *Guidance for Industry: Providing Regulatory Submissions to CBER in Electronic Format.*

☐ Electronic Submission Format conforms to approved list in Docket number 92s-0251 [see 21 CFR 11.1(d) and 11.2].

☐ **Electronic Signatures conform to emerging guidelines, or a paper copy with appropriate nonelectronic signatures is included.**

(For more details concerning electronic submissions, see ERSR guidelines.)

☐ Drug Master File completed, including information on facilities, processes, and articles used in manufacturing, processing, packaging, and storage.

☐ **CONTENT: Overview**

   ☐ 505(b)2 provides sufficient information to permit determination of whether the drug is safe and effective in its proposed use(s) and whether the benefits of the drug outweigh the risks.

   ☐ 505(b)2 provides sufficient information to permit determination of whether the drug's proposed labeling (package insert) is appropriate and what it should contain.

   ☐ 505(b)2 provides sufficient information to permit determination of whether the methods used in manufacturing the drug and the controls used to maintain the drug's quality are adequate to preserve the drug's identity, strength, quality, and purity.

☐ **CONTENT: Organizational structure**

   ☐ **Cover sheet:** Form 1571

   ☐ **Table of contents:** Indicates page and volume of each section

   ☐ **Summary of published studies/industry actions:** Complete with summary, analysis, and evaluation

   ☐ **Investigator's Brochure:** Conformity with International Conference on Harmonization (ICH) *Good Clinical Practice: Guideline for the Investigator's Brochure*

   ☐ **Protocol:** Copy of the protocol for each conducted clinical study. Note that phase 1 protocols should provide a brief outline, including estimation of number of subjects to be included, description of safety exclusions, and description of dosing plan (duration, dose, method). All protocols should address monitoring of blood chemistry and vital signs and toxicity-based modification plans.

☐ **CMC information:** Should contain sufficient detail to assure identification, quality, purity, and strength of the investigational drug and should include stability data of duration appropriate to the length of the proposed study. FDA concerns to be addressed focus on products made with unknown or impure components, products with chemical structures known to be of high likely toxicity, products know to be chemically unstable, products with an impurity profile indicative of a health hazard or insufficiently defined to assess potential health hazard, or poorly characterized master or working cell bank.

  ■ Chemistry and manufacturing introduction
  ■ Drug substance
    ○ Description: physical, chemical, or biological characteristics
    ○ Name and address of manufacturer
    ○ Method of preparation
    ○ Limits and analytical methods
    ○ Stability information
  ■ Drug product
    ○ List of components
    ○ Qualitative composition
    ○ Name and address of drug product manufacturer
    ○ Description of manufacturing and packaging procedures
    ○ Limits and analytical methods: identity, strength, quality, and purity
    ○ Stability results
  ■ Placebo
  ■ Labels and labeling
  ■ Environmental assessment (or claim for exclusion): 21 CFR 312.23(a)(7)(iv)(e)

☐ **Pharmacology and toxicology information [21 CFR 312.23(a)(8)]**
  ■ Pharmacology and drug distribution [21 CFR 312.23(a)(8)(i)]
    ○ Description of pharmacological effects and mechanisms of action
    ○ Description of absorption, distribution, metabolism, and excretion of the drug
  ■ Toxicology summary [21 CFR 312.23(a)(8)(ii)(a)]: Summary of toxicological effects in animals and *in vitro*
    ○ Description of design of toxicological trials and any deviations from design

- ○ Systematic presentation of animal toxicology studies and toxico-kinetic studies
- ▪ Toxicology full data tabulation [21 CFR 312.23(a)(8)(ii)(b)]: Data points with either
- ▪ brief description of the study or
- ▪ copy of the protocol with amendments
- ▪ Toxicology GLP Certification [21 CFR 312.23(a)(8)(iii)]
- ☐ **Previous human experience with the investigational drug:** Summary report of any U.S. or non-U.S. human experience with the drug
- ☐ **References:** Indexed copies of referenced articles with comprehensive bibliography
- ☐ **Support:** Evaluation of the referent support provided
  - ☐ **Key issues:** All key issues appropriately referenced, including
    - ☐ Investigator's Brochure
    - ☐ Protocols
    - ☐ CMC information
    - ☐ Pharmacology and toxicology information
    - ☐ Previous human experience with the investigational drug
  - ☐ **Credible:** References are from credible scientific journals and/or sources.
  - ☐ **Organized:** References are organized and tied to text.

COMMENTS:
DISPOSITION:
    Receipt date:
    Response due date:
    Disposition:
    Notification date:

GUIDANCE FOR INDUSTRY[1]—APPLICATIONS COVERED BY SECTION 505(b)(2)

DRAFT GUIDANCE[2]
Comments and suggestions regarding this draft document should be submitted within 60 days of publication of the Federal Register notice announcing the

---

[1]This guidance was prepared by CDER at the FDA. This guidance document represents the Agency's current thinking on the types of applications that may be submitted pursuant to section 505(b)(2) of the Act. It does not create or confer any rights for or on any person and does not operate to bind the FDA or the public. An alternative approach may be used if such approach satisfies the requirements of the applicable statute, regulations, or both.

[2]This guidance document is being distributed for comment purposes only.

availability of the draft guidance. Submit comments to Dockets Management Branch (HFA-305), Food and Drug Administration, 5630 Fishers Lane, Rm. 1061, Rockville, MD 20857. All comments should be identified with the docket number listed in the notice of availability that publishes in the Federal Register.

For questions on the content of the draft document, contact Virginia Beakes, (301) 594-2041.
U.S. Department of Health and Human Services
Food and Drug Administration
Center for Drug Evaluation and Research
October 1999
Guidance for Industry
Applications Covered by Section 505(b)(2)

For additional copies, contact:
Drug Information Branch
Division of Communications Management, HFD-210
Center for Drug Evaluation and Research
5600 Fishers Lane
Rockville, MD 20857
Tel: 301-827-4573
http://www.fda.gov/cder/guidance/index.htm

October 1999

What Is the Purpose of This Guidance?

This guidance identifies the types of applications that are covered by section 505(b)(2) of the Federal Food, Drug, and Cosmetic Act (the Act). A 505(b)(2) application is an NDA described in section 505(b)(2) of the Act. It is submitted under section 505(b)(1) of the Act and approved under section 505(c) of the Act. This guidance also provides further information and amplification regarding the FDA's regulations at 21 CFR 314.54.

Section 505 of the Act describes three types of new drug applications: (1) an application that contains full reports of investigations of safety and effectiveness [section 505(b)(1)], (2) an application that contains full reports of investigations of safety and effectiveness but where at least some of the information required for approval comes from studies not conducted by or for the applicant and for which the applicant has not obtained a right of reference [section 505(b)(2)], and (3) an application that contains information to show that the proposed product is identical in active ingredient, dosage form, strength, route of administration, labeling, quality, performance characteristics, and intended use, among other things, to a previously approved product [section 505(j)]. Note that a supplement to an application is an NDA.

Section 505(b)(2) was added to the Act by the Drug Price Competition and Patent Term Restoration Act of 1984 (Hatch–Waxman Amendments). This provision expressly permits the FDA to rely, for approval of an NDA, on data not developed by the applicant. Sections 505(b)(2) and (j) together replaced the FDA's *paper NDA policy*, which had permitted an applicant to rely on studies published in the scientific literature to demonstrate the safety and effectiveness of duplicates of certain post-1962 pioneer drug products [see 46 Federal Register (FR) 27396, May 19, 1981]. Enactment of the generic drug approval provision of the Hatch–Waxman Amendments ended the need for approvals of duplicate drugs through the paper NDA process by permitting approval under 505(j) of duplicates of approved drugs (listed drugs) on the basis of chemistry and BE data, without the need for evidence from literature of effectiveness and safety. Section 505(b)(2) permits approval of applications other than those for duplicate products and permits reliance for such approvals on literature or on an Agency finding of safety and/or effectiveness for an approved drug product.

Definitions for specific terms used throughout this guidance are given in the Glossary.

What Is a 505(b)(2) Application?

A 505(b)(2) application is one for which one or more of the investigations relied upon by the applicant for approval "were not conducted by or for the applicant and for which the applicant has not obtained a right of reference or use from the person by or for whom the investigations were conducted" [21 U.S.C. 355(b)(2)].

What Type of Information Can an Applicant Rely On? What type of information can an applicant rely on in an application that is based upon studies "not conducted by or for the applicant and for which the applicant has not obtained a right of reference"?

1. *Published literature*   An applicant should submit a 505(b)(2) application if approval of an application will rely to any extent on published literature [a *literature-based* 505(b)(2)]. If the applicant has not obtained a right of reference to the raw data underlying the published study or studies, the application is a 505(b)(2) application; if the applicant obtains a right of reference to the raw data, the application may be a full NDA [i.e., one submitted under section 505(b)(1)]. An NDA will be a 505(b)(2) application if any of the specific information necessary for approval is obtained from literature or from another source to which the applicant does not have a right of reference, even if the applicant also conducted

clinical studies to support approval. Note, however, that this does not mean **any** reference to published general information (e.g., about disease etiology, support for particular end points, methods of analysis) or to general knowledge causes the application to be a 505(b)(2) application. Rather, reference should be to specific information (clinical trials, animal studies) necessary to the approval of the application.

2. *The Agency's finding of safety and effectiveness for an approved drug*   An applicant should submit a 505(b)(2) application for a change in a drug when approval of the application relies on the Agency's previous finding of safety and/or effectiveness for a drug. This mechanism, which is embodied in a regulation at 21 CFR 314.54, essentially makes the Agency's conclusions that would support the approval of a 505(j) application available to an applicant who develops a modification of a drug. Section 314.54 permits a 505(b)(2) applicant to rely on the Agency's finding of safety and effectiveness for an approved drug to the extent such reliance would be permitted under the generic drug approval provisions at section 505(j). This approach is intended to encourage innovation in drug development without requiring duplicative studies to demonstrate what is already known about a drug while protecting the patent and exclusivity rights for the approved drug.

It is possible that an applicant could submit a 505(b)(2) application that relies both on literature and upon the Agency's finding of safety and effectiveness for a previously approved drug product (e.g., to support a new claim).

What Kind of Application Can Be Submitted as a 505(b)(2) Application?

1. *New chemical entity (NCE)/new molecular entity (NME)*   A 505(b)(2) application may be submitted for an NCE when some part of the data necessary for approval is derived from studies not conducted by or for the applicant and to which the applicant has not obtained a right of reference. For an NCE, this data is likely to be derived from published studies, rather than the FDA's previous finding of safety and effectiveness of a drug. If the applicant had a right of reference to all of the information necessary for approval, even if the applicant had not conducted the studies, the application would be a considered a 505(b)(1) application.

2. *Changes to previously approved drugs*   For changes to a previously approved drug product, an application may rely on the Agency's finding of safety and effectiveness of the previously approved product, coupled with the information needed to support the change from the approved product. The additional information could be new studies conducted by the applicant or published data. This use of section 505(b)(2), described in the regulations at 21 CFR 314.54, was intended to encourage innova-

tion without creating duplicate work and reflects the same principle as the 505(j) application: it is wasteful and unnecessary to carry out studies to demonstrate what is already known about a drug. The approach was described in a letter to industry dated April 10, 1987, from Dr. Paul D. Parkman, then Acting Director of the Center for Drugs and Biologics. This guidance helps to clarify and amplify the approaches stated in the April 10, 1987 letter and in the regulations.

An applicant should file a 505(b)(2) application if it is seeking approval of a change to an approved drug that would not be permitted under section 505(j), because approval will require the review of clinical data. However, section 505(b)(2) applications should not be submitted for duplicates of approved products that are eligible for approval under 505(j) [see 21 CFR 314.101(d)(9)].

In addition, an applicant may submit a 505(b)(2) application for a change in a drug product that is eligible for consideration pursuant to a suitability petition under Section 505(j)(2)(C) of the Act. In the preamble to the implementing regulations for the Hatch–Waxman amendments to the Act, the Agency noted that an application submitted pursuant to section 505(b)(2) of the Act is appropriate even when it could also be submitted in accordance with a suitability petition as defined at section 505(j)(2)(C) of the Act (see 57 FR 17950; April 28, 1992).

What Are Some Examples of 505(b)(2) Applications?

Following are examples of changes to approved drugs for which 505(b)(2) applications should be submitted. Please note that in particular cases, changes of the type described immediately below may not require review of information other than BA or BE studies or data from limited confirmatory testing.[3] In those particular cases, approval of the drug may also be sought in a 505(j) application based on an approved suitability petition as described in section 505(j)(2)(C) of the Act. The descriptions below address the situation in which the application should be filed as a 505(b)(2) application because approval of the application will require review of studies beyond those that can be considered under section 505(j). Some or all of the additional information could be provided by literature or reference to past FDA findings of safety and effectiveness for approved drugs, or it could be based upon studies conducted by or for the applicant or to which it has obtained a right of reference.

Dosage Form. An application for a change of dosage form, such as a change from a solid oral dosage form to a transdermal patch, that relies to some extent upon the Agency's finding of safety and/or effectiveness for an approved drug.

---

[3] Limited confirmatory testing is explained in further detail in 54 FR 288872, 28880 (July 10, 1989) and 57 FR 17950, 17957-58 (April 28, 1992).

Strength. An application for a change to a lower or higher strength.

Route of Administration. An application for a change in the route of administration, such as a change from an intravenous to intrathecal route.

Substitution of an Active Ingredient in a Combination Product. An application for a change in one of the active ingredients of an approved combination product for another active ingredient that has or has not been previously approved.

Following are additional examples of applications that may be accepted pursuant to section 505(b)(2) of the Act. Some or all of the additional information could be provided by the literature or reference to past FDA findings of safety and effectiveness for approved drugs, or it could be based on studies conducted by or for the applicant or to which it has obtained a right of reference.

Formulation. An application for a proposed drug product that contains a different quality or quantity of an excipient(s) than the listed drug where the studies required for approval are beyond those considered limited confirmatory studies appropriate to a 505(j) application.

Dosing Regimen. An application for a new dosing regimen, such as a change from twice daily to once daily.

Active Ingredient. An application for a change in an active ingredient such as a different salt, ester, complex, chelate, clathrate, racemate, or enantiomer of an active ingredient in a listed drug containing the same active moiety.

NME. In some cases, an NME may have been studied by parties other than the applicant, and published information may be pertinent to the new application. This is particularly likely if the NME is the prodrug of an approved drug or the active metabolite of an approved drug. In some cases, data on a drug with similar pharmacological effects could be considered critical to approval.

Combination Product. An application for a new combination product in which the active ingredients have been previously approved individually.

Indication. An application for a not previously approved indication for a listed drug.

Prescription/Over-the-Counter (OTC) Switch. An application to change a prescription indication to an OTC indication.

OTC Monograph. An application for a drug product that differs from a product described in an OTC monograph (21 CFR 330.11), such as a non-monograph indication or a new dosage form.

Naturally Derived or Recombinant Active Ingredient. An application for a drug product containing an active ingredient(s) derived from animal or botanical sources or recombinant technology where clinical investigations are necessary to show that the active ingredient is the same as an active ingredient in a listed drug.

Bioinequivalence. Generally, an application for a pharmaceutically equivalent drug product must be submitted under section 505(j) of the Act, and the proposed product must be shown to be bioequivalent to the reference-listed drug [21 CFR 314.101(d)(9)]. Applications for proposed drug products where the rate [21 CFR 314.54(b)(2)] and/or extent [21 CFR 314.54(b)(1)] of absorption exceed, or are otherwise different from, the 505(j) standards for BE compared with a listed drug may be submitted pursuant to section 505(b)(2) of the Act. Such a proposed product may require additional clinical studies to document safety and efficacy at the different rate and extent of delivery. Generally, the differences in rate and extent of absorption should be reflected in the labeling of the 505(b)(2) product. The proposed product does not need to be shown to be clinically *better* than the previously approved product; however, a 505(b)(2) application should not be used as a route of approval for poorly bioavailable generic drug products unable to meet the 505(j) standards for BE. If the proposed product is a duplicate of an already approved product, it should not be submitted as a 505(b)(2) application [21 CFR 314.101(d)(9)].

For example, a 505(b)(2) application would be appropriate for a controlled release product that is bioinequivalent to a reference listed drug where

1. the proposed product is at least as bioavailable as the approved pharmaceutically equivalent product (unless it has some other advantage, such as smaller peak/trough ratio) or
2. the pattern of release of the proposed product, although different, is at least as favorable as the approved pharmaceutically equivalent product.

What Cannot be Submitted as 505(b)(2) Applications?

- An application that is a duplicate of a listed drug and eligible for approval under section 505(j) [see 21 CFR 314.101(d)(9)];
- An application in which the *only* difference from the reference-listed drug is that the extent to which the active ingredient(s) is absorbed or otherwise made available to the site of action is less than the listed drug [21 CFR 314.54(b)(1)]; or
- An application in which the *only* difference from the reference listed drug is that the rate at which its active ingredient(s) is absorbed or otherwise made available to the site of action is *unintentionally* less than that of the listed drug [21 CFR 314.54(b)(2)].

Why Does It Matter If an NDA Is a 505(b)(2) Application?

Unlike a full NDA for which the sponsor has conducted or obtained a right of reference to all the data essential to approval, the filing or approval of a 505(b)(2) application may be delayed due to patent or exclusivity protections covering an approved product. Section 505(b)(2) applications must include patent certifications described at 21 CFR 314.50(i) and must provide notice of certain patent certifications to the NDA holder and patent owner under 21 CFR 314.52.

Patent and Exclusivity Protections that Could Affect a 505(b)(2) Application

A. What Type of Patent and/or Exclusivity Protection Is a 505(b)(2) Application Eligible For? A 505(b)(2) application may itself be granted three years of Waxman–Hatch exclusivity if one or more of the clinical investigations, other than BA/BE studies, was essential to approval of the application and was conducted or sponsored by the applicant [21 CFR 314.50(j); 314.108(b)(4) and (5)]. A 505(b)(2) application may also be granted 5 years of exclusivity if it is for a NCE [21 CFR 314.50(j); 314.108(b)(2)]. A 505(b)(2) application may also be eligible for orphan-drug exclusivity (21 CFR 314.20-316.36) or pediatric exclusivity (section 505A of the Act).

A 505(b)(2) application must contain information on patents claiming the drug or its method of use [21 CFR 314.54(a)(1)(v)].

B. What Could Delay the Approval or Filing of a 505(b)(2) Application? Approval or filing of a 505(b)(2) application, like a 505(j) application, may be delayed because of patent and exclusivity rights that apply to the listed drug [21 CFR 314.50(i), 314.107, and 314.108 and section 505A of the Act]. This is the case even if the application also includes clinical investigations supporting approval of the application.

What Should Be Included in 505(b)(2) Applications?

The Act [sections 505(b)(1) and (b)(2)] and FDA regulations (21 CFR 314.54) distinguish between 505(b)(1) and (b)(2) applications. Although the two types of applications must meet the same standards for approval (see section 505(b) and (c) of the Act), they differ in source of information to support safety and effectiveness, the patent certification requirements, BA/BE evidence, exclusivity bars, and processing within the FDA. The requirements for 505(b)(1) and 505(b)(2) applications are described at 21 CFR 314.50. Additional requirements for certain 505(b)(2) applications are described at 21 CFR 314.54.

A 505(b)(2) application should include the following:

- Identification of those portions of the application that rely on information the applicant does not own or to which the applicant does not have a right of reference (e.g., for reproductive toxicity studies)

- If the 505(b)(2) seeks to rely on the Agency's previous finding of safety or efficacy for a listed drug or drugs, identification of any and all listed drugs by established name, proprietary name (if any), dosage form, strength, route of administration, name of the listed drug's sponsor, and the application number [21 CFR 314.54(a)(1)(iii)]. Even if the 505(b)(2) application is based solely upon literature and does not rely expressly on an Agency finding of safety and effectiveness for a listed drug, the applicant must identify the listed drug(s) on which the studies were conducted, if there are any. If the 505(b)(2) application is for an NCE and the 505(b)(2) applicant is not relying on literature derived from studies of an approved drug, there may not be a listed drug. If there is a listed drug that is the pharmaceutical equivalent to the drug proposed in the 505(b)(2) application, that drug should be identified as the listed drug.
- Information with respect to any patents that claim the drug or the use of the drug for which approval is sought [21 CFR 314.50(h)]. This patent information will be published in the Orange Book when the application is approved.
- Information required under 314.50(j) if the applicant believes it is entitled to marketing exclusivity [21 CFR 314.54(a)(1)(vii)]
- A patent certification or statement as required under section 505(b)(2) of the Act with respect to any relevant patents that claim the listed drug and that claim any other drugs which the investigations relied on by the applicant for approval of the application were conducted, or that claim a use for the listed or other drug [21 CFR 314.54(a)(1)(vi)]

If there is a listed drug that is the pharmaceutical equivalent of the drug proposed in the 505(b)(2) application, the 505(b)(2) applicant should provide patent certifications for the patents listed for the pharmaceutically equivalent drug. Patent certifications should specify the exact patent number(s) and the exact name of the listed drug or other drug even if all relevant patents have expired.

- If an application is for approval of a new indication and not for the indications approved for the listed drug, a certification so stating [21 CFR 314.54(a)(1)(iv)]
- A statement as to whether the listed drug(s) identified above has received a period of marketing exclusivity [21 CFR 314.108(b)]. If a listed drug is protected by exclusivity, filing or approval of the 505(b)(2) application may be delayed.
- A BA/BE study comparing the proposed product to the listed drug (if any)
- Studies necessary to support the change or modification from the listed drug or drugs (if any). Complete studies of safety and effectiveness may not be necessary if appropriate bridging studies are found to provide an

adequate basis for reliance upon the FDA's finding of safety and effectiveness of the listed drug(s).

Before submitting the application, the applicant should submit a plan to the
appropriate new-drug evaluation division identifying the types of bridging
studies that should be conducted. The applicant should also identify those
components of its application for which it expects to rely on the FDA's finding
of safety and effectiveness of a previously approved drug product. The division
will critique the plan and provide guidance.

NEW DRUGS

SEC. 505. [21 U.S.C. 355]

(a) No person shall introduce or deliver for introduction into interstate commerce any new drug, unless an approval of an application filed pursuant
to subsection (b) or (j) is effective with respect to such drug.

(b)

(1) Any person may file with the Secretary an application with respect to
any drug subject to the provisions of subsection (a). Such persons shall
submit to the Secretary as a part of the application

(A) full reports of investigations which have been made to show
whether or not such drug is safe for use and whether such drug
is effective in use;

(B) a full list of the articles used as components of such drug;

(C) a full statement of the composition of such drug;

(D) a full description of the methods used in, and the facilities and
controls used for, the manufacture, processing, and packing of
such drug;

(E) such samples of such drug and of the articles used as components
thereof as the Secretary may require;

(F) specimens of the labeling proposed to be used for such drug;
and

(G) any assessments required under section 505B. The applicant shall
file with the application the patent number and the expiration
date of any patent which claims the drug for which the applicant
submitted the application or which claims a method of using such
drug and with respect to which a claim of patent infringement
could reasonably be asserted if a person not licensed by the
owner engaged in the manufacture use or sale of the drug. If an
application is filed under this subsection for a drug and a patent

which claims such drug or a method of using such drug is issued after the filing date but before approval of the application, the applicant shall amend the application to include the information required by the preceding sentence. Upon approval of the application, the Secretary shall publish information submitted under the two preceding sentences. The Secretary shall, in consultation with the Director of the National Institutes of Health and with representatives of the drug manufacturing industry, review and develop guidance, as appropriate, on the inclusion of women and minorities in clinical trials required by clause (A).

(2) An application submitted under paragraph (1) for a drug for which the investigations described in clause (A) of such paragraph and relied upon by the applicant for approval of the application were not conducted by or for the applicant and for which the applicant has not obtained a right of reference or use from the person by or for whom the investigations were conducted shall also include

  (A) a certification, in the opinion of the applicant and to the best of his knowledge, with respect to each patent which claims the drug for which such investigations were conducted or which claims a use for such drug for which the applicant is seeking approval under this subsection and for which information is required to be filed under paragraph (1) or subsection (c)

    (i) that such patent information has not been filed,

    (ii) that such patent has expired,

    (iii) of the date on which such patent will expire, or

    (iv) that such patent is invalid or will not be infringed by the manufacture, use, or sale of the new drug for which the application is submitted; and

  (B) if with respect to the drug for which investigations described in paragraph (1)(A) were conducted, information was filed under paragraph (1) or subsection (c) for a method of use patent which does not claim a use for which the applicant is seeking approval under this subsection, a statement that the method of use patent does not claim such a use.

(3) Notice of opinion that patent is invalid or will not be infringed.

  (A) Agreement to give notice. An applicant that makes a certification described in paragraph (2)(A)(iv) shall include in the application a statement that the applicant will give notice as required by this paragraph.

  (B) Timing of notice. An applicant that makes a certification described in paragraph (2)(A)(iv) shall give notice as required under this paragraph

(i) if the certification is in the application, not later than 20 days after the date of the postmark on the notice with which the Secretary informs the applicant that the application has been filed; or

(ii) if the certification is in an amendment or supplement to the application, at the time at which the applicant submits the amendment or supplement, regardless of whether the applicant has already given notice with respect to another such certification contained in the application or in an amendment or supplement to the application.

(C) Recipients of notice. An applicant required under this paragraph to give notice shall give notice to

(i) each owner of the patent that is the subject of the certification (or a representative of the owner designated to receive such a notice); and

(ii) the holder of the approved application under this subsection for the drug that is claimed by the patent or a use of which is claimed by the patent (or a representative of the holder designated to receive such a notice).

(D) Contents of notice. A notice required under this paragraph shall

(i) state that an application that contains data from bioavailability or bioequivalence studies has been submitted under this subsection for the drug with respect to which the certification is made to obtain approval to engage in the commercial manufacture, use, or sale of the drug before the expiration of the patent referred to in the certification; and

(ii) include a detailed statement of the factual and legal basis of the opinion of the applicant that the patent is invalid or will not be infringed.

(4)

(A) An applicant may not amend or supplement an application referred to in paragraph (2) to seek approval of a drug that is a different drug than the drug identified in the application as submitted to the Secretary.

(B) With respect to the drug for which such an application is submitted, nothing in this subsection or subsection (c)(3) prohibits an applicant from amending or supplementing the application to seek approval of a different strength.

(5)

(A) The Secretary shall issue guidance for the individuals who review applications submitted under paragraph (1) or under section 351 of the Public Health Service Act, which shall relate to promptness in conducting the review, technical excellence, lack of bias and conflict of interest, and knowledge of regulatory and scientific standards, and which shall apply equally to all individuals who review such applications.

(B) The Secretary shall meet with a sponsor of an investigation or an applicant for approval for a drug under this subsection or section 351 of the Public Health Service Act if the sponsor or applicant makes a reasonable written request for a meeting for the purpose of reaching agreement on the design and size of clinical trials intended to form the primary basis of an effectiveness claim. The sponsor or applicant shall provide information necessary for discussion and agreement on the design and size of the clinical trials. Minutes of any such meeting shall be prepared by the Secretary and made available to the sponsor or applicant upon request.

(C) Any agreement regarding the parameters of the design and size of clinical trials of a new drug under this paragraph that is reached between the Secretary and a sponsor or applicant shall be reduced to writing and made part of the administrative record by the Secretary. Such agreement shall not be changed after the testing begins, except

  (i) with the written agreement of the sponsor or applicant, or

  (ii) pursuant to a decision made in accordance with subparagraph (D) by the director of the reviewing division, that a substantial scientific issue essential to determining the safety or effectiveness of the drug has been identified after the testing has begun.

(D) A decision under subparagraph (C)(ii) by the director shall be in writing and the Secretary shall provide to the sponsor or applicant an opportunity for a meeting at which the director and the sponsor or applicant will be present and at which the director will document the scientific issue involved.

(E) The written decisions of the reviewing division shall be binding upon, and may not directly or indirectly be changed by, the field or compliance division personnel unless such field or compliance division personnel demonstrate to the reviewing division why such decision should be modified.

(F) No action by the reviewing division may be delayed because of the unavailability of information from or action by field personnel unless the reviewing division determines that a delay is necessary to assure the marketing of a safe and effective drug.

(G) For purposes of this paragraph, the reviewing division is the division responsible for the review of an application for approval of a drug under this subsection or section 351 of the Public Health Service Act (including all scientific and medical matters, chemistry, manufacturing, and controls).

(c)

(1) Within 180 days after the filing of an application under subsection (b), or such additional period as may be agreed upon by the Secretary and the applicant, the Secretary shall either

(A) approve the application if he then finds that none of the grounds for denying approval specified in subsection (d) apply, or

(B) give the applicant notice of an opportunity for a hearing before the Secretary under subsection (d) on the question whether such application is approvable. If the applicant elects to accept the opportunity for hearing by written request within 30 days after such notice, such hearing shall commence not more than 90 days after the expiration of such 30 days unless the Secretary and the applicant otherwise agree. Any such hearing shall thereafter be conducted on an expedited basis and the Secretary's order thereon shall be issued within 90 days after the date fixed by the Secretary for filing final briefs.

(2) If the patent information described in subsection (b) could not be filed with the submission of an application under subsection (b) because the application was filed before the patent information was required under subsection (b) or a patent was issued after the application was approved under such subsection, the holder of an approved application shall file with the Secretary, the patent number and the expiration date of any patent which claims the drug for which the application was submitted or which claims a method of using such drug and with respect to which a claim of patent infringement could reasonably be asserted if a person not licensed by the owner engaged in the manufacture, use, or sale of the drug. If the holder of an approved application could not file patent information under subsection (b) because it was not required at the time the application was approved, the holder shall file such information under this subsection not later than 30 days after the date of the enactment of this sentence, and if the holder of an approved application could not file patent information under subsection (b) because no patent had been issued when an application was filed or approved, the holder shall file such information under this subsection not later than 30 days after the date the patent involved is issued. Upon the submission of patent information under this subsection, the Secretary shall publish it.

(3) The approval of an application filed under subsection (b) which contains a certification required by paragraph (2) of such subsection shall be made effective on the last applicable date determined by applying the following to each certification made under subsection (b)(2)(A):

(A) If the applicant only made a certification described in clause (i) or (ii) of subsection (b)(2)(A) or in both such clauses, the approval may be made effective immediately.

(B) If the applicant made a certification described in clause (iii) of subsection (b)(2)(A), the approval may be made effective on the date certified under clause (iii).

(C) If the applicant made a certification described in clause (iv) of subsection (b)(2)(A), the approval shall be made effective immediately unless, before the expiration of 45 days after the date on which the notice described in subsection (b)(3) is received, an action is brought for infringement of the patent that is the subject of the certification and for which information was submitted to the Secretary under paragraph (2) or subsection (b)(1) before the date on which the application (excluding an amendment or supplement to the application) was submitted. If such an action is brought before the expiration of such days, the approval may be made effective upon the expiration of the 30-month period beginning on the date of the receipt of the notice provided under subsection (b)(3) or such shorter or longer period as the court may order because either party to the action failed to reasonably cooperate in expediting the action, except that

(i) if before the expiration of such period the district court decides that the patent is invalid or not infringed (including any substantive determination that there is no cause of action for patent infringement or invalidity), the approval shall be made effective on

(I) the date on which the court enters judgment reflecting the decision; or

(II) the date of a settlement order or consent decree signed and entered by the court stating that the patent that is the subject of the certification is invalid or not infringed;

(ii) if before the expiration of such period the district court decides that the patent has been infringed

(I) if the judgment of the district court is appealed, the approval shall be made effective

(aa) the date on which the court of appeals decides that the patent is invalid or not infringed (including any substantive determination that there is no cause of action for patent infringement or invalidity); or

(bb) the date of a settlement order or consent decree signed and entered by the court of appeals stating that the patent that is the subject of the certification is invalid or not infringed; or

(II) if the judgment of the district court is not appealed or is affirmed, the approval shall be made effective on the date specified by the district court in a court order under section 271(e)(4)(A) of title 35, United States Code;

(iii) if before the expiration of such period the court grants a preliminary injunction prohibiting the applicant from engaging in the commercial manufacture or sale of the drug until the court decides the issues of patent validity and infringement and if the court decides that such patent is invalid or not infringed, the approval shall be made effective as provided in clause (i); or

(iv) if before the expiration of such period the court grants a preliminary injunction prohibiting the applicant from engaging in the commercial manufacture or sale of the drug until the court decides the issues of patent validity and infringement and if the court decides that such patent has been infringed, the approval shall be made effective as provided in clause (ii).

In such an action, each of the parties shall reasonably cooperate in expediting the action.

(D) Civil action to obtain patent certainty.

(i) Declaratory judgment absent infringement action.

(I) In general. No action may be brought under section 2201 of title 28, United States Code, by an applicant referred to in subsection (b)(2) for a declaratory judgment with respect to a patent which is the subject of the certification referred to in subparagraph (C) unless

(aa) the 45-day period referred to in such subparagraph has expired;

(bb) neither the owner of such patent nor the holder of the approved application under subsection (b) for the drug that is claimed by the patent or a use of which is claimed by the patent brought a civil action against the applicant for infringement of the patent before the expiration of such period; and

(cc) in any case in which the notice provided under paragraph (2)(B) relates to noninfringement, the notice was accompanied by a document described in subclause (III).

(II) Filing of civil action. If the conditions described in items (aa), (bb), and as applicable, (cc) of subclause (I) have been met, the applicant referred to in such subclause may, in accordance with section 2201 of title 28, United States Code, bring a civil action under such section against the owner or holder referred to in such subclause (but not against any owner or holder that has brought such a civil action against the applicant, unless that civil action was dismissed without prejudice) for a declaratory judgment that the patent is invalid or will not be infringed by the drug for which the applicant seeks approval, except that such civil action may be brought for a declaratory judgment that the patent will not be infringed only in a case in which the condition described in subclause (I)(cc) is applicable. A civil action referred to in this subclause shall be brought in the judicial district where the defendant has its principal place of business or a regular and established place of business.

(III) Offer of confidential access to application. For purposes of subclause (I)(cc), the document described in this subclause is a document providing an offer of confidential access to the application that is in the custody of the applicant referred to in subsection (b)(2) for the purpose of determining whether an action referred to in subparagraph (C) should be brought. The document providing the offer of confidential access shall contain such restrictions as to persons entitled to access, and on the use and disposition of any information accessed, as would apply had a protective order been entered for the purpose of protecting trade secrets and other confidential business information. A request for access to an application under an offer of confidential access shall be considered acceptance of the offer of confidential access with the restrictions as to persons entitled to access, and on the use and disposition of any information accessed, contained in the offer of confidential access, and those restrictions and other terms of the offer of confidential access shall be considered terms of an enforceable contract. Any person provided an offer of confidential access shall review the application for the sole and limited purpose of evaluating possible infringement of the patent that is the subject of the certification under subsection (b)(2)(A)(iv) and for no other purpose, and may not disclose information of no relevance to any issue of patent infringement to any person other than a person provided an offer of confidential access. Further, the application may be redacted by the applicant to remove any information of no relevance to any issue of patent infringement.

(ii) Counterclaim to infringement action.

    (I) In general. If an owner of the patent or the holder of the approved application under subsection (b) for the drug that is claimed by the patent or a use of which is claimed by the patent brings a patent infringement action against the applicant, the applicant may assert a counterclaim seeking an order requiring the holder to correct or delete the patent information submitted by the holder under subsection (b) or this subsection on the ground that the patent does not claim either

        (aa) the drug for which the application was approved, or

        (bb) an approved method of using the drug.

    (II) No independent cause of action. Subclause (I) does not authorize the assertion of a claim described in subclause (I) in any civil action or proceeding other than a counterclaim described in subclause (I).

(iii) No damages. An applicant shall not be entitled to damages in a civil action under clause (i) or a counterclaim under clause (ii).

(E)

    (i) If an application (other than an abbreviated new drug application) submitted under subsection (b) for a drug, no active ingredient (including any ester or salt of the active ingredient) of which has been approved in any other application under subsection (b), was approved during the period beginning January 1, 1982, and ending on the date of the enactment of this subsection, the Secretary may not make the approval of another application for a drug for which the investigations described in clause (A) of subsection (b)(1) and relied upon by the applicant for approval of the application were not conducted by or for the applicant and for which the applicant has not obtained a right of reference or use from the person by or for whom the investigations were conducted effective before the expiration of ten years from the date of the approval of the application previously approved under subsection (b).

(ii) If an application submitted under subsection (b) for a drug, no active ingredient (including any ester or salt of the active ingredient) of which has been approved in any other application under subsection (b), is approved after the date of the enactment of this clause, no application which refers to the drug for which the subsection (b) application was submitted and for which the investigations described in clause (A) of subsection (b)(1) and relied upon by the applicant for approval of the application were not conducted by or for the applicant and for which the applicant has not obtained a right of reference or use from the person by or for whom the investigations were conducted may be submitted under subsection (b) before the expiration of five years from the date of the approval of the application under subsection (b), except that such an application may be submitted under subsection (b) after the expiration of four years from the date of the approval of the subsection (b) application if it contains a certification of patent invalidity or noninfringement described in clause (iv) of subsection (b)(2)(A). The approval of such an application shall be made effective in accordance with this paragraph except that, if an action for patent infringement is commenced during the one-year period beginning forty-eight months after the date of the approval of the subsection (b) application, the 30-month period referred to in subparagraph (C) shall be extended by such amount of time (if any) which is required for seven and one-half years to have elapsed from the date of approval of the subsection (b) application.

(iii) If an application submitted under subsection (b) for a drug, which includes an active ingredient (including any ester or salt of the active ingredient) that has been approved in another application approved under subsection (b), is approved after the date of the enactment of this clause and if such application contains reports of new clinical investigations (other than bioavailability studies) essential to the approval of the application and conducted or sponsored by the applicant, the Secretary may not make the approval of an application submitted under subsection (b) for the conditions of approval of such drug in the approved subsection (b) application effective before the expiration of three years from the date of the approval of the application under subsection (b) if the investigations described in clause (A) of subsection (b)(1) and relied upon by the applicant for approval of the application were not conducted by or for the applicant and if the applicant has not obtained a right of reference or use from the person by or for whom the investigations were conducted.

(iv) If a supplement to an application approved under subsection (b) is approved after the date of enactment of this clause and the supplement contains reports of new clinical investigations (other than bioavailability studies) essential to the approval of the supplement and conducted or sponsored by the person submitting the supplement, the Secretary may not make the approval of an application submitted under subsection (b) for a change approved in the supplement effective before the expiration of three years from the date of the approval of the supplement under subsection (b) if the investigations described in clause (A) of subsection (b)(1) and relied upon by the applicant for approval of the application were not conducted by or for the applicant and if the applicant has not obtained a right of reference or use from the person by or for whom the investigations were conducted.

(v) If an application (or supplement to an application) submitted under subsection (b) for a drug, which includes an active ingredient (including any ester or salt of the active ingredient) that has been approved in another application under subsection (b), was approved during the period beginning January 1, 1982, and ending on the date of the enactment of this clause, the Secretary may not make the approval of an application submitted under this subsection and for which the investigations described in clause (A) of subsection (b)(1) and relied upon by the applicant for approval of the application were not conducted by or for the applicant and for which the applicant has not obtained a right of reference or use from the person by or for whom the investigations were conducted and which refers to the drug for which the subsection (b) application was submitted effective before the expiration of two years from the date of enactment of this clause.

(4) A drug manufactured in a pilot or other small facility may be used to demonstrate the safety and effectiveness of the drug and to obtain approval for the drug prior to manufacture of the drug in a larger facility, unless the Secretary makes a determination that a full scale production facility is necessary to ensure the safety or effectiveness of the drug.

(d) If the Secretary finds, after due notice to the applicant in accordance with subsection (c) and giving him an opportunity for a hearing, in accordance with said subsection, that

(1) the investigations, reports of which are required to be submitted to the Secretary pursuant to subsection (b), do not include adequate tests by all methods reasonably applicable to show whether or not such drug is safe for use under the conditions prescribed, recommended, or suggested in the proposed labeling thereof;

(2) the results of such tests show that such drug is unsafe for use under such conditions or do not show that such drug is safe for use under such conditions;

(3) the methods used in, and the facilities and controls used for, the manufacture, processing, and packing of such drug are inadequate to preserve its identity, strength, quality, and purity;

(4) upon the basis of the information submitted to him as part of the application, or upon the basis of any other information before him with respect to such drug, he has insufficient information to determine whether such drug is safe for use under such conditions; or

(5) evaluated on the basis of the information submitted to him as part of the application and any other information before him with respect to such drug, there is a lack of substantial evidence that the drug will have the effect it purports or is represented to have under the conditions of use prescribed, recommended, or suggested in the proposed labeling thereof; or

(6) the application failed to contain the patent information prescribed by subsection (b); or

(7) based on a fair evaluation of all material facts, such labeling is false or misleading in any particular; he shall issue an order refusing to approve the application. If, after such notice and opportunity for hearing, the Secretary finds that clauses (1) through (6) do not apply, he shall issue an order approving the application. As used in this subsection and subsection (e), the term "substantial evidence" means evidence consisting of adequate and well-controlled investigations, including clinical investigations, by experts qualified by scientific training and experience to evaluate the effectiveness of the drug involved, on the basis of which it could fairly and responsibly be concluded by such experts that the drug will have the effect it purports or is represented to have under the conditions of use prescribed, recommended, or suggested in the labeling or proposed labeling thereof. If the Secretary determines, based on relevant science, that data from one adequate and well-controlled clinical investigation and confirmatory evidence (obtained prior to or after such investigation) are sufficient to establish effectiveness, the Secretary may consider such data and evidence to constitute substantial evidence for purposes of the preceding sentence.

(e) The Secretary shall, after due notice and opportunity for hearing to the applicant, withdraw approval of an application with respect to any drug under this section if the Secretary finds

   (1) that clinical or other experience, tests, or other scientific data show that such drug is unsafe for use under the conditions of use upon the basis of which the application was approved;

   (2) that new evidence of clinical experience, not contained in such application or not available to the Secretary until after such application was approved, or tests by new methods, or tests by methods not deemed reasonably applicable when such application was approved, evaluated together with the evidence available to the Secretary when the application was approved, shows that such drug is not shown to be safe for use under the conditions of use upon the basis of which the application was approved; or

   (3) on the basis of new information before him with respect to such drug, evaluated together with the evidence available to him when the application was approved, that there is a lack of substantial evidence that the drug will have the effect it purports or is represented to have under the conditions of use prescribed, recommended, or suggested in the labeling thereof; or

   (4) the patent information prescribed by subsection (c) was not filed within 30 days after the receipt of written notice from the Secretary specifying the failure to file such information; or

   (5) that the application contains any untrue statement of a material fact: *Provided,* that if the Secretary (or, in his absence, the officer acting

as Secretary) finds that there is an imminent hazard to the public health, he may suspend the approval of such application immediately, and give the applicant prompt notice of his action and afford the applicant the opportunity for an expedited hearing under this subsection; but the authority conferred by this proviso to suspend the approval of an application shall not be delegated. The Secretary may also, after due notice and opportunity for hearing to the applicant, withdraw the approval of an application submitted under subsection (b) or (j) with respect to any drug under this section if the Secretary finds (1) that the applicant has failed to establish a system for maintaining required records, or has repeatedly or deliberately failed to maintain such records or to make required reports, in accordance with a regulation or order under subsection (k) or to comply with the notice requirements of section 510(k)(2), or the applicant has refused to permit access to, or copying or verification of, such records as required by paragraph (2) of such subsection; or (2) that on the basis of new information before him, evaluated together with the evidence before him when the application was approved, the methods used in, or the facilities and controls used for, the manufacture, processing, and packing of such drug are inadequate to assure and preserve its identity, strength, quality, and purity and were not made adequate within a reasonable time after receipt of written notice from the Secretary specifying the matter complained of; or (3) that on the basis of new information before him, evaluated together with the evidence before him when the application was approved, the labeling of such drug, based on a fair evaluation of all material facts, is false or misleading in any particular and was not corrected within a reasonable time after receipt of written notice from the Secretary specifying the matter complained of. Any order under this subsection shall state the findings upon which it is based.

(f) Whenever the Secretary finds that the facts so require, he shall revoke any previous order under subsection (d) or (e) refusing, withdrawing, or suspending approval of an application and shall approve such application or reinstate such approval, as may be appropriate.

(g) Orders of the Secretary issued under this section shall be served (1) in person by any officer or employee of the Department designated by the Secretary or (2) by mailing the order by registered mail or by certified mail addressed to the applicant or respondent at his last-known address in the records of the Secretary.

(h) An appeal may be taken by the applicant from an order of the Secretary refusing or withdrawing approval of an application under this section. Such appeal shall be taken by filing in the United States court of appeals for the circuit wherein such applicant resides or has his principal place of business, or in the United States Court of Appeals for the District of

Columbia Circuit, within 60 days after the entry of such order, a written petition praying that the order of the Secretary be set aside. A copy of such petition shall be forthwith transmitted by the clerk of the court to the Secretary, or any officer designated by him for that purpose, and thereupon the Secretary shall certify and file in the court the record upon which the order complained of was entered, as provided in section 2112 of title 28, United States Code. Upon the filing of such petition, such court shall have exclusive jurisdiction to affirm or set aside such order, except that until the filing of the record, the Secretary may modify or set aside his order. No objection to the order of the Secretary shall be considered by the court unless such objection shall have been urged before the Secretary or unless there were reasonable grounds for failure so to do. The finding of the Secretary as to the facts, if supported by substantial evidence, shall be conclusive. If any person shall apply to the court for leave to adduce additional evidence, and shall show to the satisfaction of the court that such additional evidence is material and that there were reasonable grounds for failure to adduce such evidence in the pro-ceeding before the Secretary, the court may order such additional evi-dence to be taken before the Secretary and to be adduced upon the hearing in such manner and upon such terms and conditions as to the court may seem proper. The Secretary may modify his findings as to the facts by reason of the additional evidence so taken, and he shall file with the court such modified findings which, if supported by substantial evidence, shall be conclusive, and his recommendation, if any, for the setting aside of the original order. The judgment of the court affirming or setting aside any such order of the Secretary shall be final, subject to review by the Supreme Court of the United States upon certiorari or certification as provided in section 1254 of title 28 of the United States Code. The commencement of proceedings under this subsection shall not, unless specifically ordered by the court to the contrary, operate as a stay of the Secretary's order.

(i)

    (1) The Secretary shall promulgate regulations for exempting from the operation of the foregoing subsections of this section drugs intended solely for investigational use by experts qualified by scientific training and experience to investigate the safety and effectiveness of drugs. Such regulations may, within the discretion of the Secretary, among other conditions relating to the protection of the public health, provide for conditioning such exemption upon

        (A) the submission to the Secretary, before any clinical testing of a new drug is undertaken, of reports, by the manufacturer or the sponsor of the investigation of such drug, or preclinical tests (including tests on animals) of such drug adequate to justify the proposed clinical testing;

(B) the manufacturer or the sponsor of the investigation of a new drug proposed to be distributed to investigators for clinical testing obtaining a signed agreement from each of such investigators that patients to whom the drug is administered will be under his personal supervision, or under the supervision of investigators responsible to him, and that he will not supply such drug to any other investigator, or to clinics, for administration to human beings;

(C) the establishment and maintenance of such records, and the making of such reports to the Secretary, by the manufacturer or the sponsor of the investigation of such drug, of data (including but not limited to analytical reports by investigators) obtained as the result of such investigational use of such drug, as the Secretary finds will enable him to evaluate the safety and effectiveness of such drug in the event of the filing of an application pursuant to subsection (b); and

(D) the submission to the Secretary by the manufacturer or the sponsor of the investigation of a new drug of a statement of intent regarding whether the manufacturer or sponsor has plans for assessing pediatric safety and efficacy.

(2) Subject to paragraph (3), a clinical investigation of a new drug may begin 30 days after the Secretary has received from the manufacturer or sponsor of the investigation a submission containing such information about the drug and the clinical investigation, including

(A) information on design of the investigation and adequate reports of basic information, certified by the applicant to be accurate reports, necessary to assess the safety of the drug for use in clinical investigation; and

(B) adequate information on the chemistry and manufacturing of the drug, controls available for the drug, and primary data tabulations from animal or human studies.

(3)

(A) At any time, the Secretary may prohibit the sponsor of an investigation from conducting the investigation (referred to in this paragraph as a "clinical hold") if the Secretary makes a determination described in subparagraph (B). The Secretary shall specify the basis for the clinical hold, including the specific information available to the Secretary, which served as the basis for such clinical hold, and confirm such determination in writing.

(B) For purposes of subparagraph (A), a determination described in this subparagraph with respect to a clinical hold is that

      (i) the drug involved represents an unreasonable risk to the safety of the persons who are the subjects of the clinical investigation, taking into account the qualifications of the clinical investigators, information about the drug, the design of the clinical investigation, the condition for which the drug is to be investigated, and the health status of the subjects involved; or

      (ii) the clinical hold should be issued for such other reasons as the Secretary may by regulation establish (including reasons established by regulation before the date of the enactment of the Food and Drug Administration Modernization Act of 1997).

  (C) Any written request to the Secretary from the sponsor of an investigation that a clinical hold be removed shall receive a decision, in writing and specifying the reasons therefor, within 30 days after receipt of such request. Any such request shall include sufficient information to support the removal of such clinical hold.

(4) Regulations under paragraph (1) shall provide that such exemption shall be conditioned upon the manufacturer, or the sponsor of the investigation, requiring that experts using such drugs for investigational purposes certify to such manufacturer or sponsor that they will inform any human beings to whom such drugs, or any controls used in connection therewith, are being administered, or their representatives, that such drugs are being used for investigational purposes and will obtain the consent of such human beings or their representatives, except where it is not feasible or it is contrary to the best interests of such human beings. Nothing in this subsection shall be construed to require any clinical investigator to submit directly to the Secretary reports on the investigational use of drugs.

(j)

  (1) Any person may file with the Secretary an abbreviated application for the approval of a new drug.

  (2)

    (A) An abbreviated application for a new drug shall contain

      (i) information to show that the conditions of use prescribed, recommended, or suggested in the labeling proposed for the new drug have been previously approved for a drug listed under paragraph (7) (hereinafter in this subsection referred to as a "listed drug");

      (ii)

        (I) if the listed drug referred to in clause (i) has only one active ingredient, information to show that the active ingredient of the new drug is the same as that of the listed drug;

(II) if the listed drug referred to in clause (i) has more than one active ingredient, information to show that the active ingredients of the new drug are the same as those of the listed drug; or

(III) if the listed drug referred to in clause (i) has more than one active ingredient and if one of the active ingredients of the new drug is different and the application is filed pursuant to the approval of a petition filed under subparagraph (C), information to show that the other active ingredients of the new drug are the same as the active ingredients of the listed drug, information to show that the different active ingredient is an active ingredient of a listed drug or of a drug which does not meet the requirements of section 201(p), and such other information respecting the different active ingredient with respect to which the petition was filed as the Secretary may require;

(iii) information to show that the route of administration, the dosage form, and the strength of the new drug are the same as those of the listed drug referred to in clause (i), or, if the route of administration, the dosage form, or the strength of the new drug is different and the application is filed pursuant to the approval of a petition filed under subparagraph (C), such information respecting the route of administration, dosage form, or strength with respect to which the petition was filed as the Secretary may require;

(iv) information to show that the new drug is bioequivalent to the listed drug referred to in clause (i), except that if the application is filed pursuant to the approval of a petition filed under subparagraph (C), information to show that the active ingredients of the new drug are of the same pharmacological or therapeutic class as those of the listed drug referred to in clause (i) and the new drug can be expected to have the same therapeutic effect as the listed drug when administered to patients for a condition of use referred to in clause (i);

(v) information to show that the labeling proposed for the new drug is the same as the labeling approved for the listed drug referred to in clause (i) except for changes required because of differences approved under a petition filed under subparagraph (C) or because the new drug and the listed drug are produced or distributed by different manufacturers;

(vi) the items specified in clauses (B) through (F) of subsection (b)(1);

(vii) a certification, the opinion of the applicant and to the best of his knowledge, with respect to each patent which claims the listed drug referred to in clause (i) or which claims a use for such listed drug for which the applicant is seeking approval under this subsection and for which information is required to be filed under subsection (b) or (c)

   (I) that such patent information has not been filed,

   (II) that such patent has expired,

   (III) of the date on which such patent will expire, or

   (IV) that such patent is invalid or will not be infringed by the manufacture, use, or sale of the new drug for which the application is submitted; and

(viii) if with respect to the listed drug referred to in clause (i) information was filed under subsection (b) or (c) for a method of use patent which does not claim a use for which the applicant is seeking approval under this subsection, a statement that the method of use patent does not claim such a use. The Secretary may not require that an abbreviated application contain information in addition to that required by clauses (i) through (viii).

(B) Notice of opinion that patent is invalid or will not be infringed.

(i) Agreement to give notice. An applicant that makes a certification described in subparagraph (A)(vii)(IV) shall include in the application a statement that the applicant will give notice as required by this subparagraph.

(ii) Timing of notice. An applicant that makes a certification described in subparagraph (A)(vii)(IV) shall give notice as required under this subparagraph

   (I) if the certification is in the application, not later than 20 days after the date of the postmark on the notice with which the Secretary informs the applicant that the application has been filed; or

   (II) if the certification is in an amendment or supplement to the application, at the time at which the applicant submits the amendment or supplement, regardless of whether the applicant has already given notice with respect to another such certification contained in the application or in an amendment or supplement to the application.

(iii) Recipients of notice. An applicant required under this subparagraph to give notice shall give notice to

(I) each owner of the patent that is the subject of the certification (or a representative of the owner designated to receive such a notice); and

(II) the holder of the approved application under subsection (b) for the drug that is claimed by the patent or a use of which is claimed by the patent (or a representative of the holder designated to receive such a notice).

(iv) Contents of notice. A notice required under this subparagraph shall

(I) state that an application that contains data from bioavailability or bioequivalence studies has been submitted under this subsection for the drug with respect to which the certification is made to obtain approval to engage in the commercial manufacture, use, or sale of the drug before the expiration of the patent referred to in the certification; and

(II) include a detailed statement of the factual and legal basis of the opinion of the applicant that the patent is invalid or will not be infringed.

(C) If a person wants to submit an abbreviated application for a new drug which has a different active ingredient or whose route of administration, dosage form, or strength differ from that of a listed drug, such person shall submit a petition to the Secretary seeking permission to file such an application. The Secretary shall approve or disapprove a petition submitted under this subparagraph within 90 days of the date the petition is submitted. The Secretary shall approve such a petition unless the Secretary finds

(i) that investigations must be conducted to show the safety and effectiveness of the drug or of any of its active ingredients, the route of administration, the dosage form, or strength which differ from the listed drug; or

(ii) that any drug with a different active ingredient may not be adequately evaluated for approval as safe and effective on the basis of the information required to be submitted in an abbreviated application.

(D)

(i) An applicant may not amend or supplement an application to seek approval of a drug referring to a different listed drug from the listed drug identified in the application as submitted to the Secretary.

(ii) With respect to the drug for which an application is submitted, nothing in this subsection prohibits an applicant from amending or supplementing the application to seek approval of a different strength.

(iii) Within 60 days after the date of the enactment of the Medicare Prescription Drug, Improvement, and Modernization Act of 2003, the Secretary shall issue guidance defining the term "listed drug" for purposes of this subparagraph.

(3)

(A) The Secretary shall issue guidance for the individuals who review applications submitted under paragraph (1), which shall relate to promptness in conducting the review, technical excellence, lack of bias and conflict of interest, and knowledge of regulatory and scientific standards, and which shall apply equally to all individuals who review such applications.

(B) The Secretary shall meet with a sponsor of an investigation or an applicant for approval for a drug under this subsection if the sponsor or applicant makes a reasonable written request for a meeting for the purpose of reaching agreement on the design and size of bioavailability and bioequivalence studies needed for approval of such application. The sponsor or applicant shall provide information necessary for discussion and agreement on the design and size of such studies. Minutes of any such meeting shall be prepared by the Secretary and made available to the sponsor or applicant.

(C) Any agreement regarding the parameters of design and size of bioavailability and bioequivalence studies of a drug under this paragraph that is reached between the Secretary and a sponsor or applicant shall be reduced to writing and made part of the administrative record by the Secretary. Such agreement shall not be changed after the testing begins, except

(i) with the written agreement of the sponsor or applicant; or

(ii) pursuant to a decision, made in accordance with subparagraph (D) by the director of the reviewing division, that a substantial scientific issue essential to determining the safety or effectiveness of the drug has been identified after the testing has begun.

(D) A decision under subparagraph (C)(ii) by the director shall be in writing and the Secretary shall provide to the sponsor or applicant an opportunity for a meeting at which the director and the sponsor or applicant will be present and at which the director will document the scientific issue involved.

(E) The written decisions of the reviewing division shall be binding upon, and may not directly or indirectly be changed by, the field or compliance office personnel unless such field or compliance office personnel demonstrate to the reviewing division why such decision should be modified.

(F) No action by the reviewing division may be delayed because of the unavailability of information from or action by field personnel unless the reviewing division determines that a delay is necessary to assure the marketing of a safe and effective drug.

(G) For purposes of this paragraph, the reviewing division is the division responsible for the review of an application for approval of a drug under this subsection (including scientific matters, chemistry, manufacturing, and controls).

(4) Subject to paragraph (5), the Secretary shall approve an application for a drug unless the Secretary finds

(A) the methods used in, or the facilities and controls used for, the manufacture, processing, and packing of the drug are inadequate to assure and preserve its identity, strength, quality, and purity;

(B) information submitted with the application is insufficient to show that each of the proposed conditions of use have been previously approved for the listed drug referred to in the application;

(C)

(i) If the listed drug has only one active ingredient, information submitted with the application is insufficient to show that the active ingredient is the same as that of the listed drug;

(ii) if the listed drug has more than one active ingredient, information submitted with the application is insufficient to show that the active ingredients are the same as the active ingredients of the listed drug; or

(iii) if the listed drug has more than one active ingredient and if the application is for a drug which has an active ingredient different from the listed drug, information submitted with the application is insufficient to show

(I) that the other active ingredients are the same as the active ingredients of the listed drug, or

(II) that the different active ingredient is an active ingredient of a listed drug or a drug which does not meet the requirements of section 201(p) or no petition to file an application for the drug with the different ingredient was approved under paragraph (2)(C);

(D)

    (i) if the application is for a drug whose route of administration, dosage form, or strength of the drug is the same as the route of administration, dosage form, or strength of the listed drug referred to in the application, information submitted in the application is insufficient to show that the route of administration, dosage form, or strength is the same as that of the listed drug, or

    (ii) if the application is for a drug whose route of administration, dosage form, or strength of the drug is different from that of the listed drug referred to in the application, no petition to file an application for the drug with the different route of administration, dosage form, or strength was approved under paragraph (2)(C);

(E) if the application was filed pursuant to the approval of a petition under paragraph (2)(C), the application did not contain the information required by the Secretary respecting the active ingredient, route of administration, dosage form, or strength which is not the same;

(F) information submitted in the application is insufficient to show that the drug is bioequivalent to the listed drug referred to in the application or, if the application was filed pursuant to a petition approved under paragraph (2)(C) information submitted in the application is insufficient to show that the active ingredients of the new drug are of the same pharmacological or therapeutic class as those of the listed drug referred to in paragraph (2)(A)(i) and that the new drug can be expected to have the same therapeutic effect as the listed drug when administered to patients for a condition of use referred to in such paragraph;

(G) information submitted in the application is insufficient to show that the labeling proposed for the drug is the same as the labeling approved for the listed drug referred to in the application except for changes required because of differences approved under a petition filed under paragraph (2)(C) or because the drug and the listed drug are produced or distributed by different manufacturers;

(H) information submitted in the application or any other information available to the Secretary shows that

    (i) the inactive ingredients of the drug are unsafe for use under the conditions prescribed, recommended, or suggested in the labeling proposed for the drug; or

      (ii) the composition of the drug is unsafe under such conditions because of the type or quantity of inactive ingredients included or the manner in which the inactive ingredients are included;

          (I) the approval under subsection (c) of the listed drug referred to in the application under this subsection has been withdrawn or suspended for grounds described in the first sentence of subsection (e), the Secretary has published a notice of opportunity for hearing to withdraw approval of the listed drug under subsection (c) for grounds described in the first sentence of subsection (e), the approval under this subsection of the listed drug referred to in the application under this subsection has been withdrawn or suspended under paragraph (6), or the Secretary has determined that the listed drug has been withdrawn from sale for safety or effectiveness reasons;

  (J) the application does not meet any other requirement of paragraph (2)(A); or

  (K) the application contains an untrue statement of material fact.

(5)

  (A) Within 180 days of the initial receipt of an application under paragraph (2) or within such additional period as may be agreed upon by the Secretary and the applicant, the Secretary shall approve or disapprove the application.

  (B) The approval of an application submitted under paragraph (2) shall be made effective on the last applicable date determined by applying the following to each certification made under paragraph (2)(A)(vii):

      (i) If the applicant only made a certification described in subclause (I) or (II) of paragraph (2)(A)(vii) or in both such subclauses, the approval may be made effective immediately.

      (ii) If the applicant made a certification described in subclause (III) of paragraph (2)(A)(vii), the approval may be made effective on the date certified under subclause (III).

      (iii) If the applicant made a certification described in subclause (IV) of paragraph (2)(A)(vii), the approval shall be made effective immediately unless, before the expiration of 45 days after the date on which the notice described in paragraph (2)(B) is received, an action is brought for infringement of the patent that is the subject of the certification and for which information was submitted to the Secretary under subsection (b)(1) or (c)(2) before the date on which the application (excluding an amendment or supplement to the application), which the Secretary later determines to be substantially complete, was submitted. If such an action is brought before the expiration of such days, the approval shall be made effective upon the expiration of the 30-month period beginning on the date of the receipt of the notice provided under paragraph (2)(B)(i) or such shorter or longer period as the court may order because either party to the action failed to reasonably cooperate in expediting the action, except that

(I) if before the expiration of such period the district court decides that the patent is invalid or not infringed (including any substantive determination that there is no cause of action for patent infringement or invalidity), the approval shall be made effective on

(aa) the date on which the court enters judgment reflecting the decision; or

(bb) the date of a settlement order or consent decree signed and entered by the court stating that the patent that is the subject of the certification is invalid or not infringed;

(II) if before the expiration of such period the district court decides that the patent has been infringed

(aa) if the judgment of the district court is appealed, the approval shall be made effective on

(AA) the date on which the court of appeals decides that the patent is invalid or not infringed (including any substantive determination that there is no cause of action for patent infringement or invalidity); or

(BB) the date of a settlement order or consent decree signed and entered by the court of appeals stating that the patent that is the subject of the certification is invalid or not infringed; or

(bb) if the judgment of the district court is not appealed or is affirmed, the approval shall be made effective on the date specified by the district court in a court order under section 271(e)(4)(A) of title 35, United States Code;

(III) if before the expiration of such period the court grants a preliminary injunction prohibiting the applicant from engaging in the commercial manufacture or sale of the drug until the court decides the issues of patent validity and infringement and if the court decides that such patent is invalid or not infringed, the approval shall be made effective as provided in subclause (I); or

(IV) if before the expiration of such period the court grants a preliminary injunction prohibiting the applicant from engaging in the commercial manufacture or sale of the drug until the court decides the issues of patent validity and infringement and if the court decides that such patent has been infringed, the approval shall be made effective as provided in subclause (II).

In such an action, each of the parties shall reasonably cooperate in expediting the action.

(iv) 180-day exclusivity period.

(I) Effectiveness of application. Subject to subparagraph (D), if the application contains a certification described in paragraph (2)(A)(vii)(IV) and is for a drug for which a first applicant has submitted an application containing such a certification, the application shall be made effective on the date that is 180 days after the date of the first commercial marketing of the drug (including the commercial marketing of the listed drug) by any first applicant.

(II) Definitions. In this paragraph:

(aa) 180-day exclusivity period. The term "180-day exclusivity period" means the 180-day period ending on the day before the date on which an application submitted by an applicant other than a first applicant could become effective under this clause.

(bb) First applicant. As used in this subsection, the term "first applicant" means an applicant that, on the first day on which a substantially complete application containing a certification described in paragraph (2)(A)(vii)(IV) is submitted for approval of a drug, submits a substantially complete application that contains and lawfully maintains a certification described in paragraph (2)(A)(vii)(IV) for the drug.

(cc) Substantially complete application. As used in this subsection, the term "substantially complete application" means an application under this subsection that on its face is sufficiently complete to permit a substantive review and contains all the information required by paragraph (2)(A).

(dd) Tentative approval.

(AA) In general. The term "tentative approval" means notification to an applicant by the Secretary that an application under this subsection meets the requirements of paragraph (2)(A), but cannot receive effective approval because the application does not meet the requirements of this subparagraph, there is a period of exclusivity for the listed drug under subparagraph (F) or section 505A, or there is a seven-year period of exclusivity for the listed drug under section 527.

(BB) Limitation. A drug that is granted tentative approval by the Secretary is not an approved drug and shall not have an effective approval until the Secretary issues an approval after any necessary additional review of the application.

(C) Civil action to obtain patent certainty.

(i) Declaratory judgment absent infringement action.

(I) In general. No action may be brought under section 2201 of title 28, United States Code, by an applicant under paragraph (2) for a declaratory judgment with respect to a patent which is the subject of the certification referred to in subparagraph (B)(iii) unless

(aa) the 45-day period referred to in such subparagraph has expired;

(bb) neither the owner of such patent nor the holder of the approved application under subsection (b) for the drug that is claimed by the patent or a use of which is claimed by the patent brought a civil action against the applicant for infringement of the patent before the expiration of such period; and (cc) in any case in which the notice provided under paragraph (2)(B) relates to noninfringement, the notice was accompanied by a document described in subclause (III).

(II) Filing of civil action. If the conditions described in items (aa), (bb), and as applicable, (cc) of subclause (I) have been met, the applicant referred to in such subclause may, in accordance with section 2201 of title 28, United States Code, bring a civil action under such section against the owner or holder referred to in such subclause (but not against any owner or holder that has brought such a civil action against the applicant, unless that civil action was dismissed without prejudice) for a declaratory judgment that the patent is invalid or will not be infringed by the drug for which the applicant seeks approval, except that such civil action may be brought for a declaratory judgment that the patent will not be infringed only in a case in which the condition described in subclause (I)(cc) is applicable. A civil action referred to in this subclause shall be brought in the judicial district where the defendant has its principal place of business or a regular and established place of business.

(III) Offer of confidential access to application. For purposes of subclause (I)(cc), the document described in this subclause is a document providing an offer of confidential access to the application that is in the custody of the applicant under paragraph (2) for the purpose of determining whether an action referred to in subparagraph (B)(iii) should be brought. The document providing the offer of confidential access shall contain such restrictions as to persons entitled to access, and on the use and disposition of any information accessed, as would apply had a protective order been entered for the purpose of protecting trade secrets and other confidential business information. A request for access to an application under an offer of confidential access shall be considered acceptance of the offer of confidential access with the restrictions as to persons entitled to access, and on the use and disposition of any information accessed, contained in the offer of confidential access, and those restrictions and other terms of the offer of confidential access shall be considered terms of an enforceable contract. Any person provided an offer of confidential access shall review the application for the sole and limited purpose of evaluating possible infringement of the patent that is the subject of the certification under paragraph (2)(A)(vii)(IV) and for no other purpose, and may not disclose information of no relevance to any issue of patent infringement to any person other than a person provided an offer of confidential access. Further, the application may be redacted by the applicant to remove any information of no relevance to any issue of patent infringement.

(ii) Counterclaim to infringement action.

    (I) In general. If an owner of the patent or the holder of the approved application under subsection (b) for the drug that is claimed by the patent or a use of which is claimed by the patent brings a patent infringement action against the applicant, the applicant may assert a counterclaim seeking an order requiring the holder to correct or delete the patent information submitted by the holder under subsection (b) or (c) on the ground that the patent does not claim either

        (aa) the drug for which the application was approved, or

        (bb) an approved method of using the drug.

    (II) No independent cause of action. Subclause (I) does not authorize the assertion of a claim described in subclause (I) in any civil action or proceeding other than a counterclaim described in subclause (I).

(iii) No damages. An applicant shall not be entitled to damages in a civil action under clause (i) or a counterclaim under clause (ii).

(D) Forfeiture of 180-day exclusivity period.

    (i) Definition of forfeiture event. In this subparagraph, the term "forfeiture event," with respect to an application under this subsection, means the occurrence of any of the following:

        (I) Failure to market. The first applicant fails to market the drug by the later of

        (aa) the earlier of the date that is

(AA) 75 days after the date on which the approval of the application of the first applicant is made effective under subparagraph (B)(iii), or

(BB) 30 months after the date of submission of the application of the first applicant; or

(bb) with respect to the first applicant or any other applicant (which other applicant has received tentative approval), the date that is 75 days after the date as of which, as to each of the patents with respect to which the first applicant submitted and lawfully maintained a certification qualifying the first applicant for the 180-day exclusivity period under subparagraph (B)(iv), at least one of the following has occurred:

(AA) In an infringement action brought against that applicant with respect to the patent or in a declaratory judgment action brought by that applicant with respect to the patent, a court enters a final decision from which no appeal (other than a petition to the Supreme Court for a writ of certiorari) has been or can be taken that the patent is invalid or not infringed.

(BB) In an infringement action or a declaratory judgment action described in subitem (AA), a court signs a settlement order or consent decree that enters a final judgment that includes a finding that the patent is invalid or not infringed.

(CC) The patent information submitted under subsection (b) or (c) is withdrawn by the holder of the application approved under subsection (b).

(II) Withdrawal of application. The first applicant withdraws the application or the Secretary considers the application to have been withdrawn as a result of a determination by the Secretary that the application does not meet the requirements for approval under paragraph (4).

(III) Amendment of certification. The first applicant amends or withdraws the certification for all of the patents with respect to which that applicant submitted a certification qualifying the applicant for the 180-day exclusivity period.

(IV) Failure to obtain tentative approval. The first applicant fails to obtain tentative approval of the application within 30 months after the date on which the application is filed, unless the failure is caused by a change in or a review of the requirements for approval of the application imposed after the date on which the application is filed.

(V) Agreement with another applicant, the listed drug application holder, or a patent owner. The first applicant enters into an agreement with another applicant under this subsection for the drug, the holder of the application for the listed drug, or an owner of the patent that is the subject of the certification under paragraph (2)(A)(vii)(IV), the Federal Trade Commission or the Attorney General files a complaint, and there is a final decision of the Federal Trade Commission or the court with regard to the complaint from which no appeal (other than a petition to the Supreme Court for a writ of certiorari) has been or can be taken that the agreement has violated the antitrust laws (as defined in section 1 of the Clayton Act (15 U.S.C. 12), except that the term includes section 5 of the Federal Trade Commission Act (15 U.S.C. 45) to the extent that that section applies to unfair methods of competition).

(VI) Expiration of all patents. All of the patents as to which the applicant submitted a certification qualifying it for the 180-day exclusivity period have expired.

(ii) Forfeiture. The 180-day exclusivity period described in subparagraph (B)(iv) shall be forfeited by a first applicant if a forfeiture event occurs with respect to that first applicant.

(iii) Subsequent applicant. If all first applicants forfeit the 180-day exclusivity period under clause (ii)

(I) approval of any application containing a certification described in paragraph (2)(A)(vii)(IV) shall be made effective in accordance with subparagraph (B)(iii); and

(II) no applicant shall be eligible for a 180-day exclusivity period.

(E) If the Secretary decides to disapprove an application, the Secretary shall give the applicant notice of an opportunity for a hearing before the Secretary on the question of whether such application is approvable. If the applicant elects to accept the opportunity for hearing by written request within 30 days after such notice, such hearing shall commence not more than 90 days after the expiration of such 30 days unless the Secretary and the applicant otherwise agree. Any such hearing shall thereafter be conducted on an expedited basis and the Secretary's order thereon shall be issued within 90 days after the date fixed by the Secretary for filing final briefs.

(F)

    (i) If an application (other than an abbreviated new drug application) submitted under subsection (b) for a drug, no active ingredient (including any ester or salt of the active ingredient) of which has been approved in any other application under subsection (b), was approved during the period beginning January 1, 1982, and ending on the date of the enactment of this subsection, the Secretary may not make the approval of an application submitted under this subsection which refers to the drug for which the subsection (b) application was submitted effective before the expiration of 10 years from the date of the approval of the application under subsection (b).

    (ii) If an application submitted under subsection (b) for a drug, no active ingredient (including any ester or salt of the active ingredient) of which has been approved in any other application under subsection (b), is approved after the date of the enactment of this subsection, no application may be submitted under this subsection which refers to the drug for which the subsection (b) application was submitted before the expiration of five years from the date of the approval of the application under subsection (b), except that such an application may be submitted under this subsection after the expiration of four years from the date of the approval of the subsection (b) application if it contains a certification of patent invalidity or noninfringement described in subclause (IV) of paragraph (2)(A)(vii). The approval of such an application shall be made effective in accordance with subparagraph (B) except that, if an action for patent infringement is commenced during the one-year period beginning forty-eight months after the date of the approval of the subsection (b) application, the 30-month period referred to in subparagraph (B)(iii) shall be extended by such amount of time (if any) which is required for seven and one-half years to have elapsed from the date of approval of the subsection (b) application.

(iii) If an application submitted under subsection (b) for a drug, which includes an active ingredient (including any ester or salt of the active ingredient) that has been approved in another application approved under subsection (b), is approved after the date of enactment of this subsection[10] and if such application contains reports of new clinical investigations (other than bioavailability studies) essential to the approval of the application and conducted or sponsored by the applicant, the Secretary may not make the approval of an application submitted under this subsection for the conditions of approval of such drug in the subsection (b) application effective before the expiration of three years from the date of the approval of the application under subsection (b) for such drug.

(iv) If a supplement to an application approved under subsection (b) is approved after the date of enactment of this subsection[10] and the supplement contains reports of new clinical investigations (other than bioavailability studies) essential to the approval of the supplement and conducted or sponsored by the person submitting the supplement, the Secretary may not make the approval of an application submitted under this subsection for a change approved in the supplement effective before the expiration of three years from the date of the approval of the supplement under subsection (b).

(v) If an application (or supplement to an application) submitted under subsection (b) for a drug, which includes an active ingredient (including any ester or salt of the active ingredient) that has been approved in another application under subsection (b), was approved during the period beginning January 1, 1982, and ending on the date of the enactment of this subsection, the Secretary may not make the approval of an application submitted under this subsection which refers to the drug for which the subsection

(b) application was submitted or which refers to a change approved in a supplement to the subsection (b) application effective before the expiration of two years from the date of enactment of this subsection.

(6) If a drug approved under this subsection refers in its approved application to a drug the approval of which was withdrawn or suspended for grounds described in the first sentence of subsection (e) or was withdrawn or suspended under this paragraph or which, as determined by the Secretary, has been withdrawn from sale for safety or effectiveness reasons, the approval of the drug under this subsection shall be withdrawn or suspended

(A) for the same period as the withdrawal or suspension under subsection (e) or this paragraph, or

(B) if the listed drug has been withdrawn from sale, for the period of withdrawal from sale or, if earlier, the period ending on the date the Secretary determines that the withdrawal from sale is not for safety or effectiveness reasons.

(7)

(A)

(i) Within 60 days of the date of the enactment of this subsection,[12] the Secretary shall publish and make available to the public

(I) a list in alphabetical order of the official and proprietary name of each drug which has been approved for safety and effectiveness under subsection (c) before the date of the enactment of this subsection.[11]

(II) the date of approval if the drug is approved after 1981 and the number of the application which was approved; and

(III) whether *in vitro* or *in vivo* bioequivalence studies, or both such studies, are required for applications filed under this subsection which will refer to the drug published.

(ii) Every 30 days after the publication of the first list under clause (i) the Secretary shall revise the list to include each drug which has been approved for safety and effectiveness under subsection (c) or approved under this subsection during the 30-day period.

(iii) When patent information submitted under subsection (b) or (c) respecting a drug included on the list is to be published by the Secretary, the Secretary shall, in revisions made under clause (ii), include such information for such drug.

(B) A drug approved for safety and effectiveness under subsection (c) or approved under this subsection shall, for purposes of this subsection, be considered to have been published under subparagraph (A) on the date of its approval or the date of enactment, whichever is later.

(C) If the approval of a drug was withdrawn or suspended for grounds described in the first sentence of subsection (e) or was withdrawn or suspended under paragraph (6) or if the Secretary determines that a drug has been withdrawn from sale for safety or effectiveness reasons, it may not be published in the list under subparagraph (A) or, if the withdrawal or suspension occurred after its publication in such list, it shall be immediately removed from such list

   (i) for the same period as the withdrawal or suspension under subsection (e) or paragraph (6), or

   (ii) if the listed drug has been withdrawn from sale, for the period of withdrawal from sale or, if earlier, the period ending on the date the Secretary determines that the withdrawal from sale is not for safety or effectiveness reasons.

   A notice of the removal shall be published in the Federal Register.

(8) For purposes of this subsection:

   (A)

      (i) The term "bioavailability" means the rate and extent to which the active ingredient or therapeutic ingredient is absorbed from a drug and becomes available at the site of drug action.

      (ii) For a drug that is not intended to be absorbed into the bloodstream, the Secretary may assess bioavailability by scientifically valid measurements intended to reflect the rate and extent to which the active ingredient or therapeutic ingredient becomes available at the site of drug action.

   (B) A drug shall be considered to be bioequivalent to a listed drug if

      (i) the rate and extent of absorption of the drug do not show a significant difference from the rate and extent of absorption of the listed drug when administered at the same molar dose of the therapeutic ingredient under similar experimental conditions in either a single dose or multiple doses; or

   (ii) the extent of absorption of the drug does not show a significant difference from the extent of absorption of the listed drug when administered at the same molar dose of the therapeutic ingredient under similar experimental conditions in either a single dose or multiple doses and the difference from the listed drug in the rate of absorption of the drug is intentional, is reflected in its proposed labeling, is not essential to the attainment of effective body drug concentrations on chronic use, and is considered medically insignificant for the drug.

  (C) For a drug that is not intended to be absorbed into the bloodstream, the Secretary may establish alternative, scientifically valid methods to show bioequivalence if the alternative methods are expected to detect a significant difference between the drug and the listed drug in safety and therapeutic effect.

(9) The Secretary shall, with respect to each application submitted under this subsection, maintain a record of

  (A) the name of the applicant,

  (B) the name of the drug covered by the application,

  (C) the name of each person to whom the review of the chemistry of the application was assigned and the date of such assignment, and

  (D) the name of each person to whom the bioequivalence review for such application was assigned and the date of such assignment.

      The information the Secretary is required to maintain under this paragraph with respect to an application submitted under this subsection shall be made available to the public after the approval of such application.

(k)

(1) In the case of any drug for which an approval of an application filed under subsection (b) or (j) is in effect, the applicant shall establish and maintain such records, and make such reports to the Secretary, of data relating to clinical experience and other data or information, received or otherwise obtained by such applicant with respect to such drug, as the Secretary may by general regulation, or by order with respect to such application, prescribe on the basis of a finding that such records and reports are necessary in order to enable the Secretary to determine, or facilitate a determination, whether there is or

may be ground for invoking subsection (e) of this section. Regulations and orders issued under this subsection and under subsection (i) shall have due regard for the professional ethics of the medical profession and the interests of patients and shall provide, where the Secretary deems it to be appropriate, for the examination, upon request, by the persons to whom such regulations or orders are applicable, of similar information received or otherwise obtained by the Secretary.

(2) Every person required under this section to maintain records, and every person in charge or custody thereof, shall, upon request of an officer or employee designated by the Secretary, permit such officer or employee at all reasonable times to have access to and copy and verify such records.

(l) Safety and effectiveness data and information which has been submitted in an application under subsection (b) for a drug and which has not previously been disclosed to the public shall be made available to the public, upon request, unless extraordinary circumstances are shown

(1) if no work is being or will be undertaken to have the application approved,

(2) if the Secretary has determined that the application is not approvable and all legal appeals have been exhausted,

(3) if approval of the application under subsection (c) is withdrawn and all legal appeals have been exhausted,

(4) if the Secretary has determined that such drug is not a new drug, or

(5) upon the effective date of the approval of the first application under subsection (j) which refers to such drug or upon the date upon which the approval of an application under subsection (j) which refers to such drug could be made effective if such an application had been submitted.

(m) For purposes of this section, the term "patent" means a patent issued by the United States Patent and Trademark Office.

(n)

(1) For the purpose of providing expert scientific advice and recommendations to the Secretary regarding a clinical investigation of a drug or the approval for marketing of a drug under section 505 or section 351 of the Public Health Service Act, the Secretary shall establish panels of experts or use panels of experts established before the date of enactment of the Food and Drug Administration Modernization Act of 1997, or both.

(2) The Secretary may delegate the appointment and oversight authority granted under section 904 to a director of a center or successor entity within the Food and Drug Administration.

(3) The Secretary shall make appointments to each panel established under paragraph (1) so that each panel shall consist of

   (A) members who are qualified by training and experience to evaluate the safety and effectiveness of the drugs to be referred to the panel and who, to the extent feasible, possess skill and experience in the development, manufacture, or utilization of such drugs;

   (B) members with diverse expertise in such fields as clinical and administrative medicine, pharmacy, pharmacology, pharmacoeconomics, biological and physical sciences, and other related professions;

   (C) a representative of consumer interests, and a representative of interests of the drug manufacturing industry not directly affected by the matter to be brought before the panel; and

   (D) two or more members who are specialists or have other expertise in the particular disease or condition for which the drug under review is proposed to be indicated.Scientific, trade, and consumer organizations shall be afforded an opportunity to nominate individuals for appointment to the panels. No individual who is in the regular full-time employ of the United States and engaged in the administration of this Act may be a voting member of any panel. The Secretary shall designate one of the members of each panel to serve as chairman thereof.

(4) Each member of a panel shall publicly disclose all conflicts of interest that member may have with the work to be undertaken by the panel. No member of a panel may vote on any matter where the member or the immediate family of such member could gain financially from the advice given to the Secretary. The Secretary may grant a waiver of any conflict of interest requirement upon public disclosure of such conflict of interest if such waiver is necessary to afford the panel essential expertise, except that the Secretary may not grant a waiver for a member of a panel when the member's own scientific work is involved.

(5) The Secretary shall, as appropriate, provide education and training to each new panel member before such member participates in a panel's activities, including education regarding requirements under this Act and related regulations of the Secretary, and the administrative processes and procedures related to panel meetings.

(6) Panel members (other than officers or employees of the United States), while attending meetings or conferences of a panel or otherwise engaged in its business, shall be entitled to receive compensation for each day so engaged, including travel time, at rates to be fixed by the Secretary, but not to exceed the daily equivalent of the rate in

effect for positions classified above grade GS–15 of the General Schedule. While serving away from their homes or regular places of business, panel members may be allowed travel expenses (including per diem in lieu of subsistence) as authorized by section 5703 of title 5, United States Code, for persons in the Government service employed intermittently.

(7) The Secretary shall ensure that scientific advisory panels meet regularly and at appropriate intervals so that any matter to be reviewed by such a panel can be presented to the panel not more than 60 days after the matter is ready for such review. Meetings of the panel may be held using electronic communication to convene the meetings.

(8) Within 90 days after a scientific advisory panel makes recommendations on any matter under its review, the Food and Drug Administration official responsible for the matter shall review the conclusions and recommendations of the panel, and notify the affected persons of the final decision on the matter, or of the reasons that no such decision has been reached. Each such final decision shall be documented including the rationale for the decision.

SEC. 505A. [21 U.S.C. 355a] PEDIATRIC STUDIES OF DRUGS.

(a) DEFINITIONS. As used in this section, the term "pediatric studies" or "studies" means at least one clinical investigation (that, at the Secretary's discretion, may include pharmacokinetic studies) in pediatric age groups (including neonates in appropriate cases) in which a drug is anticipated to be used.

(b) MARKET EXCLUSIVITY FOR NEW DRUGS. If, prior to approval of an application that is submitted under section 505(b)(1), the Secretary determines that information relating to the use of a new drug in the pediatric population may produce health benefits in that population, the Secretary makes a written request for pediatric studies (which shall include a timeframe for completing such studies), and such studies are completed within any such timeframe and the reports thereof submitted in accordance with subsection (d)(2) or accepted in accordance with subsection (d)(3)

(1)

   (A)

      (i) the period referred to in subsection (c)(3)(D)(ii) of section 505, and in subsection (j)(5)(F)(ii) of such section, is deemed to be five years and six months rather than five years, and the references in subsections (c)(3)(D)(ii) and (j)(5)(F)(ii) of such section to four years, to forty-eight months, and to seven and one-half years are deemed to be four and one-half years, fifty-four months, and eight years, respectively; or

(ii) the period referred to in clauses (iii) and (iv) of subsection (c)(3)(D) of such section, and in clauses (iii) and (iv) of subsection (j)(5)(F) of such section, is deemed to be three years and six months rather than three years; and

(B) if the drug is designated under section 526 for a rare disease or condition, the period referred to in section 527(a) is deemed to be seven years and six months rather than seven years; and

(2)

(A) if the drug is the subject of

(i) a listed patent for which a certification has been submitted under subsection (b)(2)(A)(ii) or (j)(2)(A)(vii)(II) of section 505 and for which pediatric studies were submitted prior to the expiration of the patent (including any patent extensions); or

(ii) a listed patent for which a certification has been submitted under subsections (b)(2)(A)(iii) or (j)(2)(A)(vii)(III) of section 505, the period during which an application may not be approved under section 505(c)(3) or section 505(j)(5)(B) shall be extended by a period of six months after the date the patent expires (including any patent extensions); or

(B) if the drug is the subject of a listed patent for which a certification has been submitted under subsection (b)(2)(A)(iv) or (j)(2)(A)(vii)(IV) of section 505, and in the patent infringement litigation resulting from the certification the court determines that the patent is valid and would be infringed, the period during which an application may not be approved under section 505(c)(3) or section 505(j)(5)(B) shall be extended by a period of six months after the date the patent expires (including any patent extensions).

(C) MARKET EXCLUSIVITY FOR ALREADY-MARKETED DRUGS. If the Secretary determines that information relating to the use of an approved drug in the pediatric population may produce health benefits in that population and makes a written request to the holder of an approved application under section 505(b)(1) for pediatric studies (which shall include a timeframe for completing such studies), the holder agrees to the request, the studies are completed within any such timeframe, and the reports thereof are submitted in accordance with subsection (d)(2) or accepted in accordance with subsection (d)(3)

(1)

    (A) (i) the period referred to in subsection (c)(3)(D)(ii) of section 505, and in subsection (j)(5)(F)(ii) of such section, is deemed to be five years and six months rather than five years, and the references in subsections (c)(3)(D)(ii) and (j)(5)(F)(ii) of such section to four years, to forty-eight months, and to seven and one-half years are deemed to be four and one-half years, fifty-four months, and eight years, respectively; or (ii) the period referred to in clauses (iii) and (iv) of subsection (c)(3)(D) of such section, and in clauses (iii) and (iv) of subsection (j)(5)(F) of such section, is deemed to be three years and six months rather than three years; and

    (B) if the drug is designated under section 526 for a rare disease or condition, the period referred to in section 527(a) is deemed to be seven years and six months rather than seven years; and

(2)

    (A) if the drug is the subject of

        (i) a listed patent for which a certification has been submitted under subsection (b)(2)(A)(ii) or (j)(2)(A)(vii)(II) of section 505 and for which pediatric studies were submitted prior to the expiration of the patent (including any patent extensions); or

        (ii) a listed patent for which a certification has been submitted under subsection (b)(2)(A)(iii) or (j)(2)(A)(vii)(III) of section 505, the period during which an application may not be approved under section 505(c)(3) or section 505(j)(5)(B)(ii) shall be extended by a period of six months after the date the patent expires (including any patent extensions); or

    (B) if the drug is the subject of a listed patent for which a certification has been submitted under subsection (b)(2)(A)(iv) or (j)(2)(A)(vii)(IV) of section 505, and in the patent infringement litigation resulting from the certification the court determines that the patent is valid and would be infringed, the period during which an application may not be approved under section 505(c)(3) or section 505(j)(5)(B) shall be extended by a period of six months after the date the patent expires (including any patent extensions).

(d) CONDUCT OF PEDIATRIC STUDIES.

    (1) AGREEMENT FOR STUDIES. The Secretary may, pursuant to a written request from the Secretary under subsection (b) or (c), after consultation with

(A) the sponsor of an application for an investigational new drug under section 505(i);

(B) the sponsor of an application for a new drug under section 505(b)(1); or

(C) the holder of an approved application for a drug under section 505(b)(1),agree with the sponsor or holder for the conduct of pediatric studies for such drug. Such agreement shall be in writing and shall include a timeframe for such studies.

(2) WRITTEN PROTOCOLS TO MEET THE STUDIES REQUIRE-MENT. If the sponsor or holder and the Secretary agree upon written protocols for the studies, the studies requirement of subsection (b) or (c) is satisfied upon the completion of the studies and submission of the reports thereof in accordance with the original written request and the written agreement referred to in paragraph (1). In reaching an agreement regarding written protocols, the Secretary shall take into account adequate representation of children of ethnic and racial minorities. Not later than 60 days after the submission of the report of the studies, the Secretary shall determine if such studies were or were not conducted in accordance with the original written request and the written agreement and reported in accordance with the requirements of the Secretary for filing and so notify the sponsor or holder.

(3) OTHER METHODS TO MEET THE STUDIES REQUIREMENT. If the sponsor or holder and the Secretary have not agreed in writing on the protocols for the studies, the studies requirement of subsection (b) or (c) is satisfied when such studies have been completed and the reports accepted by the Secretary. Not later than 90 days after the submission of the reports of the studies, the Secretary shall accept or reject such reports and so notify the sponsor or holder. The Secretary's only responsibility in accepting or rejecting the reports shall be to determine, within the 90 days, whether the studies fairly respond to the written request, have been conducted in accordance with commonly accepted scientific principles and protocols, and have been reported in accordance with the requirements of the Secretary for filing.

(4) WRITTEN REQUEST TO HOLDERS OF APPROVED APPLICATIONS FOR DRUGS THAT HAVE MARKET EXCLUSIVITY

(A) REQUEST AND RESPONSE. If the Secretary makes a written request for pediatric studies (including neonates, as appropriate) under subsection (c) to the holder of an application approved under section 505(b)(1), the holder, not later than 180 days after receiving the written request, shall respond to the Secretary as to the intention of the holder to act on the request by

(i) indicating when the pediatric studies will be initiated, if the holder agrees to the request; or

(ii) indicating that the holder does not agree to the request.

(B) NO AGREEMENT TO REQUEST

(i) REFERRAL. If the holder does not agree to a written request within the time period specified in subparagraph (A), and if the Secretary determines that there is a continuing need for information relating to the use of the drug in the pediatric population (including neonates, as appropriate), the Secretary shall refer the drug to the Foundation for the National Institutes of Health established under section 499 of the Public Health Service Act (42 U.S.C. 290b) (referred to in this paragraph as the "Foundation") for the conduct of the pediatric studies described in the written request.

(ii) PUBLIC NOTICE. The Secretary shall give public notice of the name of the drug, the name of the manufacturer, and the indications to be studied made in a referral under clause (i).

(C) LACK OF FUNDS. On referral of a drug under subparagraph (B)(i), the Foundation shall issue a proposal to award a grant to conduct the requested studies unless the Foundation certifies to the Secretary, within a timeframe that the Secretary determines is appropriate through guidance, that the Foundation does not have funds available under section 499(j)(9)(B)(i) to conduct the requested studies. If the Foundation so certifies, the Secretary shall refer the drug for inclusion on the list established under section 409I of the Public Health Service Act for the conduct of the studies.

(D) EFFECT OF SUBSECTION. Nothing in this subsection (including with respect to referrals from the Secretary to the Foundation) alters or amends section 301(j) of this Act or section 552 of title 5 or section 1905 of title 18, United States Code.

(E) NO REQUIREMENT TO REFER. Nothing in this subsection shall be construed to require that every declined written request shall be referred to the Foundation.

(F) WRITTEN REQUESTS UNDER SUBSECTION (b). For drugs under subsection (b) for which written requests have not been accepted, if the Secretary determines that there is a continuing need for information relating to the use of the drug in the pediatric population (including neonates, as appropriate), the Secretary shall issue a written request under subsection (c) after the date of approval of the drug.

(e) DELAY OF EFFECTIVE DATE FOR CERTAIN APPLICATION. If the Secretary determines that the acceptance or approval of an application under section 505(b)(2) or 505(j) for a new drug may occur after submission of reports of pediatric studies under this section, which were submitted prior to the expiration of the patent (including any patent extension) or the applicable period under clauses (ii) through (iv) of section 505(c)(3)(D) or clauses (ii) through (iv) of section 505(j)(5)(F), but before the Secretary has determined whether the requirements of subsection (d) have been satisfied, the Secretary shall delay the acceptance or approval under section 505(b)(2) or 505(j) until the determination under subsection (d) is made, but any such delay shall not exceed 90 days. In the event that requirements of this section are satisfied, the applicable six month period under subsection (b) or (c) shall be deemed to have been running during the period of delay.

(f) NOTICE OF DETERMINATIONS ON STUDIES REQUIREMENT. The Secretary shall publish a notice of any determination that the requirements of subsection (d) have been met and that submissions and approvals under subsection (b)(2) or (j) of section 505 for a drug will be subject to the provisions of this section.

(g) LIMITATIONS. A drug to which the six-month period under subsection (b) or (c) has already been applied

(1) may receive an additional six-month period under subsection (c)(1)(A)(ii) for a supplemental application if all other requirements under this section are satisfied, except that such a drug may not receive any additional such period under subsection (c)(2); and

(2) may not receive any additional such period under subsection (c)(1)(B).

(h) RELATIONSHIP TO PEDIATRIC RESEARCH REQUIREMENTS. Notwithstanding any other provision of law, if any pediatric study is required by a provision of law (including a regulation) other than this section and such study meets the completeness, timeliness, and other requirements of this section, such study shall be deemed to satisfy the requirement for market exclusivity pursuant to this section.

(i) LABELING SUPPLEMENTS

(1) PRIORITY STATUS FOR PEDIATRIC SUPPLEMENTS. Any supplement to an application under section 505 proposing a labeling change pursuant to a report on a pediatric study under this section

(A) shall be considered to be a priority supplement, and

(B) shall be subject to the performance goals established by the Commissioner for priority drugs.

(2) DISPUTE RESOLUTION

    (A) REQUEST FOR LABELING CHANGE AND FAILURE TO AGREE. If the Commissioner determines that an application with respect to which a pediatric study is conducted under this section is approvable and that the only open issue for final action on the application is the reaching of an agreement between the sponsor of the application and the Commissioner on appropriate changes to the labeling for the drug that is the subject of the application, not later than 180 days after the date of submission of the application

        (i) the Commissioner shall request that the sponsor of the application make any labeling change that the Commissioner determines to be appropriate; and

        (ii) if the sponsor of the application does not agree to make a labeling change requested by the Commissioner, the Commissioner shall refer the matter to the Pediatric Advisory Committee.

    (B) ACTION BY THE PEDIATRIC ADVISORY SUBCOMMITTEE OF THE ANTI-INFECTIVE DRUGS ADVISORY COMMITTEE. Not later than 90 days after receiving a referral under subparagraph (A)(ii), the Pediatric Advisory Committee shall

        (i) review the pediatric study reports, and

        (ii) make a recommendation to the Commissioner concerning appropriate labeling changes, if any.

    (C) CONSIDERATION OF RECOMMENDATIONS. The Commissioner shall consider the recommendations of the Pediatric Advisory Committee and, if appropriate, not later than 30 days after receiving the recommendation, make a request to the sponsor of the application to make any labeling change that the Commissioner determines to be appropriate.

    (D) MISBRANDING. If the sponsor of the application, within 30 days after receiving a request under subparagraph (C), does not agree to make a labeling change requested by the Commissioner, the Commissioner may deem the drug that is the subject of the application to be misbranded.

    (E) NO EFFECT ON AUTHORITY. Nothing in this subsection limits the authority of the United States to bring an enforcement action under this Act when a drug lacks appropriate pediatric labeling. Neither course of action (the Pediatric Advisory Committee process or an enforcement action referred to in the preceding sentence) shall preclude, delay, or serve as the basis to stay the other course of action.

(j)   DISSEMINATION OF PEDIATRIC INFORMATION

    (1)   IN GENERAL. Not later than 180 days after the date of submission of a report on a pediatric study under this section, the Commissioner shall make available to the public a summary of the medical and clinical pharmacology reviews of pediatric studies conducted for the supplement, including by publication in the Federal Register.

    (2)   EFFECT OF SUBSECTION. Nothing in this subsection alters or amends section 301(j) of this Act or section 552 of title 5 or section 1905 of title 18, United States Code.

(k)   CLARIFICATION OF INTERACTION OF MARKET EXCLUSIVITY UNDER THIS SECTION AND MARKET EXCLUSIVITY AWARDED TO AN APPLICANT FOR APPROVAL OF A DRUG UNDER SECTION 505(j). If a 180-day period under section 505(j)(5)(B)(iv) overlaps with a 6-month exclusivity period under this section, so that the applicant for approval of a drug under section 505(j) entitled to the 180-day period under that section loses a portion of the 180-day period to which the applicant is entitled for the drug, the 180-day period shall be extended from

    (1)   the date on which the 180-day period would have expired by the number of days of the overlap, if the 180-day period would, but for the application of this subsection, expire after the 6-month exclusivity period; or

    (2)   the date on which the 6-month exclusivity period expires, by the number of days of the overlap if the 180-day period would, but for the application of this subsection, expire during the six-month exclusivity period.

(l)   PROMPT APPROVAL OF DRUGS UNDER SECTION 505(j) WHEN PEDIATRIC INFORMATION IS ADDED TO LABELING.

    (1)   GENERAL RULE. A drug for which an application has been submitted or approved under section 505(j) shall not be considered ineligible for approval under that section or misbranded under section 502 on the basis that the labeling of the drug omits a pediatric indication or any other aspect of labeling pertaining to pediatric use when the omitted indication or other aspect is protected by patent or by exclusivity under clause (iii) or (iv) of section 505(j)(5)(F).

    (2)   LABELING. Notwithstanding clauses (iii) and (iv) of section 505(j)(5)(F), the Secretary may require that the labeling of a drug approved under section 505(j) that omits a pediatric indication or other aspect of labeling as described in paragraph (1) include

        (A)   a statement that, because of marketing exclusivity for a manufacturer

            (i)   the drug is not labeled for pediatric use; or

            (ii)   in the case of a drug for which there is an additional pediatric use not referred to in paragraph (1), the drug is not labeled for the pediatric use under paragraph (1); and

(B) a statement of any appropriate pediatric contraindications, warnings, or precautions that the Secretary considers necessary.

(3) PRESERVATION OF PEDIATRIC EXCLUSIVITY AND OTHER PROVISIONS. This subsection does not affect

(A) the availability or scope of exclusivity under this section,

(B) the availability or scope of exclusivity under section 505 for pediatric formulations,

(C) the question of the eligibility for approval of any application under section 505(j) that omits any other conditions of approval entitled to exclusivity under clause (iii) or (iv) of section 505(j)(5)(F), or

(D) except as expressly provided in paragraphs (1) and (2), the operation of section 505.

(m) REPORT. The Secretary shall conduct a study and report to Congress not later than January 1, 2001, based on the experience under the program established under this section. The study and report shall examine all relevant issues, including

(1) the effectiveness of the program in improving information about important pediatric uses for approved drugs;

(2) the adequacy of the incentive provided under this section;

(3) the economic impact of the program on taxpayers and consumers, including the impact of the lack of lower cost generic drugs on patients, including on lower income patients; and

(4) any suggestions for modification that the Secretary determines to be appropriate.

(n) SUNSET. A drug may not receive any six-month period under subsection (b) or (c) unless

(1) on or before October 1, 2007, the Secretary makes a written request for pediatric studies of the drug;

(2) on or before October 1, 2007, an application for the drug is accepted for filing under section 505(b); and

(3) all requirements of this section are met.

SEC. 505B. (21 U.S.C. 355C) RESEARCH INTO PEDIATRIC USES FOR DRUGS AND BIOLOGICAL PRODUCTS

(a) NEW DRUGS AND BIOLOGICAL PRODUCTS

(1) IN GENERAL. A person that submits an application (or supplement to an application)

    (A) under section 505 for a new active ingredient, new indication, new dosage form, new dosing regimen, or new route of administration; or

    (B) under section 351 of the Public Health Service Act (42 U.S.C. 262) for a new active ingredient, new indication, new dosage form, new dosing regimen, or new route of administration shall submit with the application the assessments described in paragraph (2).

(2) ASSESSMENTS

    (A) IN GENERAL. The assessments referred to in paragraph (1) shall contain data, gathered using appropriate formulations for each age group for which the assessment is required, that are adequate

        (i) to assess the safety and effectiveness of the drug or the biological product for the claimed indications in all relevant pediatric subpopulations; and

        (ii) to support dosing and administration for each pediatric subpopulation for which the drug or the biological product is safe and effective.

    (B) SIMILAR COURSE OF DISEASE OR SIMILAR EFFECT OF DRUG OR BIOLOGICAL PRODUCT-

        (i) IN GENERAL. If the course of the disease and the effects of the drug are sufficiently similar in adults and pediatric patients, the Secretary may conclude that pediatric effectiveness can be extrapolated from adequate and well-controlled studies in adults, usually supplemented with other information obtained in pediatric patients, such as pharmacokinetic studies.

        (ii) EXTRAPOLATION BETWEEN AGE GROUPS. A study may not be needed in each pediatric age group if data from 1 age group can be extrapolated to another age group.

(3) DEFERRAL. On the initiative of the Secretary or at the request of the applicant, the Secretary may defer submission of some or all assessments required under paragraph (1) until a specified date after approval of the drug or issuance of the license for a biological product if

    (A) the Secretary finds that

        (i) the drug or biological product is ready for approval for use in adults before pediatric studies are complete,

        (ii) pediatric studies should be delayed until additional safety or effectiveness data have been collected, or

        (iii) there is another appropriate reason for deferral, and

(B) the applicant submits to the Secretary
   (i) certification of the grounds for deferring the assessments,
   (ii) a description of the planned or ongoing studies, and
   (iii) evidence that the studies are being conducted or will be conducted with due diligence and at the earliest possible time.

(4) WAIVERS

(A) FULL WAIVER. On the initiative of the Secretary or at the request of an applicant, the Secretary shall grant a full waiver, as appropriate, of the requirement to submit assessments for a drug or biological product under this subsection if the applicant certifies and the Secretary finds that
   (i) necessary studies are impossible or highly impracticable (because, for example, the number of patients is so small or the patients are geographically dispersed);
   (ii) there is evidence strongly suggesting that the drug or biological product would be ineffective or unsafe in all pediatric age groups; or
   (iii) the drug or biological product
      (I) does not represent a meaningful therapeutic benefit over existing therapies for pediatric patients; and
      (II) is not likely to be used in a substantial number of pediatric patients.

(B) PARTIAL WAIVER. On the initiative of the Secretary or at the request of an applicant, the Secretary shall grant a partial waiver, as appropriate, of the requirement to submit assessments for a drug or biological product under this subsection with respect to a specific pediatric age group if the applicant certifies and the Secretary finds that
   (i) necessary studies are impossible or highly impracticable (because, for example, the number of patients in that age group is so small or patients in that age group are geographically dispersed);
   (ii) there is evidence strongly suggesting that the drug or biological product would be ineffective or unsafe in that age group;
   (iii) the drug or biological product
      (I) does not represent a meaningful therapeutic benefit over existing therapies for pediatric patients in that age group; and
      (II) is not likely to be used by a substantial number of pediatric patients in that age group; or

(iv) the applicant can demonstrate that reasonable attempts to produce a pediatric formulation necessary for that age group have failed

(C) PEDIATRIC FORMULATION NOT POSSIBLE. If a waiver is granted on the ground that it is not possible to develop a pediatric formulation, the waiver shall cover only the pediatric groups requiring that formulation.

(D) LABELING REQUIREMENT. If the Secretary grants a full or partial waiver because there is evidence that a drug or biological product would be ineffective or unsafe in pediatric populations, the information shall be included in the labeling for the drug or biological product.

(b) MARKETED DRUGS AND BIOLOGICAL PRODUCTS

(1) IN GENERAL. After providing notice in the form of a letter and an opportunity for written response and a meeting, which may include an advisory committee meeting, the Secretary may (by order in the form of a letter) require the holder of an approved application for a drug under section 505 or the holder of a license for a biological product under section 351 of the Public Health Service Act (42 U. S.C. 262) to submit by a specified date the assessments described in subsection (a)(2) if the Secretary finds that

(A)

(i) the drug or biological product is used for a substantial number of pediatric patients for the labeled indications; and

(ii) the absence of adequate labeling could pose significant risks to pediatric patients; or

(B)

(i) there is reason to believe that the drug or biological product would represent a meaningful therapeutic benefit over existing therapies for pediatric patients for 1 or more of the claimed indications; and

(ii) the absence of adequate labeling could pose significant risks to pediatric patients.

(2) WAIVERS

(A) FULL WAIVER. At the request of an applicant, the Secretary shall grant a full waiver, as appropriate, of the requirement to submit assessments under this subsection if the applicant certifies and the Secretary finds that

(i) necessary studies are impossible or highly impracticable (because, for example, the number of patients in that age group is so small or patients in that age group are geographically dispersed); or

      (ii) there is evidence strongly suggesting that the drug or bio-logical product would be ineffective or unsafe in all pediatric age groups.

  (B) PARTIAL WAIVER. At the request of an applicant, the Secretary shall grant a partial waiver, as appropriate, of the requirement to submit assessments under this subsection with respect to a specific pediatric age group if the applicant certifies and the Secretary finds that

      (i) necessary studies are impossible or highly impracticable (because, for example, the number of patients in that age group is so small or patients in that age group are geographically dispersed);

      (ii) there is evidence strongly suggesting that the drug or bio-logical product would be ineffective or unsafe in that age group;

      (iii)

         (I) the drug or biological product

            (aa) does not represent a meaningful therapeutic benefit over existing therapies for pediatric patients in that age group; and

            (bb) is not likely to be used in a substantial number of pediatric patients in that age group; and

         (II) the absence of adequate labeling could not pose significant risks to pediatric patients; or

      (iv) the applicant can demonstrate that reasonable attempts to produce a pediatric formulation necessary for that age group have failed.

  (C) PEDIATRIC FORMULATION NOT POSSIBLE. If a waiver is granted on the ground that it is not possible to develop a pediatric formulation, the waiver shall cover only the pediatric groups requiring that formulation.

  (D) LABELING REQUIREMENT. If the Secretary grants a full or partial waiver because there is evidence that a drug or biological product would be ineffective or unsafe in pediatric populations, the information shall be included in the labeling for the drug or biological product.

(3) RELATIONSHIP TO OTHER PEDIATRIC PROVISIONS

  (A) NO ASSESSMENT WITHOUT WRITTEN REQUEST. No assessment may be required under paragraph (1) for a drug subject to an approved application under section 505 unless

      (i) the Secretary has issued a written request for a related pediatric study under section 505A(c) of this Act or section 409I of the Public Health Service Act (42 U.S.C. 284m);

(ii)

    (I) if the request was made under section 505A(c)

        (aa) the recipient of the written request does not agree to the request; or

        (bb) the Secretary does not receive a response as specified under section 505A(d)(4)(A); or

    (II) if the request was made under section 409I of the Public Health Service Act (42 U.S.C. 284m)

        (aa) the recipient of the written request does not agree to the request; or

        (bb) the Secretary does not receive a response as specified under section 409I(c)(2) of that Act; and

(iii) (I) the Secretary certifies under subparagraph (B) that there are insufficient funds under sections 409I and 499 of the Public Health Service Act (42 U.S.C. 284m, 290b) to conduct the study; or

    (II) the Secretary publishes in the Federal Register a certification that certifies that

        (aa) no contract or grant has been awarded under section 409I or 499 of the Public Health Service Act (42 U.S.C. 284m, 290b); and

        (bb) not less than 270 days have passed since the date of a certification under subparagraph (B) that there are sufficient funds to conduct the study.

(B) NO AGREEMENT TO REQUEST. Not later than 60 days after determining that no holder will agree to the written request (including a determination that the Secretary has not received a response specified under section 505A(d) of this Act or section 409I of the Public Health Service Act (42 U.S.C. 284m), the Secretary shall certify whether the Secretary has sufficient funds to conduct the study under section 409I or 499 of the Public Health Service Act (42 U.S.C. 284m, 290b), taking into account the prioritization under section 409I.

(c) MEANINGFUL THERAPEUTIC BENEFIT. For the purposes of paragraph (4)(A)(iii)(I) and (4)(B)(iii)(I) of subsection (a) and paragraphs (1)(B)(i) and (2)(B)(iii)(I)(aa) of subsection (b), a drug or biological product shall be considered to represent a meaningful therapeutic benefit over existing therapies if the Secretary estimates that

      (1) if approved, the drug or biological product would represent a significant improvement in the treatment, diagnosis, or prevention of a disease, compared with marketed products adequately labeled for that use in the relevant pediatric population; or

      (2) the drug or biological product is in a class of products or for an indication for which there is a need for additional options.

(d) SUBMISSION OF ASSESSMENTS. If a person fails to submit an assessment described in subsection (a)(2), or a request for approval of a pediatric formulation described in subsection (a) or (b), in accordance with applicable provisions of subsections (a) and (b)

      (1) the drug or biological product that is the subject of the assessment or request may be considered misbranded solely because of that failure and subject to relevant enforcement action (except that the drug or biological product shall not be subject to action under section 303); but

      (2) the failure to submit the assessment or request shall not be the basis for a proceeding

         (A) to withdraw approval for a drug under section 505(e); or

         (B) to revoke the license for a biological product under section 351 of the Public Health Service Act (42 U.S.C. 262).

(e) MEETINGS. Before and during the investigational process for a new drug or biological product, the Secretary shall meet at appropriate times with the sponsor of the new drug or biological product to discuss

      (1) information that the sponsor submits on plans and timelines for pediatric studies; or

      (2) any planned request by the sponsor for waiver or deferral of pediatric studies.

(f) SCOPE OF AUTHORITY. Nothing in this section provides to the Secretary any authority to require a pediatric assessment of any drug or biological product, or any assessment regarding other populations or uses of a drug or biological product, other than the pediatric assessments described in this section.

(g) ORPHAN DRUGS. Unless the Secretary requires otherwise by regulation, this section does not apply to any drug for an indication for which orphan designation has been granted under section 526.

(h) INTEGRATION WITH OTHER PEDIATRIC STUDIES. The authority under this section shall remain in effect so long as an application subject to this section may be accepted for filing by the Secretary on or before the date specified in section 505A(n).

REFERENCES

April 10, 1987, letter from then Acting Director of the Center for Drugs and Biologics to all NDA and ANDA holders and applicants.

"Abbreviated New Drug Application Regulations; Proposed Rule," *Federal Register* 54, no. 130, (Monday, July 10, 1989): 28872.

"Abbreviated New Drug Regulations; Final Rule," *Federal Register* 57, no. 82, (Tuesday, April 28, 1992): 17950.sss

"Abbreviated New Drug Application Regulations; Patent and Exclusivity Provisions; Final Rule," *Federal Register* 59, no. 190, (Monday, October 3, 1994): 50338.

Glossary

505(b)(2) application. an application submitted under section 505(b)(1) of the Act for a drug for which one or more of the investigations relied on by the applicant for approval of the "application were not conducted by or for the applicant and for which the applicant has not obtained a right of reference or use from the person by or for whom the investigations were conducted" [21 U.S.C. 355(b)(2)].

active ingredient. "any component that is intended to furnish pharmacological activity or other direct effect in the diagnosis, cure, mitigation, treatment, or prevention of disease, or to affect the structure or any function of the body of man or of animals. The term includes those components that may undergo chemical change in the manufacture of the drug product and be present in the drug product in a modified form intended to furnish the specified activity or effect" [21 CFR 60.3(b)(2)].

active moiety. "the molecule or ion, excluding those appended portions of the molecule that cause the drug to be an ester, salt (including a salt with hydrogen or coordination bonds), or other noncovalent derivative (such as a complex, chelate, or clathrate) of the molecule, responsible for the physiological or pharmacological action of the drug substance" [21 CFR 314.108(a)].

investigations relied on for approval. those without which the application cannot be approved (i.e., animal and human safety tests as well as clinical investigations of effectiveness).

listed drug. "a new drug product that has an effective approval under section 505(c) of the act for safety and effectiveness or under section 505(j) of the act, which has not been withdrawn or suspended under section 505(e)(1) through (e)(5) or (j)(5) of the act, and which has not been withdrawn from sale for what the FDA has determined are reasons of safety or effectiveness. Listed drug status is evidenced by the drug product's identification as a drug with an effective approval in the current edition of FDA's 'Approved Drug Products with Therapeutic Equivalence Evaluations' (the list) or any current supplement thereto, as a drug with an effective approval. A drug product is deemed to be a listed drug on the date of effective approval of the application or abbreviated application for that drug product" [21 CFR 314.3(b)].

literature. published reports of well-controlled studies that support safety or effectiveness; proposed and final monographs published in the Federal Register; the data supporting a Federal Register notice announcing a product's safety and/or effectiveness.

Orange Book. *Approved Drug Products with Therapeutic Equivalence Evaluations* and any current supplement to the publication.

pharmaceutical equivalent or duplicate. "drug products that contain identical amounts of the identical active drug ingredient, i.e., the same salt or ester of the same therapeutic moiety, in identical dosage forms, but not necessarily containing the same inactive ingredients, and that meet the identical compendial or other applicable standard of identity, strength, quality, and purity, including potency and, where applicable, content uniformity disintegration times and/or dissolution rates" [21 CFR 320.1(c)]. Products with different mechanisms of release can be considered to be pharmaceutical equivalents or duplicates.

referenced-listed drug. "the listed drug identified by the FDA as the drug product upon which an applicant relies in seeking approval of its abbreviated application" [21 CFR 314.3(b)].

right of reference or use. "the authority to rely upon, and otherwise use, an investigation for the purpose of obtaining approval of an application, including the ability to make available the underlying raw data from the investigation for FDA audit, if necessary" [21 CFR 314.3(b)].

Sponsors have the right of reference to any studies (1) they conduct, (2) that are conducted for them, or (3) for which they formally obtain a documented *right of reference.*

An applicant is not considered to have a *right of reference* to published studies because the applicant does not have access to the raw data. However, if the raw data are in the public domain, a right of reference is unnecessary.

suitability petition. a citizen petition submitted to the Agency seeking permission to file an abbreviated new drug application for a change from a listed drug in dosage form, strength, route of administration, or active ingredient in a combination product [See section 505(j)(2)(C) of the Act]

CHAPTER 7

Abbreviated New Drug Applications (ANDAs)

The ANDA is intended to streamline the review process for genetic versions of approved drug products. It was originally designed with two complimentary intents: to reduce the review time and work effort involved in review of New Drug Applications and to provide a simplified pathway for submission of applications for generic versions of already approved drugs. The ANDA has earned a positive track record in both of these areas.

Yet, despite the simplified process, ANDAs have swamped the FDA in recent years. In 2000, approximately 300 ANDAs were submitted. By 2006, the annual ANDA count had increased to almost 800 applications. And there has been no sign of the growth curve decreasing. No doubt, without the shortened ANDA process, the wave would be even more daunting, but, even with the simplified version, the FDA is fighting a constant battle to keep up with a rapidly rising tide.

Despite this dilemma and its streamlining response, the focus and intent of ANDA has remained constant: to provide data demonstrating the safety and effectiveness of an applicant drug. While the ANDA strives to establish that safety and efficacy for a generic version of an existing drug, the goal is fully compatible with the New Drug Application (NDA) [and the with 505(b)2 version of the NDA]. This intent and process are established in 21 Code of Federal Regulations (CFR) 314.94 (ANDA for Drug Product) and in 21 CFR 314.420 [Drug Master File (DMF) for Drug Substances].

ANDA CONTENT

An ANDA relies heavily on the previously approved NDA for evidence of efficacy and ultimate safety and concentrates instead on the manufacturing issues related to the specific generic formulation. Specifically, the ANDA focuses on three areas: Formulation and manufacturing, container integrity

---

Guidebook for Drug Regulatory Submissions, by Sandy Weinberg
Copyright © 2009 John Wiley & Sons, Inc.

and packaging, and stability and expiration. More specifically, it focuses on the DMF portion of the ANDA details.

Characterization of the DMF: specifications of the DMF content

Synthesis process: chemical formulae and process for synthesizing the drug product

In-process quality and safety controls:

Process Analytical Technology or conventional periodic production checks on quality, purity, contaminants, and safety controls

Analytical methods: technical tests used to determine analytical characteristics

Specifications: detailed chemical description of product

Stability data: shelf life and storage condition stability information

The Drug Product sections describe the following:

Formulation of the drug product: methodology for formulating, including intermediate steps and incipients

Manufacturing process: pilot and full production plans

In-process quality and safety controls: Process Analytical Technology or conventional periodic production checks on quality, purity, contaminants, and safety controls

Analytical methods: technical tests used to determine analytical characteristics

Specifications: detailed chemical description of product

Stability data: shelf life and storage condition stability information

In all of these areas, the ANDA incorporates and makes reference to elements common to the original NDA and describes and explicates areas of difference from the NDA. A tacit FDA review criterion is whether or not the ANDA drug represents sufficient overlap with the original NDA to characterize and incorporate the original NDA-approved product rather than a new drug itself.

DIFFERENCES WITH 505(b)2

Because of the "Abbreviated" nomenclature in the ANDA title and because of the often shortened form of the NDA represented by the 505(b)2 NDA, there has been some confusion between the two applications. Perhaps the ANDA should have been called the "Abbreviated Generic Drug Application" form: it is appropriate only as an application for a manufacturing variant of an approved (via an NDA) new drug, presumably off patent or exclusivity. The

505(b)2 NDA, on the other hand, is an application describing a new drug never before approved, albeit one for which research independent of the applicant has been conducted and is referenced.

The 505(b)2 abbreviates the NDA by incorporating outside research; the ANDA abbreviates the process by incorporating data in a previously approved NDA.

EMERGING INITIATIVES

As an unprecedented number of drugs go off patent, as the individualized drug reactions represented by variants in gender, age, and genetics are better understood, and as the modifications of side effect profiles represented by even minor changes in manufacturing processes and in-process controls are more tightly measured, the number of ANDAs submitted is expected to continue to rise dramatically. Here are clearly strong economic and reaction pressures encouraging and rewarding companies that focus their energies on the development of generic versions of blockbuster drugs.

With FDA resources ever under triage, the Agency is intensely seeking ways to improve the ANDA review process. There are three strategies—two official, one *sub rosa*—in process.

First, the FDA is in the process of revising the basic current Good Manufacturing Practices (cGMP) to better reflect current industry automation and procedural realities. This initiative, titled "CGMP for the 21st Century" is an attempt to catch up with the European Medicines Agency (EMEA) GAMP4-GAMP5 (General Assistance Medical Programs) series. While a final version is still several years away, preliminary indications are that it will incorporate key automation elements of 21 CFR Part 11; will better harmonize with GAMP and International Conference on Harmonization (ICH) guidelines; and will address active pharmaceutical ingredient (API) and formulation issues in greater detail.

Second, the ICH is itself issuing revised (and improved) guidelines that should clarify several ANDA issues. ICH Q10 is available in draft form and is now under final review, providing greater clarification of DMF-related manufacturing issues. In addition, four ICH quality-related guidelines—Q1ARs, Q3AR, Q3BR, and Q3C—have been released with strong guidance to more tightly define appropriate in-process control procedures. Together, these ICH guidelines provide clear direction for manufacturing control in an ANDA (or other) environment.

Finally, and less formally, the FDA is increasing pressure on and inspection of international manufacturers of API and final drug product, particularly in China and India. This new pressure, largely a result of the alleged heparin contamination, will likely have the *sub rosa* effect of slowing down the process of developing new generic drugs while both reducing the number and increasing the quality of ANDAs. Generic drug companies producing in whole or part in Asia will be forced in invest in top-level quality controls and in the documentation of those controls, likely reducing the number of ANDAs and improving the quality of those submitted.

Together, these three initiatives should reduce the ANDA workload over the next three to five years, though they do not represent long-term solutions to the processing effort problem. In many ways, the ANDA situation is simply a reflection of the problems in NDA review and will ultimately be solved only through a significant expansion of the FDA and its resources, a shifting of some FDA responsibility to other agencies (for example, moving Vaccine review to the National Institutes of Health or Centers for Disease Control), or greater reliance on the private sector (perhaps subcontracting site audits).

SUMMARY

The ANDA is itself an attempt to reduce the submission and review workload required with an NDA. The ANDA builds upon the safety and effectiveness data in the NDA and focuses on the unique formulation and manufacturing process used in producing the generic version. An increase in the number of ANDAs, however, has created a new pressure, forcing the FDA to seek methods—largely based upon new ICH guidelines, updated cGMPs, and increasingly stringent scrutiny of international generic drug production facilities—to cope with a sharp increase in the number of ANDAs.

While these techniques should provide some sort term relief, they do not address the fundamental problems of relative decreasing of FDA resources even as Agency responsibilities are increasing. Until this fundamental problem is addressed, the review process for ANDAs—and for NDAs—will grow increasingly lengthy, inefficient, and frustrating.

ANDA SUBMISSION CHECKLIST

This checklist is intended for use in the preparation and submission of ANDA. It is recommended that, prior to transmission to the FDA, a second internal review should be conducted by an individual or department not involved in the preparation of the submission (presumably Quality Assurance).

The checklist was developed through discussions with consultants and Quality Assurance directors and has been field-tested in final form with three successful submissions.

Note that since an ANDA is intended to reference and incorporate the research findings (safety and efficacy) of the original product applicant, other specific issues may arise depending upon the details of that original NDA. ANDA applicants should carefully review the requirements and recommendations of the NDA and/or the 505(b)2 NDA in preparation for the ANDA.

☐ Form 1571 completed
☐ Cover letter
  ☐ Name and address of sponsor
  ☐ Name, address, title, telephone, and e-mail of contact person
  ☐ Generic and trade name of drug or drug product
  ☐ FDA Code Number (assigned at time of pre-conference)
☐ Form 3674 "Certification of Compliance with Requirements of Clinical-Trails.gov Data Bank" completed (if clinical trials have been conducted)
☐ Three copies of application in indexed binders
☐ Pagination: All pages included and properly numbered
☐ Headings: Section headings confirming to submission subparagraphs, with initial Table of Contents
☐ Integrated references: All referenced articles included in final section, internally referenced in text
☐ Bibliography: Complete standard format bibliography listing all referenced articles
☐ Container closure and packaging system information provided
☐ Microbiological analysis provided
☐ Human pharmacokinetics and bioavailability information provided
☐ Complete Chemistry, Manufacturing, and Control (CMC) Information provided, including evidence of purity, stability, toxicology testing, and integrity of API, placebo, and final product.
☐ Analysis of all cited published studies and of all cited FDA findings, summarizing relevance and results
☐ Complete study protocol of bioequivalence (BE)/bioavailability (BA) study and for any additional studies conducted by applicant
☐ Raw data for all applicant-conducted studies
☐ DMF completed, including information on facilities, processes, and articles used in manufacturing, processing, packaging, and storage
☐ Analysis of all applicant-conducted studies and summaries of all relevant studies conducted by original product applicant
☐ Investigator's Brochure for all applicant-conducted studies included with detailed information for investigators and Institutional Review Board records
☐ Review of literature address all available prior instances of human use of drug product with emphasis on safety, administration, and possible adverse events
☐ Complete pharmacological profile provided for API and final product
☐ Summary of regulatory status and marketing history in United States and foreign countries

☐ Summary of adverse reactions to proposed drug in any country
  ☐ NDA addresses all issues and questions raised in the pre-ANDA meeting
☐ Prescription Drug User Fee Act information provided

If ANDA is submitted electronically:

☐ Form FDA-356h, Application to Market, is included.
☐ Form FDA-3397, User Fees, is included.

[For more details concerning Electronic Submissions, see Electronic Regulatory Submission and Review (ERSR) guidelines at http://www.fda.gov/cder/regulatory/ersr/default.htm.]

FDA ANDA REVIEW CHECKLIST

This FDA ANDA Review checklist has been designed in consultation with FDA reviewers, industry consultants, and regulatory professionals to serve as a summary tool indicating the evaluative criteria used by Center for Drug Evaluation and Research (CDER) and Center fir Biologics Evaluation and Research (CBER) to critique and assess applications received. It can be used internally as a part of the Quality Assurance process, as a guideline for regulatory development of an application, and/or as a self-assessment tool to predict likely FDA response to an application.

Note that since an ANDA references and incorporates the safety and efficacy findings of the original drug product, review issues may vary, depending on the inclusions in that NDA. Review of the NDA and/or 505(b)2 NDA Review requirements is suggested.

☐ **Logistics:** Submission conforms to FDA guideline 21 CFR Part 312.23(a)(10), (11), and (b), (c), (d), and (e).
  ☐ **Receipt:** Application was received in the FDA mail room.
  ☐ **IANDA jackets:** Document is contained in one or more 3-in., three-ring binders.
  ☐ **Form 1571:** ANDA is accompanied by completed Form 1571, providing (among other data) contact information including corporate name, contact name, address, telephone number, name and address of drug source, generic and trade name of drug.
  ☐ **Cover letter:** A cover letter indicates disease and therapy names.
  ☐ **Three copies:** Photocopies are acceptable.
  ☐ **Format:** Submission conforms to FDA guideline 21 CFR Part 312.23(a)(10), (11), and (b), (c), (d), and (e) and to FDA norm standards.

☐ **Pagination:** All pages included and properly numbered

☐ **Headings:** Section headings conforming to submission subparagraphs

☐ **Integrated references:** Copies of all referenced articles, with references integrated into the body of text

☐ **Bibliography:** Complete standard format bibliography as referenced in text

NOTE: If electronic submission is selected:

☐ Advance notification letter is provided.

☐ Electronic Submission Format conforms to approved list in Docket number 92s-0251 [see 21 CFR 11.1(d) and 11.2].

☐ Electronic Signatures conform to emerging guidelines or a paper copy with appropriate nonelectronic signatures is included.

☐ **CONTENT: Organizational structure**

    ☐ **Cover sheet:** Form 1571

    ☐ **Table of contents:** indicates page and volume of each section

    ☐ **Introductory statement and general investigational plan:** Two- to three-page summary identifying sponsor needs and general (phase) plans

    ☐ **Investigator's Brochure:** Conformity with ICH *Good Clinical Practice: Guideline for the Investigator's Brochure* (if applicable)

    ☐ **Protocol:** Copy of the protocol for each proposed clinical study. Note that phase 1 protocols should provide a brief outline, including estimation of number of subjects to be included, description of safety exclusions, and description of dosing plan (duration, dose, method). All protocols should address monitoring of blood chemistry and vital signs, and toxicity-based modification plans (if applicable).

    ☐ **CMC information:** should contain sufficient detail to assure identification, quality, purity, and strength of the investigational drug and should include stability data of duration appropriate to the length of the proposed study. FDA concerns to be addressed focus on products made with unknown or impure components, products with chemical structures known to be of likely high toxicity, products know to be chemically unstable, products with an impurity profile indicative of a health hazard or insufficiently defined to assess potential health hazard, or poorly characterized master or working cell bank.

        ■ Chemistry and Manufacturing Introduction

        ■ Drug substance

            ○ Description: physical, chemical, or biological characteristics

            ○ Name and address of manufacturer

            ○ Method of preparation

- o Limits and analytical methods
- o Stability information
- ■ Drug product
  - o List of components
  - o Qualitative composition
  - o Name and address of drug product manufacturer
  - o Description of manufacturing and packaging procedures
  - o Limits and analytical methods: identity, strength, quality, and purity
  - o Stability results
- ■ Placebo
- ■ Labels and labeling
- ■ Environmental assessment (or claim for exclusion): 21 CFR 312.23(a)(7)(iv)(e)
- ☐ **Pharmacology and toxicology information [21 CFR 312.23(a)(8)]**
  - ■ Pharmacology and drug distribution [21 CFR 312.23(a)(8)(i)]
    - o Description of pharmacological effects and mechanisms of action
    - o Description of absorption, distribution, metabolism, and excretion of the drug
  - ■ Toxicology summary [21 CFR 312.23(a)(8)(ii)(a)]: summary of toxicological effects in animals and *in vitro*
    - o Description of design of toxicological trials and any deviations from design
    - o Systematic presentation of animal toxicology studies and toxicokinetic studies
  - ■ Toxicology full data tabulation [21 CFR 312.23(a)(8)(ii)(b)]: data points with either
    - ■ Brief description of the study or
    - ■ Copy of the protocol with amendments
  - ■ Toxicology GLP certification [21 CFR 312.23(a)(8)(iii)]
- ☐ **Previous human experience with the investigational drug:** Summary report of any U.S. or non-U.S. human experience with the drug
- ☐ **References:** Indexed copies of referenced articles with comprehensive bibliography
- ☐ **Support:** Evaluation of the referent support provided
- ☐ **Key Issues:** All key issues appropriately referenced, potentially including (if applicable)
  - ☐ Investigator's Brochure
  - ☐ Protocols

☐ CMC information

☐ Pharmacology and toxicology information

☐ Previous human experience with the investigational drug

☐ **Credible:** References are from credible scientific journals and/or sources

☐ **Organized:** References are organized and tied to text

COMMENTS:
DISPOSITION:
    Receipt date:
    Response due date:
    Disposition:
    Notification date:

ANDA PROCESS FOR GENERIC DRUGS

Introduction

An ANDA contains data that, when submitted to the FDA's CDER, Office of Generic Drugs, provide for the review and ultimate approval of a generic drug product. Once approved, an applicant may manufacture and market the generic drug product to provide a safe, effective, low-cost alternative to the American public.

A generic drug product is one that is comparable to an innovator drug product in dosage form, strength, route of administration, quality, performance characteristics, and intended use. All approved products, both innovator and generic, are listed in the FDA's *Approved Drug Products with Therapeutic Equivalence Evaluations* at http://www.fda.gov/cder/ob/default.htm (*Orange Book*).

Generic drug applications are termed "abbreviated" because they are generally not required to include preclinical (animal) and clinical (human) data to establish safety and effectiveness. Instead, generic applicants must scientifically demonstrate that their product is bioequivalent (i.e., performs in the same manner as the innovator drug). One of the ways scientists demonstrate bioequivalence (BE) is by measuring the time it takes the generic drug to reach the bloodstream in 24 to 36 healthy volunteers. This gives them the rate of absorption, or bioavailability (BA), of the generic drug, which they can then compare with that of the innovator drug. The generic version must deliver the same amount of active ingredients into a patient's bloodstream in the same amount of time as that of the innovator drug.

Using BE as the basis for approving generic copies of drug products was established by the Drug Price Competition and Patent Term Restoration Act of 1984, also known as the Waxman–Hatch Act. This Act expedites the availability of less costly generic drugs by permitting the FDA to approve applications to market generic versions of brand-name drugs without conducting costly and duplicative clinical trials. At the same time, the brand-name companies can apply for up to five additional years longer patent protection for the new medicines they developed to make up for time lost while their products were going through the FDA's approval process. Brand-name drugs are subject to the same BE tests as generics upon reformulation. For more information on generic drug bioequivalency requirements, please see the chapter entitled "FDA Ensures Equivalence of Generic Drugs" in *From Test Tube to Patient: Improving Health Through Human Drugs.*

The Office of Generic Drugs home page provides additional information to generic drug developers, including an interactive flowchart presentation of the ANDA review process, focusing on how CDER determines the safety and BE of generic drug products prior to approval for marketing. Generic drug application reviewers focus on BE data, chemistry and microbiology data, requests for plant inspection, and drug labeling information.

The Web site is designed for individuals from pharmaceutical companies, government agencies, academic institutions, private organizations, or other organizations interested in bringing a generic drug to market. Each of the sections below contains information from CDER to assist you in the ANDA process. Click on a link on the Web page to go directly to a section.

Resources for ANDA Submissions

The following resources have been gathered to provide you with the legal requirements of an ANDA, assistance from CDER to help you meet those requirements, and internal ANDA review principles, policies, and procedures.

Guidance Documents for ANDAs

The Agency's recent opinion of a specific subject is expressed in guidance documents. These documents are prepared to provide drug sponsors and FDA review staff guidelines for the processing, content, and evaluation of applications, and for the design, production, manufacturing, and testing of regulated products. Additionally, they provide consistency in the Agency's regulation, inspection, and enforcement procedures. Guidances are not regulation or laws and therefore they are not enforceable, but merely recommended processes. Alternative approaches may be used if it satisfies all mandatory requirements of the applicable statute, regulations, or both. For information on a specific guidance document, please contact the originating office.

The FDA has numerous guidances that relate to ANDA content and format issues. Below is a list of some recent guidances of interest. See Drug Information Branch's Guidance Documents for a complete list of available guidances online and instructions on how to obtain them. Most of these documents are in Adobe Acrobat format also known as portable document format (PDF). The free upgrade to Adobe Acrobat 3.0 or higher is recommended, especially if you have difficulty opening any of the documents below. For information on a specific guidance document, please contact the originating office.

Guidance documents to help prepare ANDAs are listed together on CDER's Guidance Document Index Web page in the following categories.

- Generics
- Generics (Draft—Distributed for comment purposes only)
- Procedural Draft: *Applications Covered by Section 505(b)(2)*_(Issued October 1999, Posted December 7, 1999), which permits the FDA to rely, for approval of an NDA, on data not developed by the applicant.
- Biopharmaceutics
- *Bioavailability and Bioequivalence Studies for Orally Administered Drug Products—General Considerations.* Optional Format: PDF (Issued October 2000, Posted October 27, 2000). Should be useful for applicants planning to conduct BA and BE studies during the IND period for an NDA, BE studies intended for submission in an ANDA, and BE studies conducted in the postapproval period for certain changes in both NDAs and ANDAs
- DMF. A submission to the FDA that may be used to provide confidential, detailed information about facilities, processes, or articles used in the manufacturing, processing, packaging, and storing of one or more human drugs
- Required Specifications for the FDA's IND, NDA, and ANDA DMF Binders
- *Guidance for Industry: Changes to an Approved NDA or ANDA*
- *Refusal to Receive* (Issued July 12, 1993, Posted November 26, 1999). Clarifies CDER's decisions to refuse to receive an incomplete application
- Inactive Ingredient Database. Contains all inactive ingredients present in approved drug products or conditionally approved drug products currently marketed for human use

Laws, Regulations, Policies, and Procedures

The mission of the FDA is to enforce laws enacted by the U.S. Congress and regulations established by the Agency to protect the consumer's health, safety, and pocketbook. The Federal Food, Drug, and Cosmetic Act is the basic food and drug law of the United States. With numerous amendments, it is the most extensive law of its kind in the world. The law is intended to assure consumers that foods are pure and wholesome, safe to eat, and produced under sanitary conditions; that drugs and devices are safe and effective for their intended uses; that cosmetics are safe and made from appropriate ingredients; and that all labeling and packaging is truthful, informative, and not deceptive.

CFR. The final regulations published in the Federal Register (daily published record of proposed rules, final rules, meeting notices, etc.) are collected in the CFR. The CFR is divided into 50 titles, which represent broad areas subject to Federal regulations. The FDA's portion of the CFR interprets the Federal Food, Drug and Cosmetic Act and related statutes. Section 21 of the CFR contains most of the regulations pertaining to food and drugs. The regulations document most actions of all drug sponsors that are required under Federal law. The following regulations apply to the ANDA process.

- 21 CFR Part 314—*Applications for FDA Approval to Market a New Drug or/and Antibiotic Drug*
- 21 CFR Part 320—*Bioavailability and Bioequivalence Requirements*. For more information on retention samples, please see Bioequivalence Study "Retention Samples."
  - Bioavailability and Bioequivalence Requirements; Abbreviated Applications; Final Rule. (TXT) (PDF) (Issued and posted December 19, 2002)
- 21 CFR Part 310—*New Drugs*

Manual of Policies and Procedures (MaPPs). CDER's MaPPs provides official instructions for internal practices and procedures followed by CDER staff to help standardize the drug review process and other activities, both internal and external. MaPPs define external activities as well. All MAPPs are available for the public to review to get a better understanding of office policies, definitions, staff responsibilities, and procedures. MaPP documents to help prepare ANDAs are listed together on CDER's MaPP Web page.

- Chapter 5200—*Generic Drugs*

ANDA Forms and Electronic Submissions

- ANDA Checklist for Completeness and Acceptability (Word) (October 17, 2007)
- FDA Form 356h. Application to Market a New Drug for Human Use/ Antibiotic Drug for Human Use

- The CDER Office of Generic Drugs has developed a guidance document entitled Providing Regulatory Submissions in Electronic Format—ANDAs (PDF version) (Issued June 6, 2002, Posted June 27, 2002) to assist applicants making regulatory submissions of ANDAs in electronic format. This guidance should be used in conjunction with the following guidances:
  - *Guidance for Industry: Providing Regulatory Submissions in Electronic Format—General Considerations*
  - *Regulatory Submissions in Electronic Format; New Drug Applications*

For more information on electronic submissions, see ERSR.

Related Topics

- IND. Provides resources to assist drug sponsors with submitting applications for approval to begin new drug experiments on human subjects.
- NDA. Provides resources to assist drug sponsors with submitting applications for approval to market a new drug.
- Drug Application Regulatory Compliance. The approval process for NDAs includes a review of the manufacturer's compliance with cGMP. This Web page provides resources to help meet compliance.
- Information for Clinical Investigators. Provides regulations and guidelines to scientists who design and run experiments (clinical trials) to test the safety and effectiveness of new drugs on human subjects.
- Small Business Assistance Program. Helps small businesses understand the Agency's structures and rules (http://www.fda.gov/ora/fed_state/Small_Business/sb_guide/smbusrep.html).
- ERSR. Provides information on electronic drug applications, application reviews, Electronic Document Room, and other ERSR projects.
- Postdrug-approval Activities. The goal of CDER's postdrug-approval activities is to monitor the ongoing safety of marketed drugs. This is accomplished by reassessing drug risks based on new data learned after the drug is marketed and recommending ways of trying to most appropriately manage that risk.

ANDA CHECKLIST FOR CTD OR ECTD FORMAT FOR COMPLETENESS AND ACCEPTABILITY OF AN APPLICATION FOR FILING

For more information on submission of an ANDA in Electronic Common Technical Document (eCTD) format, please go to http://www.fda.gov/cder/regulatory/ersr/ectd.htm.

For more CTD and eCTD informational links, see the final page of the ANDA Checklist

ANDA #: Firm name:

PIV: Electronic or paper submission:

Related application(s):

Bio Assignments:	Micro Review
□ BPH □ BCE	
□ BST □ BDI	

First Generic Product Received?

Drug name:

Dosage form:

Random queue:

Chem team leader: PM: Labeling reviewer:

Letter Date:	**Received Date:**
Comments:	**On Cards:**
Therapeutic Code:	
Archival copy:	**Sections**
Review copy:	E-Media Disposition:
Not applicable to electronic sections	
Part 3 Combination Product Category	Refer to the Part 3 Combination Algorithm
(Must be completed for ALL Original Applications)	
Reg. Support Reviewer	**Recommendation:**
	□**FILE** □**REFUSE to RECEIVE**

ADDITIONAL COMMENTS REGARDING THE ANDA:

Module 1

ADMINISTRATIVE

1.1	**1.1.2 Signed and Completed Application Form (356h) (original signature)** (Check Rx/OTC Status)
1.2	**Cover Letter**
1.2.1	**Form FDA 3674 (PDF)**
1.3.1	**Table of Contents (paper submission only)**[1]

[1] For a comprehensive table of contents headings and hierarchy, please go to http://www.fda.gov/cder/regulatory/ersr/5640CTOC-v1.2.pdf.

1.3.2	**Field Copy Certification (original signature)** **(N/A for E-Submissions)**
1.3.3	**Debarment Certification—GDEA (Generic Drug Enforcement Act)/Other:** 1. Debarment Certification (original signature) 2. List of Convictions statement (original signature)
1.3.4	**Financial Certifications** Bioavailability/Bioequivalence Financial Certification (Form FDA 3454) Disclosure Statement (Form FDA 3455, submit copy to Regulatory Branch Chief)
1.3.5	**1.3.5.1 Patent Information** Patents listed for the RLD in the Electronic Orange Book Approved Drug Products with Therapeutic Equivalence Evaluations **1.3.5.2 Patent Certification** 1. Patent number(s) 2. Paragraph: (Check all certifications that apply) MOU PI PII PIII PIV (Statement of Notification) 3. Expiration of patent(s): 　a. Pediatric exclusivity submitted? 　b. Expiration of pediatric exclusivity? 4. Exclusivity statement:
1.4.1	**References** Letters of Authorization 1. DMF letters of authorization 　a. Type II DMF authorization letter(s) or synthesis for active pharmaceutical ingredient 　b. Type III DMF authorization letter(s) for container closure 2. U.S. Agent Letter of Authorization [U.S. Agent (if needed, countersignature on 356h)]
1.12.11	**Basis for Submission** NDA#: Ref. Listed Drug: Firm: ANDA suitability petition required? If Yes, then is change subject to PREA (change in dosage form, route or active ingredient) see section 1.9.1

Module 1 *(Continued)*

ADMINISTRATIVE

1.12.12	**Comparison between Generic Drug and RLD-505(j)(2)(A)** 1. Conditions of use 2. Active ingredients 3. Inactive ingredients 4. Route of administration 5. Dosage Form 6. Strength
1.12.14	**Environmental Impact Analysis Statement**
1.12.15	**Request for Waiver** Request for Waiver of *In Vivo* BA/BE Study(ies):
1.14.1	**Draft Labeling (Multiple Copies N/A for E-Submissions)** **1.14.1.1** 4 copies of draft (each strength and container) **1.14.1.2** 1 side-by-side labeling comparison of containers and carton with all differences annotated and explained **1.14.1.3** 1 package insert (content of labeling) submitted electronically Was a proprietary name request submitted?[2] (If yes, send e-mail to Labeling Reviewer indicating such)
1.14.3	**Listed Drug Labeling** **1.14.3.1** 1 side-by-side labeling (package and patient insert) comparison with all differences annotated and explained **1.14.3.3** 1 RLD label and 1 RLD container label

---

[2]A model Quality Overall Summary for an immediate release tablet and an extended release capsule can be found on the OGD Web page: http://www.fda.gov/cder/ogd/.

Module 2

SUMMARIES

2.3	**Quality Overall Summary**
	E-Submission: PDF
	Word Processed e.g., MS Word
	A model Quality Overall Summary for an immediate release tablet and an extended release capsule can be found on the OGD Web page http://www.fda.gov/cder/ogd/
	Question-based Review
	2.3.S
	Drug Substance (Active Pharmaceutical Ingredient)
	2.3.S.1 General Information
	2.3.S.2 Manufacture
	2.3.S.3 Characterization
	2.3.S.4 Control of Drug Substance
	2.3.S.5 Reference Standards or Materials
	2.3.S.6 Container Closure System
	2.3.S.7 Stability
	2.3.P
	Drug Product
	2.3.P.1 Description and Composition of the Drug Product
	2.3.P.2 Pharmaceutical Development
	2.3.P.2.1 Components of the Drug Product
	2.3.P.2.1.1 Drug Substance
	2.3.P.2.1.2 Excipients
	2.3.P.2.2 Drug Product
	2.3.P.2.3 Manufacturing Process Development
	2.3.P.2.4 Container Closure System
	2.3.P.3 Manufacture
	2.3.P.4 Control of Excipients
	2.3.P.5 Control of Drug Product
	2.3.P.6 Reference Standards or Materials
	2.3.P.7 Container Closure System
	2.3.P.8 Stability
2.7	**Clinical Summary (Bioequivalence)**
	Model Bioequivalence Data Summary Tables
	E-Submission: PDF
	Word Processed e.g., MS Word
	2.7.1 Summary of Biopharmaceutic Studies and Associated Analytical Methods
	2.7.1.1 Background and Overview
	Table 1. Submission Summary
	Table 4. Bioanalytical Method Validation
	Table 6. Formulation Data

Module 2 *(Continued)*

SUMMARIES

      2.7.1.2 Summary of Results of Individual Studies
      Table 5. Summary of *In Vitro* Dissolution
      2.7.1.3 Comparison and Analyses of Results Across Studies
      Table 2. Summary of Bioavailability (BA) Studies
      Table 3. Statistical Summary of the Comparative BA Data
      2.7.1.4 Appendix
      2.7.4.1.3 Demographic and Other Characteristics of Study Population
      Table 7. Demographic Profile of Subjects Completing the Bioequivalence Study
      2.7.4.2.1.1 Common Adverse Events
      Table 8. Incidence of Adverse Events in Individual Studies

---

MODULE 3

3.2.S DRUG SUBSTANCE

3.2.S.1	**General Information**
	3.2.S.1.1 Nomenclature
	3.2.S.1.2 Structure
	3.2.S.1.3 General Properties
3.2.S.2	**Manufacturer**
	3.2.S.2.1
	Manufacturer(s) (This section includes contract manufacturers and testing labs)
	Drug Substance (Active Pharmaceutical Ingredient)
	1. Name and Full Address(es) of the Facility(ies)
	2. Function or Responsibility
	3. Type II DMF number for API
	4. CFN or FEI numbers
3.2.S.3	**Characterization**
3.2.S.4	**Control of Drug Substance (Active Pharmaceutical Ingredient)**
	3.2.S.4.1 Specification
	Testing specifications and data from drug substance manufacturer(s)
	3.2.S.4.2 Analytical Procedures
	3.2.S.4.3 Validation of Analytical Procedures

              1. Spectra and chromatograms for reference
                 standards and test samples
              2. Samples-Statement of Availability and
                 Identification of:
                 a. Drug Substance
                 b. Same lot number(s)
              3.2.S.4.4 Batch Analysis
              1. COA(s) specifications and test results from drug
                 substance manufacturer(s)
              2. Applicant certificate of analysis
              3.2.S.4.5 Justification of Specification

3.2.S.5	**Reference Standards or Materials**
3.2.S.6	**Container Closure Systems**
3.2.S.7	**Stability**

MODULE 3

3.2.P DRUG PRODUCT

3.2.P.1	**Description and Composition of the Drug Product**

              1. Unit composition
              2. Inactive ingredients and amounts are
                 appropriate per IIG

3.2.P.2	**Pharmaceutical Development**

              Pharmaceutical Development Report

3.2.P.3	**Manufacture**

              3.2.P.3.1 Manufacture(s) (Finished Dosage
                 Manufacturer and Outside Contract Testing
                 Laboratories)
              1. Name and Full Address(es)of the Facility(ies)
              2. cGMP Certification:
              3. Function or Responsibility
              4. CFN or FEI numbers
              3.2.P.3.2 Batch Formula
              3.2.P.3.3 Description of Manufacturing Process
                 and Process Controls
              1. Description of the Manufacturing Process
              2. Master Production Batch Record(s) for largest
                 intended production runs
              (no more than 10× pilot batch) with equipment
                 specified
              3. If sterile product: Aseptic fill / Terminal
                 sterilization
              4. Reprocessing Statement
               3.2.P.3.4 Controls of Critical Steps and
                 Intermediates
              3.2.P.3.5 Process Validation and/or Evaluation
              1. Microbiological sterilization validation
              2. Filter validation (if aseptic fill)

Module 3 *(Continued)*

3.2.S DRUG SUBSTANCE	

3.2.P.4	**Controls of Excipients (Inactive Ingredients)**
	Source of inactive ingredients identified
	3.2.P.4.1 Specifications
	1. Testing specifications (including identification and characterization)
	2. Suppliers' COA (specifications and test results)
	3.2.P.4.2 Analytical Procedures
	3.2.P.4.3 Validation of Analytical Procedures
	3.2.P.4.4 Justification of Specifications
	Applicant COA
3.2.P.5	**Controls of Drug Product**
	3.2.P.5.1 Specification(s)
	3.2.P.5.2 Analytical Procedures
	3.2.P.5.3 Validation of Analytical Procedures
	Samples-Statement of Availability and Identification of:
	1. Finished Dosage Form
	2. Same lot numbers
	3.2.P.5.4 Batch Analysis
	Certificate of Analysis for Finished Dosage Form
	3.2.P.5.5 Characterization of Impurities
	3.2.P.5.6 Justification of Specifications
3.2.P.7	**Container Closure System**
	1. Summary of Container Closure System (if new resin, provide data)
	2. Components Specification and Test Data
	3. Packaging Configuration and Sizes
	4. Container Closure Testing
	5. Source of supply and suppliers address
3.2.P.8	**3.2.P.8.1 Stability (Finished Dosage Form)**
	1. Stability Protocol submitted
	2. Expiration Dating Period
	3.2.P.8.2 Postapproval Stability and Conclusion
	Postapproval Stability Protocol and Commitments
	3.2.P.8.3 Stability Data
	1. Three-month accelerated stability data
	2. Batch numbers on stability records the same as the test batch

MODULE 3

3.2.R REGIONAL
INFORMATION

3.2.R	**3.2.R.1.S Executed Batch Records for**
(Drug Substance)	**Drug Substance (if available)**
	3.2.R.2.S Comparability Protocols
	3.2.R.3.S Methods Validation Package
	Methods Validation Package (three copies)
	(Multiple Copies N/A for E-Submissions)
	(Required for Non-USP drugs)
3.2.R	**3.2.R.1.P.1**
(Drug Product)	**Executed Batch Records**
	Copy of Executed Batch Record with
	Equipment Specified, Including
	Packaging Records (Packaging and
	Labeling Procedures)
	Batch Reconciliation and Label
	Reconciliation
	Theoretical Yield
	Actual Yield
	Packaged Yield
	3.2.R.1.P.2 Information on Components
	3.2.R.2.P Comparability Protocols
	3.2.R.3.P Methods Validation Package
	Methods Validation Package (three copies)
	(Multiple Copies N/A for E-Submissions)
	(Required for Non-USP drugs)

MODULE 5

CLINICAL
STUDY
REPORTS

5.2	**Tabular Listing of Clinical Studies**
5.3.1	**Bioavailability/Bioequivalence**
(complete	1. Formulation data same?
study data)	a. Comparison of all Strengths (check
	proportionality of multiple strengths)
	b. Parenterals, Ophthalmics, Otics, and Topicals
	per 21 CFR 314.94 (a)(9)(iii)-(v)
	2. Lot Numbers of Products used in BE Study(ies):
	3. Study Type: (Continue with the appropriate
	study type box below)
	5.3.1.2 Comparative BA/BE Study Reports
	1. Study(ies) meets BE criteria (90% CI of 80-125,
	C max, AUC)

Module 5 *(Continued)*

CLINICAL STUDY REPORTS	

	2. Summary Bioequivalence tables:
	Table 10. Study Information
	Table 12. Dropout Information
	Table 13. Protocol Deviations
	5.3.1.3
	***In Vitro–In Vivo* Correlation Study Reports**
	1. Summary Bioequivalence tables:
	Table 11. Product Information
	Table 16. Composition of Meal Used in Fed
	Bioequivalence Study
	5.3.1.4
	Reports of Bioanalytical and Analytical Methods for Human Studies
	1. Summary Bioequivalence table:
	Table 9. Reanalysis of Study Samples
	Table 14. Summary of Standard Curve and QC Data for Bioequivalence Sample Analyses
	Table 15. SOPs Dealing with Bioanalytical Repeats of Study Samples
	5.3.7
	Case Report Forms and Individual Patient Listing

5.4	**Literature References**

Possible Study Types:

Study Type	***In Vivo* BE Study(ies) with PK End Points** (i.e., fasting/fed/sprinkle)
	1. Study(ies) meets BE criteria (90% CI of 80–125, C max, AUC)
	2. EDR e-mail: Data Files Submitted: YES SENT TO EDR
	3. *In Vitro* Dissolution
Study Type	***In Vivo* BE Study with Clinical End Points**
	1. Properly defined BE end points (evaluated by Clinical Team)
	2. Summary results meet BE criteria: 90% CI of the proportional difference in success rate between test and reference must be within (−0.20, +0.20) for a binary/dichotomous end point. For a continuous end point, the test/reference ratio of the mean result must be within (0.80, 1.25).
	3. Summary results indicate superiority of active treatments (test and reference) over vehicle/placebo ($p < 0.05$) (evaluated by Clinical Team)
	4. EDR e-mail: Data Files Submitted
Study Type	***In Vitro* BE Study(ies)** (i.e., *in vitro* binding assays)
	1. Study(ies) meets BE criteria (90% CI of 80–125)
	2. EDR e-mail: Data Files Submitted:
	3. *In Vitro* Dissolution:

Study Type   **Nasally Administered Drug Products**
1. Solutions (Q1/Q2 sameness):
    a. *In Vitro* Studies (Dose/Spray Content Uniformity, Droplet/ Drug Particle Size Distribution, Spray Pattern, Plume Geometry, Priming, and Repriming)
2. Suspensions (Q1/Q2 sameness):
    a. *In Vivo* PK Study
        1. Study(ies) meets BE Criteria (90% CI of 80–125, C max, AUC)
        2. EDR e-mail: Data Files Submitted
    b. *In Vivo* BE Study with Clinical End Points
        1. Properly defined BE end points (evaluated by Clinical Team)
        2. Summary results meet BE criteria (90% CI within +/– 20% of 80–125)
        3. Summary results indicate superiority of active treatments (test and reference) over vehicle/placebo (p < 0.05) (evaluated by Clinical Team)
        4. EDR e-mail: Data Files Submitted
    c. *In Vitro* Studies (Dose/Spray Content Uniformity, Droplet/ Drug Particle Size Distribution, Spray Pattern, Plume Geometry, Priming, and Repriming)

Study Type   **In Vivo BE Study(ies) with PD End Points** (e.g., topical corticosteroid vasoconstrictor studies)
1. Pilot Study (determination of ED50)
2. Pivotal Study (study meets BE criteria 90%CI of 80–125)

Study Type   **Transdermal Delivery Systems**
1. *In Vivo* PK Study
1. Study(ies) meet BE Criteria (90% CI of 80–125, C max, AUC)
2. In Vitro Dissolution
3. EDR e-mail: Data Files Submitted
2. Adhesion Study
3. Skin Irritation/Sensitization Study

GUIDANCE FOR INDUSTRY[3] ORGANIZATION OF AN ANDA AND AN ABBREVIATED ANTIBIOTIC APPLICATION (AADA)

Introduction

This guidance describes the recommended organization of ANDAs and AADAs and related submissions. Some ANDA and AADA submissions are

---

[3]This guidance was prepared by the Office of Generic Drugs at the FDA's CDER. This guidance document represents the Agency's current thinking on the organization of an abbreviated application. It does not create or confer any rights for or on any person and does not operate to bind FDA or the public. An alternative approach may be used if such approach satisfies the requirement of the applicable statute, regulations, or both.

difficult to review because they are complex, voluminous, or poorly organized. An application submitted with the proper jacket, organized with a clear table of contents and corresponding tabs, and with correct pagination makes the review process easier and more efficient. This guide summarizes one way an application can be organized that will be acceptable to the FDA. This guidance document replaces the Office of Generic Drugs Policy and Procedure Guide 30-91.

Definitions

abbreviated application. An application described under 21 CFR § 314.94, including all amendments and supplements to the application. The term applies to both abbreviated new drug applications and abbreviated antibiotic applications.

archival copy. A complete copy of the an abbreviated application intended to serve as the official reference source for the Agency.

field copy. A duplicate of the archival copy to be submitted to the applicant's home FDA District Office.

review copy. A duplicate of the archival copy for use by Agency reviewers.

Policy

Archival, Review, and Field Copy. An ANDA and AADA applicant should submit archival, review, and field copies of the application in English.

The archival copy is a complete copy of an application and is intended to serve as the official reference source for the Agency. After an application is approved, the archival copy is retained by the Agency and serves as the sole file copy of the approved application. The review copy is destroyed. If there is a requirement for a BE study, then the review copy is divided into two parts containing the scientific information needed for FDA review of the application by different scientific reviewers. One part should contain information about CMC, and one part should contain information about BA and BE.

Each part contains sections (e.g., "Labeling") that permit concurrent review of the application by various review disciplines (see "Review Copy—Additional Guidance" for further explanation).

An applicant may submit all or portions of the archival copy of the application in any form that the applicant and the FDA agree is acceptable. Submission of electronic versions of the application are welcome but should be discussed with the Office of Generic Drugs prior to actual submission.

Each application should be submitted in color-coded jackets. Information about the volume size and identification, the jacket specifications (including color coding), the size and quality of paper for text, and mailing instructions are shown in *Appendix A*.

Cover Letter. Each submission (whether original, amendment, supplement, or annual report) should include a dated cover letter with a clear, brief introductory statement. The cover letter should be on the letterhead of the applicant or the applicant's agent. If a letterhead other than that of the applicant is used, an explanation of why the applicant's letterhead was not used should be included. The cover letter should assist the reviewer by including, at a minimum, the following:

1. Purpose of the submission
2. Type of submission (ANDA, AADA, amendment, supplement, annual report, or resubmission as a result of prior withdrawal of an application)
3. Name, title, signature, and address of the applicant
4. Proprietary name (if any) and established name of the drug product
5. Number of volumes submitted

For amendments, supplements, and annual reports, either the cover letter or the narrative for the section that was changed by the new submission should contain a description of the specific changes to previously submitted material. A comparison between the new information and the old information is preferred.

The cover letter should include a clear heading for special situations, such as: "Major" or "Minor" Amendment, or "Special Supplement—Changes Being Effected," or "Supplement—Expedited Review Requested."

Table of Contents. Each original application or other submission, as applicable, should include a table of contents. The purpose of the table of contents is to tell the reviewer where information can be found in the application. *Appendix B* provides a suggested table of contents for a typical ANDA. *Appendix B* is intended to complement the applicable regulations and can be used for general guidance in assembling the application but should not be relied on solely for determining contents of the submission. Although not all sections apply to AADAs, this table of contents may be adjusted to accommodate the specific needs of the AADA.

If a section of the suggested table of contents is not used, insert a page behind the tab for that section (see Tabs) and state "not applicable" in the table of contents and in the text. If a new subsection (line item within a section currently on the table of contents) is added to the table of contents, modify the application accordingly. Additional sections should be placed at the end of the table of contents and begin with number XXII (see *Appendix B*, "Suggested Table of Contents"). If the archival or review copy of the application requires more than one volume, the table of contents should be duplicated and placed in each volume. Thus, the same table of contents should be used in all jacketed volumes (see "Review Copy—Additional Guidance" for further explanation regarding the separation of the review copy).

Tabs. The contents of the submission should be organized by sections, and each section should be identified by a tab that corresponds to the section set forth in the table of contents. The tab shows the number and brief descriptive name of the section it identifies (e.g., *Appendix B*, "Section VI—Bioavailability/Bioequivalence").

Applicants may also use tabs for subsections within a section. In this event, use of a different color tab for subsections is useful. However, too many tabs may result in an unwieldy application.

Pagination. All pages of the archival copy of the application (except the tab pages) should be numbered in sequence. The sequence begins with page number 1 for the front side of the Application Form (Section I of *Appendix B*) and increases consecutively to the last page of the application. The sections and line items in the table of contents should accurately reflect the page numbers of the corresponding text.

The page number should be placed on the bottom center of each sheet of paper. Each submission after the original application (e.g., amendments or supplements) should also begin with page 1 and run consecutively to the end of that submission. Correct pagination is essential to the reviewer in locating material in an application. Correct, consistent pagination between the text and the table of contents is especially important when an application consists of more than one volume.

Review Copy—Additional Guidance. In addition to the archival copy, the applicant should submit a review copy. The review copy may contain two parts if BA/BE data are required, one part containing primarily chemistry, manufacturing, and controls data, and the other part containing BA/BEdata. (Note that there will be gaps in the page numbering of the review copy if a BA/BE part is required, since neither part contains all sections in the archival copy (see *Appendix C*). Each part may contain one or more volumes, depending on the size of the submission. Each volume of the review copy should contain the complete table of contents, identical to that of the archival copy. For identification purposes, the CMC review partshould be contained in a red jacket (or jackets), while the BA/BE[7] review part should be contained in an orange jacket (or jackets).

Sections contained in the review copy should be identical to those of the archival copy, including use of the same page numbers. For the typical ANDA (see *Appendix B*), both parts will contain Sections I through V, and VII. The CMC part will also contain Sections VIII through XXI, and the BA/BE part would contain Section VI (see *Appendix C*).

Field Copy—Additional Guidance. In addition to the archival copy, domestic applicants must submit a certification (21CFR 314.94) that a "true" third/field copy of the technical sections (CMC) of the application has been submitted to the appropriate FDA District Office. Foreign applicants should submit the field copy to the Office of Generic Drugs (see *Appendix A* for mailing address and specifications).

APPENDIXES

Appendix A: Suggested Specifications

1. **Volume Size and Identification**
   A. Each volume of an application should not be more than 3 in. thick.
   B. The name and address of the applicant, the name of the drug, dosage form, and strength of the drug should be displayed on the front of the jacket of each volume.
   C. Please do NOT number the volumes. The Agency will number the volumes.
   D. All original abbreviated applications should be submitted in jackets. Small amendments or supplements not contained within jackets should be bound with fasteners (NO STAPLES) rather than by three-ring binders.

2. **Jacket Color and Ordering**
   A. The volume jackets of the application should be color coded.

	Color	Form Number
Archival Copy	Blue	FDA 2626
Review Copy: (See "Review Copy—Additional Guidance" for further information.)		
(1) CMC (not containing Bio)	Red	FDA 2626a
(2) BA/BE	Orange	FDA 2626c
Field Copy: (See "Field Copy—Additional Guidance" for further information.)		
	Burgundy	FDA 2626h

   B. A limited number of jackets may be obtained free of charge by sending a Special Order form (obtained from Consolidated Forms and Publications Distribution Center) that states the form number (as shown above), quantity, name, address, and telephone number of requestor to:

Consolidated Forms and Publications Distribution Center
Washington Commerce Center
3222 Hubbard Road
Landover, MD 20785

Additional jackets, with the following specifications, may be purchased from a commercial source:

(1) Archival Copy
Polyvinyl type jacket 0.023 to 0.025 gauge
Front cover: 9″ × 11½″
Back cover: 9″ × 12″ with a full ½″ tab along the top edge.
Color: as stated aboveHidden reinforced 1″ hinges for front and back covers.
Rounded outside corners for front and back covers.

(2) Review Copy
Extra-heavy paper jacket
Front cover: 9″ × 11½″
Back cover: 9″ × 12″ with a full ½″ tab along the top edge.
Color: as stated above
Hidden reinforced 1″ hinges for front and back covers.
Rounded outside corners for front and back covers.

(3) Field Copy
Extra-heavy paper jacket
Front cover: 9″ × 11½″
Back cover: 9″ × 12″ with a full 1½″ tab along the top edge.
Color: as stated above
Hidden reinforced 1″ hinges for front and back covers.
Rounded outside corners for front and back covers.

3. **Paper Size and Quality**
   A. Good U. S. standard quality bond, 8½″ × 11″, loose leaf paper
   B. Three holes punched on left hand margin
   C. One-inch margins to accommodate readability after binding and photocopying
   D. Typing on both sides of paper is allowed if bleeding through the other side does not occur
   E. Paper should accommodate photocopying.

4. **Mailing**
   A. The packing carton should identify the contents by
   Drug name
   Applicant's name
   Applicant's address
   "Archival Copy Enclosed" or "Review Copy Enclosed" (or both)

B. Mail abbreviated applications to:
Office of Generic Drugs
CDER, FDA
MPN II, HFD-600
7500 Standish Place
Rockville, MD 20855

C. Archival and review copies of abbreviated applications sent by overnight courier service or a parcel service should be sent to:
Office of Generic Drugs
CDER, FDA
Metro Park North II
7500 Standish Place, Room 150
Rockville, MD 20855

Appendix B: Suggested Table of Contents

This suggested table of contents applies to an original ANDA. Although not all sections apply to an AADA, this table of contents may be adjusted to accommodate the specific needs of the AADA.The page numbers shown, 1–214, are for illustrative purposes only.

Appendix C: Composition of Review Copies

The following table illustrates the suggested separation of text for the "red" part of the review copy containing chemistry, and for the "orange" part of the review copy containing BA/BE. The "sections" referred to are those shown on the suggested table of contents in *Appendix B*.

Table   Composition of review copies corresponding to suggested table of contents (*Appendix B*)

Section	Red copy	Orange copy
I	X	X
II	X	X
III	X	X
IV	X	X
V	X	X
VI (BIO)	–	X
VII	X	X
VIII–XXI	X	–

The U.S. Food and Drug Administration (FDA) is an agency of the United States Department of Health and Human Services and is responsible for the safety regulation of most types of foods, dietary supplements, drugs, vaccines, biological medical products, blood products, medical devices, radiation-emitting devices, veterinary products, and cosmetics. The FDA also enfoirces section 361 of the Public Health Service Act and the associated regulations, including sanitation requirements on interstate travel as well as sepcific rules for control of disease on many U.S. products.

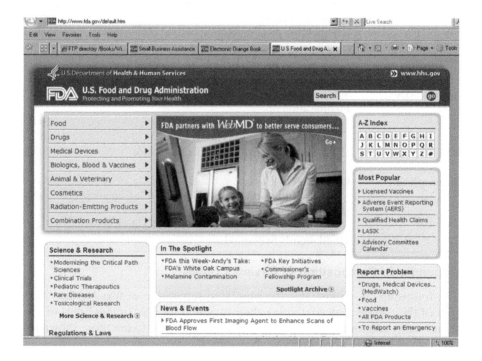

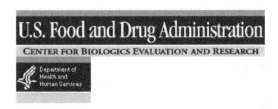

2002 Biological NDA and ANDA Approvals

This list reflects information regarding the supplements as of the approval date. It is not updated with regard to applicant or application status changes. The supplements are listed in order by date of approval.

Trade name/established name	Indication for use	NDA/ANDA number	Applicant	Approval date
Citrate phosphate Double dextrose/additive solution 3 Anticoagulant citrate phosphate 2X dextrose solution (CP2D)	Use only with automated apheresis devices for collecting human blood and blood components	000127	Haemonetics Corp. 400 Wood Road Braintree, MA 02184	January 18, 2002
Anticoagulant citrate dextrose solution	For use only with automated	980728	Haemonetics Corp. 400 Wood Road	February 6, 2002
Formula A Anticoagulant citrate dextrose solution (ACD)	Apheresis devices		Braintree, MA 02184	
ACD-A Solution Anticoagulant citrate dextrose solution (ACD)	For use only with automated apheresis devices	010228	Gambro BCT, Inc. 10811 W. Collins Ave. Lakewood, CO 80215	February 25, 2002
AS3 nutricel additive system additive solution formula 3 Anticoagulant citrate phosphate 2X dextrose solution	To provide the CP2D during collection and add AS3 to the separated red blood cells in order to extend the length of time they can be stored	001214	Gambro BCT, Inc. 10811 W. Collins Ave. Lakewood, CO 80215	May 29, 2002
Adsol with ACD-A/ Anticoagulant citrate dextrose solution (ACD)	Adsol preservation system combined with ACD-A anticoagulated red cell products	000922	Baxter Healthcare Corp. Fenwal Division Route 120 and Wilson Road Round Lake, IL 60073 USA	August 29, 2002

CHAPTER 8

Annual Reports

The FDA requires annual updating reports for investigational new drug applications (INDs), new drug applications (NDAs) [both standard and 505(b)2], Orphan Drugs, and abbreviated new drug applications (ANDA)s. These reports are among the most flexible and forgiving of all FDA submissions. There are, in fact, only two significant criteria: they must be filed without fail, as close to the annual date of initial submission as possible; and they must be accompanied by the appropriate submission form.

The reality is that the FDA does not generally track annual due dates at all, and the failure to file would not result in any short-term warning or action. At a later date, of course, when the complete document package is reviewed, a missing annual report will raise a red flag. But the responsibility to track and file annual reports rests solely with the submitting organization.

ORPHAN-DRUG ANNUAL REPORTS

An annual report is required for all designated Orphan Drugs. The objectives of the report are to (a) update the Agency on progress made toward the development, clinical testing, and eventual approval of the Orphan Drug and (b) confirm that the conditions originally qualifying the drug as an orphan have not substantially changed. For example, a drug intended for a disease that has significantly grown beyond to 200,000 case orphan limit may be reevaluated for orphan status.

Specifically, the Orphan-Drug Annual Report has three sections.

- Progress Report: The progress report summarizing any actions (successful or unsuccessful, complete or in progress) since the last submitted report (14 months after initial Orphan-Drug Status or 12 months after the last Annual Report). If no action has been taken, a statement to that effect should be included.

Guidebook for Drug Regulatory Submissions, by Sandy Weinberg
Copyright © 2009 John Wiley & Sons, Inc.

- Future Plans: The future plans section should include specific plans for the next 12 months and a more general outline of the complete drug development plan. While this outline may not change (or may be revised) from year to year, it should be incorporated each year as a yardstick for progress.
- Orphan Status: The latest estimate of number of patients (United States) suffering from the disease or condition should be included. Presumably the best source of this information is the Centers for Disease Control and Prevention, but other source estimates may be utilized if unbiased and accurate. Should the estimate rise above the 200,000 cutoff level, the continuation of orphan-drug status should be discussed.
- Note that the first Orphan-Drug Annual report is due 14 months after status approval; all other reports are due every 12 months thereafter.

IND ANNUAL REPORTS

Once an IND has been opened (submitted and approved), an annual report is required, as per 21 Code of Federal Regulations (CFR) 312.33. It is important to note that INDs are not formally "approved" by the FDA; they go into effect 30 days after submission unless a clinical hold for cause is instituted. The IND Annual Report therefore provides reinforcing information indicating that a clinical hold is (still) not appropriate.

The Annual Report should include four key elements.

- Enrollment, demographic, and conduct status information for each study conducted under the IND
- Adverse Event summaries for each study underway or completed, including safety reports and death and dropout reports
- Drug action information collected since submission (or since the last annual update)
- Preclinical study status information

As with the Orphan-Drug update, the first report is due within 60 days of the anniversary of the "in effect" date (i.e., 90 days after the anniversary of the initial submission). Other annual reports are due every 12 months thereafter.

All IND Annual Reports should be accompanied by a Form 1571.

NDA AND ANDA ANNUAL REPORTS

The end result of a successful NDA [traditional or 505(b)2] or ANDA is FDA approval to sell the drug product in the United States. The required annual reports are therefore described as Postmarketing Reports.

In 2007, the Congress of the United States directed the FDA to reevaluate, extend, and improve the process of postmarketing tracking of drug products. As a result, the FDA is spending 2008 and 2009 developing new guidelines for NDA/ANDA Annual Reports. These guidelines will likely be released for comment in late 2009 or early 2010 and will go into effect in approximately mid-2010.

Until the new guidelines are released, the FDA is operating under section 103(a) of Title I of the FDA Modernization Act of 1997, final rule on postmarketing study requirements (October 30, 2000: 65 FR 64607), which became effective on April 30, 2001.

Under the current "final rule," those applicants with a commitment to conduct postmarketing studies must submit an annual report within 60 days of the anniversary of the product approval, and annually thereafter until notified by the Agency that either (a) the study commitment has been met or (b) the study is either no longer feasible or would not provide any additional useful data.

While all speculation on yet-to-be-released future guidelines is by definition uncertain, it seems likely based upon the Congressional mandate that the new guidance will broaden the pool of products for which postmarketing studies will be required, will expand the duration of those studies, and possibly will increase the level of scrutiny of both studies and patient tracking.

Currently, the Annual Postmarketing Study Report should include the following:

1. A review of the study conducted, including field reports from the Coding Symbols for a Thesaurus of Adverse Reaction Terms (COSTART) or Medical Registration (MEDRA) systems
2. An analysis of the results of that study (or studies) with recommendations for action, if any
3. A plan for continued or future postmarketing studies and monitoring

SUMMARY

Unlike in most FDA submissions, there is a great deal of format and content flexibility in the Annual Reports. The most common problem is a failure to file or to file promptly. Generally, any reasonable summary of progress and plans filed one year and 60 days from the initial acceptance and every 12 months thereafter is likely to be acceptable.

The exception is the NDA/ANDA Postmarketing Study Reports, which are evolving and likely to become more structured and more closely scrutinized. Once those new guidelines are released, strict adherence to their requirements will be mandatory, at the ultimate risk of a withdrawing of drug approval.

ANNUAL REPORTS (ORPHAN, IND, NDA, ANDA) SUBMISSION CHECKLIST

This checklist is intended for use in the preparation and submission of Annual Reports for Orphan-Drug Applications, INDs, NDAs [standard and 505(b)2], and ANDAs. It is recommended that, prior to transmission to the FDA, a second internal review should be conducted by an individual or department not involved in the preparation of the submission (presumably Quality Assurance).

The checklist was developed through discussions with consultants and Quality Assurance directors and has been field-tested in final form with three successful submissions.

☐ For INDs and NDA/ANDAs: Form 1571 completed
☐ Cover letter
   ☐ Name and address of sponsor
   ☐ Name, address, title, telephone, and e-mail of contact person
   ☐ Generic and trade name of drug or drug product
   ☐ FDA code number (assigned at time of preconference)
☐ Letter includes summary of action to date, planned action, and summary of any adverse events or outcomes
☐ For NDAs/ANDAs: Updated Chemistry, Manufacturing, and Control (CMC) information provided, including evidence of purity, stability, toxicology testing, and integrity of active pharmaceutical ingredient (API), placebo, and final product.
☐ For NDA/ANDs: Drug Master File (DMF) updated, including information on facilities, processes, and articles used in manufacturing, processing, packaging, and storage
☐ For NDA/ANDAs: Investigator's Brochure updated for all applicant-conducted studies included with detailed information for investigators and Institutional Review Board records
☐ For NDA/ANDAs: Updated complete pharmacological profile provided for API and final product
☐ Summary of adverse reactions to proposed drug

ANNUAL REPORT REVIEW CHECKLIST

This Annual Report Review checklist for Orphan Drugs, INDs, NDAs [both standard and 505(b)2], and ANDAs has been designed in consultation with FDA reviewers, industry consultants, and regulatory professionals to serve as a summary tool indicating the evaluative criteria used by the Center for Drug Evaluation and Research (CDER) and the Center for Biologics Evaluation and Research (CBER) to critique and assess applications received. It can be used internally as a part of the Quality Assurance process, as a guideline for regulatory development of an application, and/or as a self-assessment tool to predict likely FDA response to an application.

- ☐ **Form 1571 (NDA, ANDA, IND):** NDA is accompanied by completed Form 1571, providing (among other data) contact information including corporate name, contact name, address, telephone number, name and address of drug source, and generic and trade name of drug.
- ☐ **Cover letter:** A cover letter indicates disease and therapy names.
- ☐ **Three COPIES:** Photocopies are acceptable.
- ☐ (IND, NDA, ANDA): **DMF** updated, including information on facilities, processes, and articles used in manufacturing, processing, packaging, and storage
- ☐ **Content: Overview**
  - ☐ Provides update on all activities since last Annual Report, provides plans for future activities, and provides summary of any adverse events
  - ☐ (IND): Provides updates and changes to Investigator's Brochure, Study Protocols, and CMC information
  - ☐ (NDA, ANDA): Provides update to postmarketing studies, CMC
- ☐ **Content:** Organizational structure
- ☐ **Cover sheet:** Form 1571 (IND, NDA, ANDA)

COMMENTS:
DISPOSITION:
  Receipt date:
  Response due date:
  Disposition:
  Notification date:

ORPHAN DRUG REGULATIONS

(Federal Register: May 29, 2007
(Volume 72, Number 102)]
(Notices)
(Page 29515–29517)
From the Federal Register Online via GPO Access (http://www.wais.access.gpo.gov.com/)
(DOCID:fr29my07-55)
  Department of Health and Human Services
  Food and Drug Administration
  (Docket No. 2006N-0420)

Agency Information Collection Activities; Submission for Office of Management and Budget Review; Comment Request
Orphan-Drugs Agency
Food and Drug Administration, HHS.
Action: Notice.

Summary

The FDA is announcing that a proposed collection of information has been submitted to the Office of Management and Budget (OMB) for review and clearance under the Paperwork Reduction Act of 1995.

Dates

Fax written comments on the collection of information by June 28, 2007.

Addresses

To ensure that comments on the information collection are received, OMB recommends that written comments be faxed to the Office of Information and Regulatory Affairs, [[Page 29516]] OMB, Attn: FDA Desk Officer, FAX: 202-395-6974. All comments should be identified with the OMB control number 0910-0167. Also include the FDA docket number found in brackets in the heading of this document.

For further information, contact Jonna Capezzuto, Office of the Chief Information Officer (HFA-250), Food and Drug Administration, 5600 Fishers Lane, Rockville, MD 20857, 301-827-4659.

Supplementary Information

In compliance with 44 U.S.C. 3507, the FDA has submitted the following proposed collection of information to OMB for review and clearance.

Orphan Drugs (OMB Control Number 0910-0167)—Extension. Sections 525 through 526 of the Federal Food, Drug, and Cosmetic Act (the act) (21 U.S.C. 360aa through 360dd) give the FDA statutory authority to do the following: (1) Provide recommendations on investigations required for approval of marketing applications for orphan drugs, (2) designate eligible drugs as orphan drugs, (3) set forth conditions under which a sponsor of an approved orphan drug obtains exclusive approval, and (4) encourage sponsors to make orphan drugs available for treatment on an "open protocol" basis before the drug has been approved for general marketing. The implementing regulations for these statutory requirements have been codified under Part 316 (21 CFR

Part 316) and specify procedures that sponsors of orphan drugs use in availing themselves of the incentives provided for orphan drugs in the act and sets forth procedures the FDA will use in administering the act with regard to orphan drugs. Section 316.10 specifies the content and format of a request for written recommendations concerning the non-clinical laboratory studies and clinical investigations necessary for approval of marketing applications. Section 316.12 provides that, before providing such recommendations, the FDA may require results of studies to be submitted for review. Section 316.14 contains provisions permitting the FDA to refuse to provide written recommendations under certain circumstances. Within 90 days of any refusal, a sponsor may submit additional information specified by the FDA. Section 316.20 specifies the content and format of an orphan-drug application which includes requirements that an applicant document that the disease is rare (affects fewer than 200,000 persons in the United States annually) or that the sponsor of the drug has no reasonable expectation of recovering costs of research and development of the drug. Section 316.26 allows an applicant to amend the applications under certain circumstances. Section 316.30 requires submission of annual reports, including progress reports on studies, a description of the investigational plan, and a discussion of changes that may affect orphan status. The information requested will provide the basis for an FDA determination that the drug is for a rare disease or condition and satisfies the requirements for obtaining orphan-drug status. Secondly, the information will describe the medical and regulatory history of the drug. The respondents to this collection of information are biotechnology firms, drug companies, and academic clinical researchers.

The information requested from respondents represents, for the most part, an accounting of information already in the possession of the applicant. It is estimated, based on frequency of requests over the past five years, that 171 persons or organizations per year will request orphan-drug designation and none will request formal recommendations on design of preclinical or clinical studies.

In the Federal Register of October 30, 2006 (71 FR 63325), the FDA published a 60-day notice requesting public comment on the information collection provisions. The FDA received one comment related to the information collection.

(Comment 1) The comment suggested that our burden estimate to prepare an Orphan-Drug Annual Report is too low.

(Response 1) Section 316.30 pertains to annual reporting, a brief progress report which is a requirement after orphan designation has been granted to a sponsor. We estimate this takes 1-h professional time and 1-h support time.

(Comment 2) The comment suggested that our estimate of 130 h to prepare and submit an orphan-drug application is too high.

(Response 2) We disagree with the comment because some sponsors have more experience with submitting Orphan-Drug Designation applications/ requests and, therefore, may require less human resource hours to compile all required information. Many other sponsors, which include foreign sponsors, do not have such experience.

The estimated 130 h pertains to Sec. Sec. 316.20, 316.21, and 316.26. These apply primarily to initial applications/requests seeking orphan-drug designation. Many applications/requests received in the Office of Orphan Products Development contain multiple volumes; include an exact duplicate copy of the original; and may include 50 or more documented references. Additional information is requested when an application/request is denied. The sponsor usually supplies the requested information in the form of an amendment.

The FDA estimates the burden of this collection of information as follows (Table 8.1):

TABLE 8.1   Estimated annual reporting burden[a]

21 CFR section	No. of respondents	Annual frequency per response	Total annual responses	Hours per responses	Total hours
316.10, 316.12, & 316.14	5	1	5	130	650
316.20, 316.21, & 316.26	171	2	342	130	44,460
316.22	30	1	30	2	60
316.27	25	1	25	4	100
316.30	500	1	500	2	1000
316.36	2	3	6	15	9
Total					46,279

[a]There are no capital costs or maintenance costs associated with this collection of information.

[[Page 29517]]
Dated: May 22, 2007.
Jeffrey Shuren,
Assistant Commissioner for Policy.
(FR Doc. E7-10271 Filed 5-25-07; 8:45 a.m.)

BILLING CODE 4160-01-S
Code of Federal Regulations
(Title 21, Volume 5)
(Revised as of April 1, 2007)
(CITE: 21CFR316)

Title 21: Food and Drugs
Chapter I: Food and Drug Administration
Department of Health and Human Services

Subchapter D: Drugs for Human Use
Part 316: Orphan Drugs
Subpart C; Designation of an Orphan Drug

Sec. 316.30 Annual Reports of Holder of Orphan-Drug Designation
Within 14 months after the date on which a drug was designated as an orphan drug and annually thereafter until marketing approval, the sponsor of a designated drug shall submit a brief progress report to the FDA Office of Orphan Products Development on the drug that includes

(a) a short account of the progress of drug development including a review of preclinical and clinical studies initiated, ongoing, and completed and a short summary of the status or results of such studies;
(b) a description of the investigational plan for the coming year, as well as any anticipated difficulties in development, testing, and marketing; and
(c) A brief discussion of any changes that may affect the orphan-drug status of the product. For example, for products nearing the end of the approval process, sponsors should discuss any disparity between the probable marketing indication and the designated indication as related to the need for an amendment to the orphan-drug designation pursuant to 316.26.

Authority: 21 U.S.C. 360aa, 360bb, 360cc, 360dd, 371.
Source: 57 FR 62085, Dec. 29, 1992, unless otherwise noted.

DMF

Important Guidance Information

This section contains lists of DMFs as well as information concerning submission of DMFs. See below for information regarding the current DMF Guideline.

The list of DMFs is current as of December 31, 2007, through DMF 21223. Changes to the DMF activity status, DMF type, holder name, and subjects made since the last update of September 30, 2007 are included.

For people who downloaded the previous list (through DMF 20742 August 15, 2007) and do not wish to download the entire updated lists, the following lists are available.

1. New DMFs since the last list.
2. A list of changes in DMF activity status, DMF type, holder name, and subject.

The lists are available in Microsoft Excel and in ASCII (tab delimited). Please note that only ACTIVE DMFs have been sorted into different types.

For the Excel files, the following lists are provided as different worksheets within one Excel file.

- All DMFs
- Active DMFs
- Active Type II DMFs
- Active Type III DMFs
- Active Type IV DMFs
- Active Type V DMFs

The following lists are still provided as separate files.

- New DMFs since the last list
- Changes

The following are the types of DMFs.

- Type I Manufacturing Site, Facilities, Operating Procedures, and Personnel (no longer applicable)
- Type II Drug Substance, Drug Substance Intermediate, and Material Used in Their Preparation, or Drug Product
- Type III Packaging Material
- Type IV Excipient, Colorant, Flavor, Essence, or Material Used in Their Preparation
- Type V FDA Accepted Reference Information

"A" = Active
"I" = Inactive
"N" = Not an assigned number
"P" = DMF Pending Filing Review

Inactivation and Retirement of DMFs

There are two reasons for a DMF to be listed as inactive.

1. The holder requested that the DMF be retired, closed, inactivated, or withdrawn.
2. For DMFs filed before December 31, 2004,
   a. there have been no amendments or annual reports submitted since it was filed, or
   b. there have been no amendments or annual reports submitted since December 31, 2004.

Note that the status "Inactive" in the list does not distinguish among these categories.

According to the regulations regarding DMFs [21 CFR 314.420(c)],

> any addition, change, or deletion of information in a drug master file (except the list required under paragraph (d) of this section) is required to be submitted in two copies and to describe by name, reference number, volume, and page number the information affected in the drug master file.

As discussed in the *Guideline for Drug Master Files* (September 1989, http://www.fda.gov/cder/guidance/dmf.htm), DMF holders should update their DMFs annually (see "Annual Reports").

The FDA is in the process of sending "Overdue Notification Letters" (ONLs) to DMF holders that have not been updated, i.e., no amendments or annual reports in three years. If a DMF holder does not respond to this letter within 90 days, the DMF is retired and is unavailable for review. There is a backlog in sending out ONLs. DMF holders can forestall the sending of an ONL by updating their DMFs, following the procedure below under "Reactivation."

Some DMFs may be listed as inactive which are, in fact, still active. Every effort will be made to correct any errors.

Reactivating a DMF

A DMF holder that wants to activate a DMF in response to an ONL should do so within 90 days of the letter date and should use the following decision tree.

1. Have there been changes to the technical information in the DMF? If yes, submit an amendment listing all the changes. This includes technical information usually submitted on a periodic basis (e.g., stability updates). Go to item 4 below.
2. Have there been changes to the administrative information in the DMF? Do not submit any changes to the administrative information except he name and address of the holder and the manufacturing facility and the contact person. If yes, submit an amendment listing all the changes. Go to item 4 below.
3. If there have been no changes, submit an Annual Report stating that no changes have been made to the DMF. Include a list of all companies authorized to reference the DMF. (Authorized parties)
4. If there have been changes that were reported in the amendment(s) (see item 2 above), submit an annual report listing
   a. the date(s) of the amendment(s),
   b. the subject(s) of the amendment(s), and
   c. a list of authorized parties.

DMFs that have been closed either because the holder has not responded to an ONL within the 90-day time period or because they were withdrawn by the holder may have been retired by the FDA and cannot be updated. Under such circumstances the DMF holder will need to resubmit the DMF. Note that a DMF will not be retired by the FDA unless an ONL has been sent AND there was no response within 90 days.

There may be a lag time between inactivation of a DMF (either by lack of timely response to an ONL or closure by the holder) and its retirement by the FDA. DMF holders who wish to reactivate an inactive DMF should contact dmfquestion@cder.fda.gov to determine whether the DMF has been retired by the FDA unless (a) the DMF was closed by the holder or (b) an ONL has been sent AND there was no response within 90 days.

Questions or Comments about DMFS

Please address ALL comments or questions regarding DMFs to dmfquestion@cder.fda.gov. All inquiries **must** have an entry in the "Subject" field of the e-mail. Due to concerns about viruses and the amount of "spam" received by this account, e-mails with subject fields that are blank or contain meaningless text strings or contain only question marks will not be opened.

Other inquiries unrelated to DMFs should go to druginfo@fda.hhs.gov.

Guidances

DMF Guideline. The version posted on the web is the current version. Note that the address for submitting DMF documentation to the FDA in the Guidance has been superseded by the Beltsville address below. No revision is planned for the immediate future. Please address question regarding the DMF Guideline to dmfquestion@cder.fda.gov.

Note that FDA regulations require that all submissions to INDs and NDAs that are in a foreign language have "complete and accurate translations." The same is true for DMFs. A "certified translation" is not required.

More Information about DMFs

See http://www.fda.gov/cder/Offices/ONDQA/presentations/shaw.pdf.

The recommendations in the DMF Guidance are, in general, still applicable. However the information below provides additional information or clarification of the recommendations in the Guidance. This information provided below falls into three categories.

1. Recommendations that are no longer applicable due to changes in regulations or guidances
2. Additional clarification of recommendations in the Guidance

3. New information for aspects of DMF filing that were not in effect when the Guidance was written

Address for Filing Original DMFs and Subsequent DMF Documents (Category 3)

Food and Drug Administration
Center for Drug Evaluation and Research
Central Document Room
5901-B Ammendale Road
Beltsville MD 20705-1266

Types of DMFS

Type I DMFs (Category 1). Type I DMFs are no longer accepted per a final rule published January 12, 2000 (65 FR 1776). See Type V DMFs below.

Holders of Type II, III, and IV DMFs should not place information regarding facilities, personnel or operating procedures in these DMFs. Only the addresses of the DMF holder and manufacturing site and contact personnel should be submitted.

Type II DMFs. Type II DMFs may be submitted in the format for "Drug substance" in the Guidance for Industry M4Q: The CTD—Quality (Category 3)

Module 1 should contain the following administrative information.

- Addresses of DMF holder and manufacturing and testing facilities
- Name and address of contact persons and/or agents
- Agent Appointment letters
- Letters of Authorization

Drug Substance See the current *Guideline for Submitting Supporting Documentation in Drug Applications for the Manufacture of Drug Substances.*

For Type II DMFs filed in CDT-Q format, Module 2 is expected.

Drug Product See the *Guideline for Submitting Supporting Documentation in Drug Applications for the Manufacture of Drug Products.*

Type III DMFs. The applicable Guidance for Type III DMFs is the *Guidance for Industry: Container Closure Systems for Packaging Human Drugs and Biologics: Chemistry, Manufacturing, and Controls Documentation* and *Questions and Answers. (Category 3)*

Note that certain USP chapters concerning packaging materials referenced in the Container-Closure Guidance have been amended in USP 30. These changes were discussed in the Pharmacopeial Forum Volume No. 32(4) Page 1176.

There are three new chapters.

- Containers—Plastics ⟨661⟩ retains the information about plastic containers formerly in Chapter ⟨661⟩.
- Containers—Glass ⟨660⟩ now contains the information about glass containers formerly in Chapter ⟨661⟩.
- Containers—Performance Testing ⟨671⟩ contains the standards and tests used to determine the functional properties of plastic containers (permeation test for polyethylene and polypropylene containers and the light transmission test).

Type V DMFs. The following types of DMFs may be filed as Type V DMFs without requesting prior clearance from the FDA. (Category 3).

- Manufacturing site, facilities, operating procedures, and personnel for sterile manufacturing plants. See *Guidance for Industry for the Submission Documentation for Sterilization Process Validation in Applications for Human and Veterinary Drug Products.*
- Contract facilities for the manufacture of biotech products. See *Draft Guidance for Industry: Submitting Type V Drug Master Files to the Center for Biologics Evaluation and Research*

Electronic DMFs (Category 3). See *Guidance for Industry: Providing Regulatory Submissions in Electronic Format—Human Pharmaceutical Product Applications and Related Submissions Using the eCTD Specifications.* To make sure you have the most recent versions of the specifications referenced in this guidance please check Electronic Common Technical Document (eCTD). Companies are encouraged to submit their DMFs in electronic form, including updating current paper DMFs. Note that all applications to CDER, including DMFs that are submitted in electronic format MUST be in ECTD format, unless a waiver is granted. See http://www.fda.gov/cder/regulatory/ersr/waiver.htm.

All Letters of Authorization for electronic DMFs should specify that the DMF has been submitted in electronic format.

Companies that wish to submit an annual report or amendment in electronic format may do so. However, once the DMF holder has made an electronic submission every subsequent submission must be in electronic format. In such cases DMF holders are advised to resubmit the entire DMF in CTD format as an amendment. This allows the DMF to be reviewable in its entirety using the electronic DMF rather than mixing paper and electronic formats. If there are any changes in the technical content of the DMF as a result of the reformatting, e.g. addition of new information, the cover letter for the amendment should specify what areas of technical information have been changed.

Agents (Category 2)

There is no regulatory requirement for an agent for any DMF, foreign or domestic. An agent for DMF purposes is not the same as an agent for the purposes of the Drug Listing and Registration System. According to a Federal Register Notice, November 27, 2001 (Vol. 6, No. 228), effective May 24, 2002, all foreign drug establishments are required to register with the FDA. As published, foreign firms are required to register and identify a U.S. agent.

If possible, the word "Agent" should be used for the legal entity (whether a company or an individual) who is authorized to act on behalf of the DMF holder. The word "Representative" should be used for an individual who is employed by the Agent or Holder as the contact point for the FDA. Agent Appointment Letters or notifications rescinding the appointment of an Agent should be sent as separate documents, rather than being included in an Annual Report or other amendment. If a company acting as an Agent changes its name, the DMF holder should issue a new Agent Appointment Letter. A change in Representative does not need to be reported in a separate amendment.

All "Agent Appointment Letters" for DMFs should be sent by the holder. The FDA recommends that such letters include the phrase "appoint AGENT NAME as the agent for DMF" rather than "authorize AGENT NAME to act as the agent for DMF," since the latter can be confused with a "Letter of Authorization." An "Agent Appointment Letter" may be included in an original DMF.

Holder Names (Category 2)

When the company that owns a DMF (DMF holder) changes its name, whether through sale of the company or simply a change in the company's name, the DMF holder must notify the FDA. This should be done in a separate amendment, rather than including the information in an Annual Report or other amendment. See Section VII.E. in the Guideline for DMFs for further recommendations on the procedure for transferring ownership. A change in the name of a company for registration purposes under Drug Listing and Registration System will not change the DMF holder name.

In general, the FDA expects the manufacturer to be the holder. If a manufacturer (Company A) of a MATERIAL wishes to have the DMF submitted by another company (Company B) and Company B wishes to act as the holder, the DMF must include statements from both companies that Company B takes full responsibility for all the information in the DMF and for all the processes and testing performed by the manufacturer. The title of the DMF that will appear on the list of DMFs will be "MATERIAL manufactured by COMPANY A in LOCATION OF COMPANY A for COMPANY B."

Annual Reports (Category 2)

According to the DMF Guideline, Annual Reports are **not** to be used to report changes in the DMF. Note that Annual Reports to DMFs are not REQUIRED by law or regulation.

> Section VII.C.
> The holder should provide an annual report on the anniversary date of the original submission. This report should contain the required list as described in B.1 and should also **identify all changes and additional information incorporated into the DMF since the previous annual report** on the subject matter of the DMF.

> VII. B.1.
> A DMF is required to contain a complete list of persons authorized to incorporate information in the DMF by reference [21 CFR 314.420(d)]. The holder should update the list in the annual update. The updated list should contain the holder's name, DMF number, and the date of the update. The update should identify by name (or code) the information that each person is authorized to incorporate and give the location of that information by date, volume, and page number.

The list of authorized parties in the Annual Report should be a complete list of authorized parties rather than a list of authorized parties added since the previous update. See discussion above under "reactivating a DMF" for recommendations on what information should be in an Annual Report and what information should be in an amendment.

Biologics Master Files

Master Files submitted in support of products regulated by CBER should be submitted as Biologics Master Files. See the CBER Web site for the products regulated by CBER.

Binders

See FDA IND, NDA, ANDA, or Drug Master File Binders. One copy of the DMF should use the blue binder and one should use the red binder.

GUIDANCE FOR INDUSTRY[1]—CHANGES TO AN APPROVED NDA OR ANDA; SPECIFICATIONS—USE OF ENFORCEMENT DISCRETION FOR COMPENDIAL CHANGES

U.S. Department of Health and Human Services
Food and Drug Administration

[1]This guidance was prepared by the Office of Compliance and the Office of Pharmaceutical Science in CDER at the FDA.

Center for Drug Evaluation and Research
November 2004
CMC
Additional copies are available from:
Office of Training and Communication
Division of Drug Information, HFD-240
Center for Drug Evaluation and Research
Food and Drug Administration
5600 Fishers Lane
Rockville, MD 20857
Tel: 301-827-4573
http://www.fda.gov/cder/guidance/index.htm

This guidance represents the FDA's current thinking on this topic. It does not create or confer any rights for or on any person and does not operate to bind the FDA or the public. You can use an alternative approach if the approach satisfies the requirements of the applicable statutes and regulations. If you want to discuss an alternative approach, contact the FDA staff responsible for implementing this guidance. If you cannot identify the appropriate FDA staff, call the appropriate telephone number listed on the title page of this guidance.

Introduction

This guidance is intended to inform NDA and ANDA holders of the FDA's plan to use enforcement discretion with regard to section 314.70(c)(2)(iii) of the final rule entitled Supplements and Other Changes to an Approved Application [21 CFR 314.70(c)(2)(iii)].[2] This subsection describes the filing requirement that a relaxation of acceptance criteria or deletion of a test to comply with an official compendium must be reported in a changes-being-effected-in-30-days supplement (CBE-30). In the exercise of its enforcement discretion, the FDA does not intend to take enforcement action if manufacturers continue to submit such changes in their annual reports. The use of enforcement discretion will give the Agency time to clarify that some of these types of postapproval changes can be submitted in an annual report, rather than in a CBE-30. The Agency intends to clarify this issue in an upcoming revision to the guidance for industry *Changes to an Approved NDA or ANDA: Questions and Answers.*

The FDA's guidance documents, including this guidance, do not establish legally enforceable responsibilities. Instead, guidances describe the Agency's current thinking on a topic and should be viewed only as recommendations, unless specific regulatory or statutory requirements are cited. The use of the

---

[2] See the Federal Register, Vol. 69, p. 18728, April 8, 2004.

word *should* in Agency guidances means that something is suggested or recommended, but not required.

Background

On April 8, 2004, the FDA published in the Federal Register (69 FR 18728) the final rule entitled Supplements and Other Changes to an Approved Application. In the same issue of the Federal Register (69 FR 18768), the FDA announced the availability of the guidance for industry entitled *Changes to an Approved NDA or ANDA* (the *Changes* guidance). The final rule sets forth requirements for post-approval changes.

Under section 314.70(c)(2)(iii) of the final rule, the relaxation of acceptance criteria or deletion of a test to comply with an official compendium that is consistent with FDA statutory and regulatory requirements must be submitted as a supplement—CBE-30 (see section VIII.C.1.e of the *Changes* guidance). Under 314.70(d)(2)(i) of the final rule, any change in a specification made to comply with an official compendium, except the relaxation of acceptance criteria or deletion of a test that is consistent with FDA statutory and regulatory requirements, is to be submitted as an Annual Report (see section VIII.D.1 of the *Changes* guidance).

Since publication of the final rule, the Agency has received communications from NDA and ANDA holders requesting clarification of the regulation as it applies to changes such as excipient monographs and general chapters. As written now, the regulations could be interpreted to require a CBE for any compendial change to relax or delete a test, resulting in an increase in the number of supplements, something that was not intended. The Agency plans to revise the *Guidance for Industry: Changes to an Approved NDA or ANDA; Questions and Answers* to provide more specific recommendations as to what types of changes can be submitted in an annual report instead of a CBE-30 supplement.

In addition, the Agency is aware that stakeholders have expressed concern that the final rule (i.e., 21 CFR 314.70), which published on April 8, 2004, and the accompanying *Changes* guidance do not take into consideration the recent FDA Pharmaceutical CGMP Initiative for the 21st Century. Accordingly, the Agency plans to align this guidance with the initiative in order to facilitate manufacturing changes to enhance product quality.

Exercise of Enforcement Discretion

The FDA intends to exercise enforcement discretion and does not intend to take action to enforce compliance with the compendial changes requirement as stated in 21 CFR 314.70(c)(2)(iii) if manufacturers submit such changes in their annual reports. The FDA intends to develop further guidance to clarify the requirements of 21 CFR 314.70(c)(2)(iii).

DRAFT GUIDANCE FOR INDUSTRY AND FDA STAFF—
ANNUAL REPORTS FOR APPROVED PREMARKET APPROVAL
APPLICATIONS (PMA)[3]

Comments and suggestions regarding this draft document should be submitted within 90 days of publication in the Federal Register of the notice announcing the availability of the draft guidance. Submit written comments to the Division of Dockets Management (HFA-305), Food and Drug Administration, 5630 Fishers Lane, Rm. 1061, Rockville, MD 20852. Alternatively, electronic comments may be submitted to http://www.fda.gov/dockets/ecomments. All comments should be identified with the docket number listed in the notice of availability that publishes in the Federal Register.

For questions regarding this document, contact Laura Byrd at 240-276-4040 or Laura.Byrd@fda.hhs.gov. For questions regarding the application of this guidance to devices regulated by CBER, contact Leonard Wilson at 301-827-0373 or by e-mail at leonard.wilson@fda.hhs.gov.

U.S. Department of Health and Human Services
Food and Drug Administration
Center for Devices and Radiological Health
Center for Devices and Radiological Health
Center for Biologics Evaluation and Research

Contains Nonbinding Recommendations
Draft—Not for Implementation

Additional Copies

Additional copies are available from the Internet at http://www.fda.gov/cdrh/ode/1585.pdf, or to receive this document via your fax machine, call the CDRH Facts-On-Demand system at 800-899-0381 or 301-827-0111 from a touch-tone telephone. Press 1 to enter the system. At the second voice prompt, press 1 to order a document. Enter the document number (**1585**) followed by the pound sign (#). Follow the remaining voice prompts to complete your request.

This draft guidance, when finalized, will represent the FDA's current thinking on this topic. It does not create or confer any rights for or on any person and does not operate to bind the FDA or the public. You can use an alternative approach if the approach satisfies the requirements of the applicable statutes and regulations. If you want to discuss an alternative approach, contact the FDA staff responsible for implementing this guidance. If you cannot identify the appropriate FDA staff, call the appropriate number listed on the title page of this guidance.

---

[3]This guidance document is being distributed for comment purposes only. Document issued on: October 26, 2006.

Introduction

Devices subject to premarket approval under section 515 of the Federal Food, Drug, and Cosmetic Act (the Act) are also subject to periodic reports imposed by the PMA approval order [21 CFR 814.82(a), 21 CFR 814.84(b)]. We typically specify that you submit a report one year from the date of approval of the original PMA and annually thereafter. Therefore, the periodic report is usually referred to as an annual report. Although this guidance addresses "annual reports," there may be circumstances where FDA specifies more frequent periodic reports. We believe this guidance will also be relevant to the more frequent reports.

This guidance document describes the information required by 21 CFR 814.84(b), additional information requirements that may be imposed by approval order under 21 CFR 814.82, and our recommendations for the level of detail you should provide in your annual report. It also identifies the steps FDA staff generally takes when reviewing annual reports, the resources available to assist staff in their reviews, and the actions they may recommend in their conclusions. This guidance document is intended to help ensure that your annual reports are complete and that the actions of CDRH and CBER staff are consistent.

In our efforts to bring safe and effective products to market as quickly as possible, CDRH needs to be able to rely on a variety of postmarket controls that will assure continuing safety and effectiveness after a medical device is widely distributed. We believe that data and information gathered in the postmarket setting are critical to our continued confidence in the safety and effectiveness of the marketed device. Annual reports are one of the important tools that the FDA relies upon to gather information about the device in its postapproval setting.

Annual reports currently contain a variety of information, including information about manufacturing changes, design changes, and labeling changes that were made during the preceding year for the PMA product. This guidance recommends that this and other information be analyzed and presented in a way that will be most useful to both the company and the FDA. For example, the guidance recommends that you describe in detail the rationale for changes made to your device, including whether the changes were the result of product complaints and adverse events. This will give us a more complete picture of the postmarket safety profile of the device. The guidance also recommends that you include a summary of all changes that were made to your device during the reporting period, including those that were the subject of a PMA supplement. Having the information submitted in this way will help ensure that limited Agency resources are devoted to assessing meaningful information rather than sifting through vast amounts of data that have not been systematically reviewed by the firm.

The FDA believes that the types of information that we are requesting in this guidance and the types of review, summary, and analysis we are recommending are already part of the quality system practices of companies that comply with good manufacturing practice (GMP) regulations. For example, design controls already require the type of look-back and assessment that we are suggesting to be part of the annual report.

Annual reports that contain well-developed and meaningful information will be an important tool for the Agency and the industry to assure postmarket safety and protect the public. When manufacturers prepare the type of analysis this guidance describes and provide this information to the FDA in annual reports, industry and the FDA will be better positioned to recognize and address possible safety signals.

The Least Burdensome Approach. This draft guidance document reflects our careful review of what we believe are the relevant issues related to annual reports and what we believe would be the least burdensome way of addressing these issues. If you have comments on whether there is a less burdensome approach, however, please submit your comments to CDER or CBER, as appropriate.

The FDA's guidance documents, including this guidance, do not establish legally enforceable responsibilities. Instead, guidances describe the Agency's current thinking on a topic and should be viewed only as recommendations, unless specific regulatory or statutory requirements are cited. The use of the word *should* in Agency guidances means that something is suggested or recommended, but not required.

Background

In the PMA approval order, the FDA requires that PMA sponsors submit postapproval periodic reports, i.e., annual reports to the FDA, in accordance with 21 CFR 814.82(a)(7) and 814.84(b). Section 21 CFR 814.84(b) describes the information required:
Unless the FDA specifies otherwise, a periodic report must

1. identify changes described in 21 CFR 814.39(a) and changes required to be reported to the FDA under 21 CFR 814.39(b); and
2. contain a summary and bibliography of the following information not previously submitted as part of the PMA.
   i. Unpublished reports of data from any clinical investigations or non-clinical laboratory studies involving the device or related devices and known to or that reasonably should be known to the applicant
   ii. Reports in the scientific literature concerning the device and known to or that reasonably should be known to the applicant. If, after reviewing the summary and bibliography, the FDA concludes that the Agency needs a copy of the unpublished or published reports, the

FDA will notify the applicant that copies of such reports shall be submitted.

You are primarily responsible for determining whether changes to your device, labeling, or manufacturing processes impact safety or effectiveness and, thus, require a PMA Supplement or 30-Day Notice.[4] This guidance is not intended to define when you should submit a new original PMA or any type of PMA Supplement.

In accordance with 21 CFR 814.84(a), you must also comply with **Medical Device Reporting** (MDR) requirements, 21 CFR Part 803, and any requirements made applicable by other regulations or by order approving the device, including the following.

- Post-approval study reports, if the FDA has imposed continuing evaluation (post-approval study) requirements on your device in the PMA approval order, 21 CFR 814.82(a)(2)
- Adverse reaction reports and device defect reports, if imposed in the PMA approval order, 21 CFR 814.82(a)(9) but only to the extent that such reports do not duplicate MDR reporting requirements

Post-Approval Study Reports

As provided by 21 CFR 814.82(a)(2), the FDA may require continuing evaluation (post-approval study) and periodic reporting on the safety, effectiveness, and reliability of your device (post-approval study report), in addition to requiring annual reports under 21 CFR 814.82(a)(7). If your approval order identifies post-approval studies you must conduct, the order will describe the purpose of the studies and how frequently you must submit post-approval study reports.

We recommend that you submit your annual report and post-approval study report separately, even if they are due at the same time. This will facilitate the FDA's review because different Offices in Center for Devices and Radiological Health (CDRH) review the post-approval study report and the annual report.[5] If you choose to provide a separate report as recommended, please include the date that you submitted your post-approval study report in your annual report.

If you choose to include your post-approval study report along with your annual report, we recommend that you create a separate section of the annual report for the post-approval study report.

---

[4] We recommend that you carefully assess whether a change requires a PMA Supplement, 21 CFR 814.39(a) or 30-Day Notice, 21 CFR 814.39(e). The list of examples in 21 CFR 814.39(a) illustrates the kind of changes that require a PMA Supplement; however, it is not an exhaustive list.

[5] See the draft guidance, *Procedures for Handling Post-Approval Studies Imposed by PMA Order*, issued for comment on September 15, 2005, at http://www.fda.gov/cdrh/osb/guidance/1561.html. (When final, the Internet address will link to the guidance issued for implementation.)

Contents of an Annual Report

A complete annual report should include all of the information described below. If your annual report is complete, we can review your annual report more efficiently, and it is more likely that we will not request additional information from you.

Cover Letter for an Annual Report. We recommend that you include a cover letter to your PMA annual report. Your cover letter should include the following.

PMA number
device name (including any model names and numbers)
company name
date of report
reporting period (i.e., the dates the reporting period begins and ends)
approval date (dates original PMA and any PMA Supplements were
   approved)

Manufacturing, Design, and Labeling Changes. To facilitate our review of your annual report, we recommend dividing your report into separate sections for manufacturing, design, and labeling changes.

As described below, each of the three sections should identify all changes made during the reporting period,[6] including those that were submitted in a PMA supplement or 30-Day Notice and those changes that you have not already reported in a PMA Supplement or 30-Day Notice.[7]

Identification of the Changes. For each change in your summary, we recommend you identify

- the change made;
- the rationale for making the change;
- a listing of any validation or other testing that was performed, including a description of the method and acceptance criteria (but not the data itself); and
- the implementation date.

---

[6] Please note that simple changes related to the device documentation or manufacturing process documentation, such as rewording or expanding for clarification, translating from one language to another, correcting typographical errors, and moving component characteristics from an engineering drawing note to a different document, such as a Standard Operating Procedure (SOP), do not need to be reported in the annual report. In general, such changes do not affect the design, performance, labeling, or processing of the device, only how the characteristics are documented.
[7] In accordance with 21 CFR 814.39(b), you may change your approved device without submitting a PMA Supplement, if the change does not affect the device's safety or effectiveness and you report the change to FDA in your annual report.

For changes that are the subject of an approved or pending PMA Supplement or 30-Day Notice, we recommend that you also identify the document number assigned by the FDA and, if approved, the approval date.

We recommend that you provide separate tables for manufacturing changes, design changes, and labeling changes. An example of a design changes table is provided below. We recommend that you include similar tables for manufacturing changes and labeling changes.

Design Changes Table

Change	Rationale for change	Summary of validation activities	Implementation date	PMA supplement type and number assigned by the FDA, if applicable	Approval date, if applicable

Examples of rationales for device changes we recommend you specify include whether the change was

- made as a result of a problem that resulted in an MDR [if so, we recommend that you provide the applicable MDR number(s)];
- made as a result of an adverse event, device defect, or failure reported to you or identified in the literature;
- associated with any recall or corrective action (see also 21 CFR 820.100);
- in response to any customer complaint, request, or suggestion;
- related to any public disclosure or communication on your part, i.e., "Dear Doctor" or "Dear Patient" letters or technical bulletins; or
- related to an FDA Safety Alert, Public Health Notification, or warning letter.

If any change that you have made is associated with any written communications to practitioners or patients, we recommend that you include a copy of the communication in your annual report.

Detailed Description of Changes Not Reported in Existing Supplements. For changes not reported in a PMA Supplement or a 30-Day Notice, we recommend that you describe the changes and the scientific and/or regulatory rationale basis for concluding that the change had no impact on safety or effectiveness. The description and rationale should provide sufficient detail to allow the FDA to determine that the changes did not require a PMA Supplement or 30-Day Notice. It may be helpful to link together the summary data in the tables with the detailed data by some means such as unique enumeration. That is, you may wish to number the items in the tables and then refer to those numbers in the detailed descriptions.

As part of your rationale for the changes you are reporting, we also recommend that you include a brief summary of the risk analysis performed to assess the effect of the changes made during the reporting period that were not already described in PMA supplements or 30-Day Notices. If you did not conduct system-level testing of the cumulative changes, your risk analysis should also assess whether incremental testing was adequate to assure continued safety and effectiveness of your device in the absence of system-level testing. If you performed the risk analysis in conformance to any consensus standards, these should be identified.

If any changes to the design, manufacturing, or labeling you have made during the reporting period (that did not require submission of a PMA supplement or 30-Day notice) are associated with MDRs, failures or recalls of any kind, corrective actions (21 CFR 820.100), complaints, or in response to FDA warning letters or inspection findings (FDA Form 483), we recommend that you

- describe your investigation of the cause or source of the problem
- explain your decision to change your device design, labeling, or manufacturing process by describing how the changes have corrected the problem and mitigated harm.[8]

Summary and Bibliography of Reports of Scientific Investigations and Literature. You are required to provide a summary and bibliography of reports in the scientific literature that are known, or that reasonably should be known to you, and that were not previously submitted as part of your PMA application [21 CFR 814.84(b)(2)(ii)]. If there are reports or scientific literature on clinical or nonclinical studies of similar devices, we recommend that you include them in your summary and bibliography.

The summary and bibliography must also include unpublished reports of data from any clinical investigations or nonclinical laboratory studies involving your device or related devices that are known or that reasonably should be known to you [21 CFR 814.84(b)(2)(i)].

Your summary should include a discussion of how the results and conclusions in the reports and literature could impact the known safety and effectiveness profile of your device. If, as a result of reviewing the reports and literature, you determine that changes to your device or its labeling are necessary, we recommend that you inform us of your plan for submitting a PMA supplement or 30-Day Notice for these changes or explain why you believe such a submission is not appropriate.

---

[8]Please note that any information supplied in this report related to corrective actions will be evaluated with the purpose of understanding the reason for the change to your device design, labeling, or manufacturing process. The information will not be evaluated for adequacy with respect to compliance with 21 CFR 820.100.

If, after reviewing your annual report, we conclude that we need an actual copy of a published or unpublished report, we will notify you. You must submit a copy in response, as required by 21 CFR 814.84(b)(2)(ii). However, if you anticipate that we will need a copy of any of these reports, you may, on your own initiative, provide it in your annual report.

Information on Devices Shipped or Sold. To help the FDA assess the public health impact of the previously requested information, we are also asking that you provide us with data about the number of devices shipped or sold during the reporting period. For device implants, data regarding the number of devices actually implanted should be provided, if it is available.

Posting of Reports and Option to Submit a Redacted Copy. The confidentiality of information in a PMA file, which includes information in annual reports, is governed by 21 CFR § 814.9. Consistent with this regulation and with 21 CFR Part 20, we intend to publicly post a redacted copy of your annual report on our Web site. The FDA will not make public any confidential commercial or financial information or trade secrets[9] or any information the disclosure of which might cause an unwarranted invasion of personal privacy.[10] You may, on your own initiative, include a redacted copy of your annual report for this purpose.

The FDA's Review of Your Annual Report

The FDA's review of annual reports will allow the Agency to assess several important issues related to postmarket safety of approved devices. These issues include the nature and adequacy of reported modifications and the adequacy of report documentation. If, after reviewing your annual report, we need additional information or if we believe the device modifications you have reported require a PMA Supplement or a 30-Day Notice, we will notify you in writing.

Several FDA offices may work in partnership in reviewing your annual report. In CDRH, the Office of Device Evaluation (ODE) or the Office of In Vitro Diagnostics (OIVD), depending on the device type, has the primary responsibility for reviewing the scientific information, including design and labeling changes. Generally, The Office of Compliance and ODE or OIVD review the manufacturing information. As necessary, the Office of Surveillance and Biometrics may also perform a search of the Manufacturer and User Facility Device Experience (MAUDE) database to further evaluate MDRs submitted during the reporting period. The review memo will include the findings from each Office.

The FDA intends to review most annual reports within 90 days of receipt. In general, our review memos follow the format described below.

[9] See 21 CFR 20.61.
[10] See, for example, 21 C.F.R. 20.63(a), "The names or other information which would identify patients or research subjects in any medical or similar report, test, study or other research project shall be deleted before the record is made available for public disclosure."

Reported Changes and Rationale for the Changes. Our review memo will summarize the changes described in the annual report and our evaluation of those changes. Our review memo will also describe our understanding of your rationale for the changes and our assessment of your rationale. The memo will clearly indicate whether we believe the changes you described are appropriate for an annual report or should have been described in a PMA Supplement or a 30-Day Notice.

Device Change Information. ODE or OIVD, in consultation with other Offices within CDRH, as appropriate, will evaluate your summary of the changes made to your device. As appropriate, we also plan to search the MAUDE database and review other FDA records to assess the postmarket safety profile of your device.

We will evaluate the information on the changes made to the device and the rationale for the changes, along with information you submitted from published and unpublished reports, and literature to determine if the safety and effectiveness profile of your device has changed. We can then determine whether any action (e.g., labeling change) is necessary to ensure the continued safety and effectiveness of your device.

FDA's Recommendations

Generally, our review memo will conclude with one of the following recommendations described below.

Acknowledgment of Complete Annual Report. If we determine that the annual report fulfills the requirements of 21 CFR 814.84, we will issue a letter or send an e-mail to inform you that the annual report is complete.

Request Additional Information. If you have not provided all the information required for an annual report, or we find that the information provided is not sufficient to allow a complete review, we plan to request additional information by letter or e-mail. If we only need clarification of an issue, we will either telephone or email you, whichever we believe will be the most expeditious.

Changes Not Appropriate for an Annual Report. If we determine that a change made to the device required a PMA Supplement or 30-Day Notice under 21 CFR 814.39 and you did not meet this requirement, we will notify you in writing. In general, we will issue a letter notifying you that a PMA Supplement or 30-Day Notice is required for the change and requesting that you provide the appropriate submission within a specified time frame. However, there may also be instances when The OC will review to determine if any additional regulatory actions are warranted.

CHAPTER 9

International Regulatory Submissions

CARL A. ROCKBURNE[1]

INTRODUCTION

The increase in travel brought on by globalization, markets, and human migration has made the regulator's role increasingly more complex. With the speed and commonality of airline travel, it is unlikely that a major disease outbreak can be effectively isolated in a single country or region. Public health issues including severe acute respiratory syndrome, West Nile Virus, and Bovine Spongiform Encephalopathy (mad cow disease) are fundamentally transforming the regulatory environment.

Further, technological and scientific advances are also altering the environmental landscape and changing the role played by regulatory organizations. All these changes have brought about the need for greater cooperation between countries relative to the regulation of therapeutic products and to the submissions/approval process that governs that regulation.

This essay reviews the submission requirements for the four markets of greatest interest to American companies: Canada, Australia, Japan, and the European Union (EU). Finally, the latest update on the International Conference on Harmonization (ICH) and attempts at harmonization is included.

INTERNATIONAL SUBMISSIONS

Canada

The Food and Drugs Act and Regulations authorize Health Canada to regulate the safety, efficacy, and quality of therapeutic products. The stages and

[1] Carl Rockburne is an international regulatory consultant with more than 35 years of experience in the field.

Guidebook for Drug Regulatory Submissions, by Sandy Weinberg
Copyright © 2009 John Wiley & Sons, Inc.

activities range from preclinical trials to postauthorization surveillance, inspection, and investigation. Participants in the regulatory process include patients and consumers, health-care professionals, research scientists, industry, academic institutions, pharmacies, hospitals, regulatory scientists, and policy makers.

New therapeutic products can be sold in Canada once they have successfully passed a review process to assess their safety, efficacy, and quality. Responsibility for this review process rests with Health Canada's Health Products and Food Branch (HPFB).

The HPFB evaluates and monitors the safety, efficacy, and quality of thousands of human and veterinary drugs, medical devices, natural health products, and other therapeutic products available to Canadians, as well as the safety and quality of food in Canada.

The goal of HPFB is to maintain public safety. To ensure that this objective is met, the HPFB duties include the following:

a. Premarket review—Before a therapeutic product is authorized for sale in Canada, the manufacturer must provide HPFB with scientific evidence of its safety, efficacy, and quality.
b. Postmarket surveillance, inspection, and investigation—Once therapeutic products reach the market, the Branch monitors them for safety, efficacy, and quality.

The Branch also works with international organizations, including regulatory authorities in other countries, to harmonize regulatory standards and processes for therapeutic products.

If the results of the clinical trial studies indicate that a new drug has potential therapeutic value that outweighs the risks associated with its proposed use, the manufacturer may seek authorization to sell the product in Canada by filing a New Drug Submission (NDS) with HPFB.

Normally, an NDS contains scientific data about the product's safety, efficacy, and quality. The NDS will also include the results of the preclinical and clinical studies; details pertaining to the production of the drug, its packaging and labeling; and information about its claimed therapeutic value, conditions for use, and side effects.

An Abbreviated NDS is used for a generic product. The submission must meet the same quality standards as an NDS, and the generic product must be shown to be as safe and efficacious as the brand-name product. An Abbreviated NDS includes scientific information that shows how the generic product performs compared with the brand-name product, as well as provide details on the production of the generic drug, its packaging, and labeling. The generic drug must be shown to deliver the same amount of medicinal ingredient at the same rate as the brand-name product.

A Supplemental NDS must be filed by the manufacturer if certain changes are made to already-authorized products. Such changes could include the dosage form or strength of the drug product, the formulation, method of manufacture, and labeling or recommended route of administration. A Supplemental NDS must also be submitted to HPFB if the manufacturer wants to expand the claims or conditions of use for the drug product.

If drugs are not approved for lack of evidence to support safety, efficacy, or quality claims, Health Canada will not grant a marketing authorization for the drug; however, the sponsor has the opportunity to offer additional supporting data and resubmit the submission at a later date.

The HPFB continues to ensure that the drug review process is as efficient as possible. It has taken several steps to streamline the process, including electronic submission, using a team approach, upgrading information technology, and strengthening scientific resources.

Further Sources of Information

Organizations	URL
Health Canada	http://www.hc-sc.gc.ca/
Health Products and Food Branch, Health Canada	http://www.hc-sc.gc.ca/hpfb-dgpsa/
Canada's *Food and Drugs Act* and Regulations	http://laws.justice.gc.ca/en/F-27/
Therapeutic Products Directorate	http://www.hc-sc.gc.ca/hpfb-dgpsa/tpd-dpt/aboutus_e.html
Biologics and Genetic Therapies Directorate	http://www.hc-sc.gc.ca/hpfb-dgpsa/bgtd-dpbtg/aboutus_e.html
Natural Health Products Directorate	http://www.hc-sc.gc.ca/hpfb-dgpsa/nhpd-dpsn/index_e.html
Marketed Health Products Directorate	http://www.hc-sc.gc.ca/hpfb-dgpsa/tpd-dpt/about-mhpd_e.html
Health Products and Food Branch Inspectorate	http://www.hc-sc.gc.ca/hpfb-dgpsa/inspectorate/index_e.html
Provincial and Territorial Government Health Ministries and Links	http://www.hc-sc.gc.ca/hcs-sss/medi-assur/ptrole/ptmin/index_e.html
Canadian Agency for Drugs and Technologies in Health	http://www.cadth.ca/
Patented Medicine Prices Review Board	http://www.pmprb-cepmb.gc.ca/

Australia

Within the Australian Government, the department that is responsible for monitoring therapeutic drugs is the Department of Health and Aging. The Therapeutic Goods Administration (TGA) is a unit of the Department of Health and Aging. The function of the TGA is to safeguard public health and safety in Australia by regulating medicines, medical devices, blood, and tissues. The Agency performs a range of assessment and monitoring activities to ensure that therapeutic goods are available and meet an acceptable standard.

The Australian community expects that medicines and medical devices in the marketplace are safe, of high quality, and of a high standard comparable to other countries. It is governed by the Therapeutic Goods Act of 1989, which came into effect in February 1991, to provide a national framework for the regulation of therapeutic goods ensuring the quality, safety, and efficacy of medicines.

The regulatory framework is based on a risk management approach designed to ensure public health and safety while, at the same time, freeing industry from any unnecessary regulatory burden.

Basically therapeutic goods must be entered on the Australian Register of Therapeutic Goods (ARTG) before they can be supplied in Australia. The ARTG is a computer database of information about therapeutic goods for human use approved for supply in or exported from Australia.

The Act set out the requirements for the inclusion of therapeutic goods in the ARTG, including advertising, labeling, and product appearance. Other provisions, such as the scheduling of substances and the safe storage of therapeutic goods, are covered by the relevant State or Territory legislation.

In order to be imported into, manufactured in, supplied in, or exported from Australia, medicines must be included in the ARTG. Intending sponsors of medicines must apply to the TGA for the inclusion of their product on the Register.

Guidelines have been established to assist sponsors in the preparation of applications to register new prescription or other high-risk medicines for human use. The format for applications is the Common Technical Document. It is a format that is also used in other parts of the world.

The Agency has published guidelines describing the information to be included with an application so that a new medicine can be registered. They apply to medicines that are evaluated by the Drug Safety and Evaluation Branch of the TGA, in accordance with the Therapeutic Goods Act. All prescription medicines and certain other high-risk medicines come under this category.

Guidelines used by applicants are preferred in order to maintain an element of flexibility and are not designed to place restraints on scientific progress. It is recognized that, in some cases resulting from scientific developments, an alternative approach may be appropriate. However, when an applicant chooses not to apply a guideline, then that decision must be explained and justified when submitted by the sponsor in support of the application.

This flexible approach to guidelines is unique in the sense that the Agency recognizes other reasons beyond scientific development that may be accepted as rationale for a sponsor not to follow rigid guidelines. Some of these include

a. circumstances unique to the product;
b. relevancy of a guideline;
c. new approach adopted by the sponsor; and
d. sufficient alternative studies have been conducted which satisfy the criteria of quality, safety, and efficacy.

A sponsor has the option to dispute that a particular guideline or an aspect of a guideline does not apply to a given product. However, supporting data must be provided in order to justify why the proposed alternative is valid.

Given the importance of these guidelines, sponsors should check the TGA for guidance and not rely entirely on printed matter. For complex applications, presubmission meetings between Agency personnel and sponsors wishing to submit an application to the Drug Safety and Evaluation Branch are recommended. Such meetings are encouraged to clarify particular issues or uncertainty whether the registration dossier to be submitted will meet all regulatory requirements.

Administrative guidelines, on the other hand, are generally less flexible. Examples include the number of copies of documentation to be submitted, forms to be completed for administrative purposes, and the presentation of the dossier. Once approved for marketing, medicines are included in the ARTG.

References

- Australian regulation of prescription medicine products
- The regulation of complementary medicines in Australia—an overview
- Therapeutics Goods Administration, Business plan 2007–2008

Mail: TGA Communications Section, PO Box 100, Woden ACT 2606, Australia
Phone: 1800-020-653 (free call within Australia)
02-6232-8610 (for publications enquiries)
Fax: 02-6232-8605
Email: info@tga.gov.au

Japan

The Ministry of Health, Labour and Welfare is the governmental body responsible for enacting legislation for pharmaceutical affairs. The regulation of clinical trials and new drug approval in Japan is based on the Pharmaceutical Affairs Law and related ordinances. The objective of the Ministry is to secure a safe medical environment through a consolidated structure of accurate reviews of pharmaceuticals and medical devices and postmarketing safety measure implementation.

The Pharmaceuticals and Medical Devices Agency (PMDA) is a government agency that conducts scientific review of Investigational New Drug Applications (INDs) and New Drug Applications (NDAs) using internal review teams. The role of the PMDA as a review agency has become critical in pharmaceutical research and development activities. The Agency fosters greater cooperation between the regulatory body and the pharmaceutical industry by providing consultation services for clinical development.

The Agency is also a member of the ICH of Technical Requirements for Registration of Pharmaceuticals for Human Use (ICH). It is a unique project that brings together the regulatory authorities of Europe, Japan, and the United States and experts from the pharmaceutical industry in the three regions to discuss scientific and technical aspects of product registration.

PMDA also consolidates all information regarding the quality, efficacy, and safety of pharmaceuticals and medical devices from manufacturers, medical institutions, and other sources. This information is scientifically reviewed and considered in the implementation of appropriate safety measures in collaboration with Ministry of Health, Labour and Welfare. Essential information is broadly disseminated to medical experts, manufacturers, and users of pharmaceuticals, medical devices, and others.

In order for a sponsor to have a new drug reviewed by the Agency, the format of the Agency must be followed. There are four types of reviews that take place.

1. Meetings where consultation is provided prior to clinical trials for questions regarding application materials for approval
2. Conformity audit, where the data attached to the application are reviewed to ensure their compliance with ethical and scientific standards
3. Approval review, where, based on the results of the conformity audit, the product is reviewed against the current scientific standards for efficacy, adverse drug reactions, and quality
4. Final Good Manufacturing procedure / Quality Management System audit

To ensure speed and accuracy, PMDA assigns the same team to provide clinical trials consultation and approval services throughout the entire process, from the preclinical trial stage to the approval stage.

It is apparent that PMDA wants to send a message that the Agency is striving for openness, cooperation, and timeliness to promote Japan's role in global drug development. The initiative will have the most immediate impact on the IND consultation process. The PMDA wants to increase the number of meetings with sponsor companies and meet with them in a timely manner. In implementing the new format, the Agency is trying to adhere to time lines. A sponsor of an IND should become aware of the schedule. The consolatory meetings will be formal from the point of view that minutes will be kept relative to discussions that take place pertaining to the IND. Using the team approach, the

Agency's goal is to have its entire New Drug Approval Process take one year between the primary meeting with the sponsor and PMDA approval.

Prior to the face-to-face meetings, there will be an inquiry and response period between sponsors and PMDA. The Agency will give its opinion, which will be open for discussion. Following the discussion, a draft of the minutes will be drawn up and finalized one month after the meeting. As an aside, the Agency is undertaking an ambitious hiring process of reviewers to address the demand for improved approval process.

In addition, the PMDA is attempting to balance the request for linguistic requirements of sponsors with the necessity of maintaining transparency with the Japanese public in order to explain the approval process for any given drug.

In conclusion, it is clear that linguistic demands are such that a prudent sponsor will require the services of a qualified translator in order to meet the demands of PMDA. In addition, it is equally important for a sponsor to engage the services of a consultant who is well versed with the new PMDA process.

References

Pharmaceuticals and Medical Devices Agency
International Affairs and Human Resources Development Division, Office of
    Planning and Coordination
Shin-Kasumigaseki Building
3-3-2 Kasumigaseki, Chiyoda-ku, Tokyo 100-0013 Japan
Tel: +81-3-3506-9456. Fax: +81-3-3506-9461
http://www.pmda.go.jp/english/operations.html

EU

Given that there are 27 independent states involved in the EU with three states, Iceland, Liechtenstein, and Norway from the European Economic Community–European Free Trade Area (EEC-EFTA), it is important that the European Medicines Agency (EMEA) and the European parliament enact regulations that will meet the needs of the peoples of the member nations relative to new medicinal advances. The founding legislation of the European Medicine Agency is found in Regulation (European Commission) No. 726/2004. The headquarters of the EMEA is located in London.

It is imperative that they continue to regulate, evaluate, and monitor the safety, efficacy, and quality of new medicines entering the European market. In addition, the EMEA must stimulate innovation and research in the pharmaceutical sector so that the sector continues to grow and meet the needs of the populace. Also, the regulatory task becomes more important as migration within the community increases.

With the large number of member countries, the EMEA has developed a pharmacovigilance regulatory control mechanism to carry out their mandate.

Accordingly, the mechanism that the Agency has found workable with its member states is to ensure that all pharmaceutical products for human use be approved through a process known as the centralized procedure. By so doing, the EMEA is able to apply efficient and transparent evaluation procedures to bring new drugs to market and initiate a process of monitoring drugs for quality, safety, and efficacy.

The Agency is utilizing modern information technology techniques to assess the quality and safety of new substance drugs that companies would like to make available within the EU. Application by a sponsor is directed to the team of experts in London following the centralized procedure. Also, if necessary, the Agency can call upon a very effective network of experts situated in 30 countries.

The extensive phamacovigilance program of collecting, monitoring, assessing, and evaluating information from pharma companies on new products ensures that the Agency meets its objective relative to the quality, safety, and efficacy of medicinal products for human use. The system involves encouraging high-quality drug applicants, with an extensive prereview period necessitating many meetings. The decision-making process has been criticized by being somewhat slow; hence, the EMEA has been working with an electronic drug submission templates to assist in accelerating the process, thereby reducing the time to bring a drug to market.

In summary, given the rigor of the centralized procedure and transparency of data required, the rationale is deemed to be important for maximizing the impact and political acceptability of the processes. It is, therefore, prudent to engage the services of a consultant who is well versed with the procedural method used by the Agency. By so doing, an applicant would be able to maximize the time and expense judiciously for all the pertinent parties concerned so that a new medicine may be brought to market within a reasonable period of time.

EMEA
7 Westferry Circus Canary Wharf
LondonE14 4HB United Kingdom
Telephone switchboard: (44-20) 74-18-84-00
Web site: www.emea.europa.eu
Contacting the EMEA by e-mail
General e-mail: mail@emea.europa.eu
General enquiries: info@emea.europa.eu

INTERNATIONAL HARMONIZATION OF REGULATORY REQUIREMENTS AND GUIDELINES

International Harmonization; Policy On Standards
Department of Health and Human Services

Food and Drug Administration
(Docket No. 94D-0300)
Agency: Food and Drug Administration, HHS.
Action: Notice.

Summary

The FDA is announcing the Agency's policy on the development and use of standards with respect to international harmonization of regulatory requirements and guidelines. Specifically, the policy is intended to address the conditions under which the FDA plans to participate with standards bodies outside of the FDA, domestic or international, in the development of standards applicable to products regulated by the FDA. The policy also covers the conditions under which the FDA intends to use the resultant standards, or other available domestic or international standards, in fulfilling its statutory mandates for safeguarding the public health.

For further information, contact Linda R. Horton, International Policy Staff (HF-23), Food and Drug Administration, 5600 Fishers Lane, Rockville, MD 20857, 301-827-3344.

Supplementary Information

In a notice published in the Federal Register of November 28, 1994 (59 FR 60870), the FDA published a draft policy on international harmonization of regulatory requirements and guidelines. The purpose of the draft policy was to articulate the FDA's policy on the development and use of standards with respect to international harmonization of regulatory requirements and guidelines. The Agency gave interested persons an opportunity to comment on the draft policy document. A discussion of the comments received and the Agency's responses is found in section III of this document.

I. Background

The purpose of this document is to articulate the FDA's policy on development and use of standards with respect to international harmonization of regulatory requirements and guidelines. As used throughout this document, the term "standards" includes what are commonly referred to as "consensus standards," "voluntary standards," and "industry standards." Also, the FDA sometimes accepts standards and makes them mandatory regulatory requirements. Although the draft policy focuses on international harmonization and international standards, its principles are applicable as well to domestic standards activities in which the FDA participates.

Statutory Mandates for FDA-Regulated Products. The FDA is the principal regulatory agency within the Public Health Service (PHS). The Agency protects the public health by, among other things, implementing statutory provisions designed to ensure that food is safe and otherwise not adulterated or misbranded; that human and veterinary drugs, human biological products, and medical devices are safe and effective; that cosmetics are safe; and that electronic product radiation is properly controlled. FDA-regulated products must be truthfully and accurately labeled and in compliance with all applicable laws and regulations. The statutory mandates for safeguarding the public health in these product sectors are prescribed in several statutes, notably in the Federal Food, Drug, and Cosmetic Act; the Public Health Service Act; and the Fair Packaging and Labeling Act.

International Harmonization of Regulatory Requirements and Guidelines. In recent decades, great changes in the world economy, together with expanded working relationships of regulatory agencies around the globe, have resulted in increased interest in international harmonization of regulatory requirements. Increased international commerce, opportunities to enhance public health through cooperative endeavors, and scarcity of government resources for regulation have resulted in efforts by the regulatory agencies of different nations to work together on standards and harmonize their regulatory requirements. Such harmonization enhances public health protection and improves government efficiencies by reducing both unwarranted contradictory regulatory requirements and redundant applications of similar requirements by multiple regulatory bodies. Harmonization facilitates cooperation in regulatory activities.

Harmonization of the FDA's regulatory requirements and guidelines with those of other countries was recently embraced as a pillar of the President's and Vice President's National Performance Review. In Reinventing Drug and Device Regulation (April 1995), international harmonization was identified as a high-priority initiative across FDA programs. Recognizing the considerable synergy between its domestic policy and its international policy priorities, the FDA is sharpening and focusing its planning for enhanced alignment of FDA and international standards.

In 1992, an FDA Task Force on International Harmonization had provided a broad assessment of the goals, scope, and direction of the FDA's international activities. These activities were found to comprise a wide variety of efforts by the FDA to retain and strengthen its public health safeguards, while striving toward common ground with its foreign government counterparts on product standards, criteria for the assessment of test data, and enforcement procedures. The task force's recommendations for the Agency included an overall FDA policy on international harmonization, which is to encourage the initiation and support of efforts, consistent with the Agency's goals and principles, that will further the international harmonization of standards and policies for the regulation of products for which the FDA has authority. Soon thereafter, the FDA's strategic plan began to recognize standards as the premier focus of the Agency's international activities.

Goals The FDA's goals in participating in international harmonization are

- to safeguard U.S. public health,
- to assure that consumer protection standards and requirements are met,
- to facilitate the availability of safe and effective products,
- to develop and utilize product standards and other requirements more effectively, and
- to minimize or eliminate inconsistent standards internationally.

General Principles FDA participation in international harmonization efforts should be guided by the following general principles.

- The harmonization activity should be consistent with U.S. Government policies and procedures and should promote U.S. interests with foreign countries.
- The harmonization activity should further the FDA's mission to protect the public health by, among other things, ensuring that food is safe and otherwise not adulterated or misbranded; that human and veterinary drugs, human biological products, and medical devices are safe and effective as required by law and are not adulterated or misbranded; that cosmetics are not adulterated or misbranded; that electronic product radiation is properly controlled; and that all of these products are labeled truthfully and informatively.
- The FDA's input into international standard-setting activities should be open to public scrutiny and should provide the opportunity for the consideration of views of all parties concerned.
- The FDA should accept, where legally permissible, the equivalent standards, compliance activities, and enforcement programs of other countries, provided that the FDA is satisfied that such standards, activities, and programs meet the FDA's level of public health protection.
- Scientific and regulatory information and knowledge should be exchanged with foreign government officials, to the extent possible within legal constraints, to expedite the approval of products and protect public health.

Thus, the Agency's primary goal in all of its international harmonization activities is to preserve and enhance its ability to accomplish its public health mission. Global harmonization is also approached with the aim of enhancing regulatory effectiveness, by providing more consumer protection with scarce government resources, and increasing worldwide consumer access to safe, effective, and high-quality products.

Other Obligations and Policies.

International Agreements The U.S. Government is a party to international trade agreements. In the United States, such trade agreements become effective only after implementing legislation is signed into law. The FDA has participated in recent international trade negotiations to ensure that the FDA's requirements are preserved and that regulatory practices can remain focused on fulfilling the Agency's mission to protect the public health while being supportive of emerging, broader U.S. Government obligations and policies. In addition, the FDA continues to be involved in work of the World Trade Organization (WTO), as well as the North American Free Trade Agreement (NAFTA) committees on sanitary and phytosanitary measures, and on technical barriers to trade, in order to foster international harmonization of regulatory requirements and to facilitate consultation on trade issues. Recently, the FDA has begun to be involved in other regional activities, e.g., the Forum on Asia Pacific Economic Cooperation, work on initial steps toward a Free Trade Area of the Americas, and work toward a Transatlantic Area that strengthens our ties with Europe.

The principal international trade agreement is the General Agreement on Tariffs and Trade (GATT), which entered into force on January 1, 1948. GATT has since been amended several times following negotiation sessions known as rounds.

The GATT Agreement on Technical Barriers to Trade (TBT), popularly known as the Standards Code, was negotiated during the Tokyo Round of the GATT in the 1970s and entered into force on January 1, 1980. As part of a general effort to reduce unnecessary nontariff barriers to trade, the TBT agreement was intended to promote use by countries of standards, technical regulations, and conformity assessment procedures that are based on work done by international standards bodies. The implementing legislation for the TBT agreement, provided in the Trade Agreements Act of 1979 as amended in 1994 [Pub. L. 103-465; 19 U.S.C. 2531-2582], has thus provided additional authority for the FDA's international standards activity. To assure that harmonization does not result in lowering safety or quality standards for U.S. consumers, this law contains the safeguard that

> no standard-related activity of any private person, Federal agency, or State agency shall be deemed to constitute an unnecessary obstacle to the foreign commerce of the United States if the demonstrable purpose of the standards-related activity is to achieve a legitimate domestic objective including, but not limited to, the protection of legitimate health or safety, essential security, environmental, or consumer interests and if such activity does not operate to exclude imported products which fully meet the objectives of such activity.

The most recent GATT round, the Uruguay Round, was concluded on December 15, 1993, and was formally signed at the Marrakech Ministerial Meeting on April 15, 1994. The new WTO will administer the new GATT and other Uruguay Round agreements, and every country that is a member of the WTO will be required to adhere to all of these agreements. On December 8, 1994, Pub. L. 103-465 was enacted in the United States to approve and implement the Uruguay Round agreements. This law included updating changes in the Trade Agreements Act that reaffirmed the duty of Federal agencies to participate in international standards activities, subject to available resources.

One of the agreements of the Uruguay Round administered by the WTO is the new agreement on TBT, which is similar in many respects to the 1980 TBT agreement. As with the 1980 TBT agreement, the purpose of the new TBT agreement is to ensure that product standards, technical regulations, and related procedures do not create unnecessary obstacles to trade. The new TBT agreement ensures and clearly states that each country has the right to establish and maintain technical regulations for the protection of human, animal, and plant life and health and the environment and for prevention against deceptive practices.

In the new TBT agreement, the term "standard" is defined as

[A] document approved by a recognized body, that provides, for common and repeated use, rules, guidelines or characteristics for products or related processes and production methods, with which compliance is not mandatory [emphasis added]. It may also include or deal exclusively with terminology, symbols, packaging, marking or labelling requirements as they apply to a product, process or production method.

Also, "technical regulation" is defined as

[A] document which lays down product characteristics or their related processes and production methods, including applicable administrative provisions, with which compliance is mandatory [emphasis added]. It may also include or deal exclusively with terminology, symbols, packaging, marking, or labelling requirements as they apply to a product, process or production method.

Thus, in the language of the new TBT agreement, when a government acts to accept a voluntary standard to make it mandatory, the resulting document is a technical regulation. A measure used to ascertain compliance with a standard or technical regulation is a conformity assessment procedure.

The new TBT agreement continues and strengthens the reference to international standards found in the 1980 TBT agreement. Specifically, the agreement states that, where technical regulations are required and relevant international standards exist or their completion is imminent, WTO-member countries shall use them or the relevant parts of them as a basis for their technical regulations, except when such international standards or relevant parts would be an ineffective or inappropriate means for the fulfillment of the legitimate objectives pursued. Further, the agreement states that, with a view toward harmonizing technical regulations on as wide a basis as possible, WTO-member countries shall play a full part within the limits of their resources in the preparation by appropriate international standards bodies of international standards for products for which they either have adopted or expect to adopt technical regulations.

Another agreement of the Uruguay Round administered by the WTO is the Agreement on the Application of Sanitary and Phytosanitary Measures (SPS agreement). This agreement pertains to those measures intended (1) to protect animal or plant life or health within a territory from risks arising from the entry, establishment, or spread of pests, diseases, disease-carrying organisms, or disease- causing organisms; (2) to protect human or animal life or health within a territory from risks arising from additives, contaminants, toxins, or disease-causing organisms in foods, beverages, or feedstuffs; (3) to protect human life or health within a territory from risks arising from diseases carried by animals, plants, or products thereof, or from entry, establishment, or spread of pests; or (4) to prevent or limit other damage within a territory from the entry, establishment, or spread of pests.

In order to harmonize SPS measures on as wide a basis as possible, the SPS agreement encourages members to base their SPS measures on international standards, guidelines, or recommendations. Thus, the SPS agreement, like the new TBT agreement, encourages use of international standards. The SPS agreement refers specifically to standards established by the Codex Alimentarius Commission, as discussed below.

NAFTA also contains TBT and SPS agreements similar to those in the new WTO agreements.

Internal U.S. Government Policy   The United States Office of Management and Budget (OMB), in its revision to OMB Circular No. A-119 (58 FR 57643, October 26, 1993), provides policy on Federal use of standards and agency participation in voluntary standards bodies and standards-developing groups: "It is the policy of the Federal Government in its procurement and regulatory activities to

a. rely on voluntary standards, both domestic and international, whenever feasible and consistent with the law and regulation pursuant to law;
b. participate in voluntary standards bodies when such participation is in the public interest and is compatible with agencies' missions, authorities, priorities, and budget resources; and
c. coordinate agency participation in voluntary standards bodies so that (1) the most effective use is made of agency resources and representatives, and (2) the views expressed by such representatives are in the public interest and, as a minimum, do not conflict with the interests and established views of the agencies."

OMB Circular No. A-119 also establishes additional policy guidance and responsibilities for U.S. Government agencies. It is applicable to all executive agency participation in voluntary standards activities, domestic and international, but not to activities carried out pursuant to treaties and international standardization agreements.

The term "standard," as defined in OMB Circular No. A-119, means

a prescribed set of rules, conditions, or requirements concerned with the definition of terms; classification of components; delineation of procedures; specification of dimensions, materials, performance, design, or operations; measurement of quality and quantity in describing materials, products, systems, services, or practices; or descriptions of fit and measurement of size.

The circular defines "voluntary standards" as

established generally by private sector bodies, both domestic and international, and are available for use by any person or organization, private or governmental. The term voluntary standard includes what are commonly referred to as "industry standards" as well as "consensus standards," but does not include professional standards of personal conduct, institutional codes of ethics, private standards of individual firms, or standards mandated by law, such as those contained in the United States Pharmacopeia and the National Formulary, as referenced in 21 U.S.C. 351. These definitions in OMB Circular No. A-119 conform to common usage and are consistent with the usage of these terms throughout this policy document. It should be noted that, under the TBT, "standards" are considered to be nonmandatory (i.e., voluntary) unless promulgated into mandatory technical regulations.

II. Standards Programs and Practices within the FDA

Purpose of FDA Involvement in Standards. The central purpose of FDA involvement in the development and use of standards is to assist the Agency in fulfilling its public health, regulatory mission. The Agency intends to participate in the development of standards, domestic or international, and adopt or use standards when such action will enhance its ability to protect consumers and the effectiveness or efficiency of its regulatory efforts. In doing so, the FDA recognizes that standards often serve as useful adjuncts to Agency regulatory controls and that economies of time and human resources are often realized in solving problems when consensus-building activities are undertaken and conducted in open, public arenas. The working together of FDA staff with other professionals outside the Agency in standards bodies effectively multiplies the technical resources available to the FDA. Further, standards bodies generally have in place procedures for periodically reviewing and updating completed standards, thus extending the resource-multiplier effect, as well as keeping the solutions current with the state of knowledge. The economy of effort translates into monetary savings to the Agency, regulated industries, and ultimately consumers. Further, using standards, especially international ones, is a means to facilitate the harmonization of FDA regulatory requirements with those of foreign governments, to better serve domestic and global public health.

Another benefit of participating in the development of standards at both domestic and international levels is that, in sharing technical information with technical groups and professionals outside the FDA, staff members have opportunities to learn of other viewpoints on an issue, to establish scientific leadership, and to remain informed of state-of-the-art science and technology.

Past and Present Activities. The FDA has been involved in standards activities for many years, and on January 25, 1977, the Agency promulgated a final regulation, now found at 21 CFR 10.95 (Sec. 10.95), covering the participation by FDA employees in standards-setting activities outside the Agency. This regulation encourages FDA participation in standard-setting activities that are in the public interest and specifies the circumstances under which FDA employees can participate in various types of standards bodies.

Standards activities of multilateral organizations such as the WHO and the Organization for Economic Cooperation and Development (OECD, an international organization with 25 member countries with advanced industrial economies) are often important to the FDA and frequently involve multiple product types. For example, the OECD is developing Genetic Toxicology Test Guidelines that are of interest to all FDA Centers. Similarly, guidelines developed under the International Programme on Chemical Safety of the WHO relate to chemicals that may be in a wide variety of FDA-regulated products, such as food additives, pesticides, drugs, animal drugs, biologics, and devices. The United States Pharmacopeia is a national standard-setting body in which FDA officials actively participate.

The principal standards organizations that are not connected with a treaty are the International Organization for Standardization (ISO) and the International Electrotechnical Commission (IEC).

Private organizations and government agencies, including the FDA, participate in the ISO and the IEC activities through the American National Standards Institute (ANSI). ANSI represents the United States in the ISO and the IEC and coordinates much of the standards development activity in the United States. As discussed below, the FDA is active in many ISO, IEC, ANSI, and standards-development organization activities. For example, the FDA is represented on the Board of Directors of ANSI and on several of its committees and working groups.

Foods and Veterinary Medicine   The FDA's Center for Food Safety and Applied Nutrition (CFSAN) and Center for Veterinary Medicine (CVM) actively participate in the development of international standards by the Codex Alimentarius Commission (Codex). Codex is an international organization formed in 1962 to facilitate world trade in foods and to promote consumer protection. It is a subsidiary of two United Nations components, the Food and Agriculture Organization (FAO) and the WHO. Codex standards cover food commodity standards (similar to FDA standards of identity), food additives, food contaminants, and residues of veterinary drugs in food. FDA officials chair two Codex committees, the Food Hygiene Committee and the Residues of Veterinary Drugs in Foods Committee, and participate in many others.

Through its involvement, the FDA has been influential in the establishment of many Codex standards. The FDA's procedures for reviewing Codex standards for purposes of regulation are codified in 21 CFR 130.6 and 564.6.

A provision of the United States implementing legislation for the Uruguay Round Agreements, Pub. L. 103-465, requires the President to designate an agency to inform the public, through a notice published in the Federal Register each year by June 1, of certain Codex Alimentarius standard-setting activities. The President, pursuant to Proclamation No. 6780 of March 23, 1995 (60 FR 15845, March 27, 1995), designated the Department of Agriculture to have this responsibility, and the first such notice of Codex activities was published in the Federal Register of May 23, 1995 (60 FR 27250).

In 1988, the governments of the United States and Canada entered into the Canada–United States Free Trade Agreement (now largely superseded by NAFTA). Since then, officials from the CFSAN and the CVM have participated in technical working groups responsible for implementation of the chapter of the agreement that deals with agriculture, food, beverage, and related goods (the Canada–United States Free Trade Agreement Technical Working Groups).

Officials from the CFSAN and the CVM also participate in the development of standards by such domestic and international groups as the Food Chemicals Codex (FCC), AOAC International (previously, the Association of Official Analytical Chemists), expert committees of the WHO, FAO, ISO, and other international consensus standards bodies. Standards developed by these organizations are used by industry, both in the United States and abroad. These standards provide industry with guidance for food grade materials and processes, and thus help elevate the quality of food and food chemicals in domestic and international trade.

The CFSAN has adopted many FCC and American Society for Testing and Materials standards and AOAC methods, incorporating them into regulations for both food additives and generally recognized as safe food ingredients. The CFSAN also refers industry to relevant FCC, Codex, or American Society for Testing and Materials standards when discussing particular issues related to good manufacturing practices. The CFSAN accepts many AOAC and equivalent methods for use by laboratories in assaying food and in testing for contaminants in food.

The CVM accepts many AOAC and equivalent methods for use by laboratories in testing for drug residues in animal tissues. The CVM has adopted the consumption estimates used by the FAO/WHO Joint Expert Committee on Food Additives in the development of standards for drug residues in animal tissues.

The CVM is also an active participant in a new harmonization effort under the auspices of the Office of International Epizooties. This activity is known as the Veterinary International Cooperation on Harmonisation (VICH) (of Technical Requirements for Registration of Veterinary Medicinal Products–EU).

Biologics and Drugs   There has been active international standard setting for biological products for more than 50 years. Officials from the FDA's CBER serve as experts or members of a variety of international committees that perform standard-setting functions. Activities have encompassed collaborative studies to establish international units of measure and to develop internationally accepted standards for control of biologics, including WHO standards. Efforts have been directed to many kinds of biological products, including vaccines, human blood and plasma products, blood testing reagents, and allergenic extracts, and have extended to biotechnology-derived growth factors, cytokines, and monoclonal antibody products.

The FDA's CDER, CBER, and the National Center for Toxicological Research actively participate in the ICH of Technical Requirements for Registration of Pharmaceuticals for Human Use (ICH). This ongoing project, begun in 1989, has been undertaken by governmental agencies responsible for regulation of drugs and by industry trade organizations from the EU, Japan, and the United States. Specifically, ICH is sponsored jointly by the Commission of the European Communities, the Japanese Ministry of Health, Labour and Welfare, the FDA, the European Federation of Pharmaceutical Industries' Associations (EFPIA), the Japan Pharmaceutical Manufacturers Association, and the Pharmaceutical Research and Manufacturers Association of the United States. In addition, the International Federation of Pharmaceutical Manufacturers Associations (IFPMA) participates as an umbrella organization for the pharmaceutical industry and provides the secretariat function for ICH. ICH operates under the direction of the ICH Steering Committee, which is comprised of representatives of these organizations. Official observer status has been given to WHO, the European Free Trade Area (EFTA), and the Health Protection Branch of Canada.

The aims of ICH are to (1) provide a forum for a dialog between regulatory agencies and the pharmaceutical industry on differences in the technical requirements for product registration (i.e., requirements for product marketing) in the EU, Japan, and the United States; (2) identify areas where modifications in technical requirements or greater mutual acceptance of research and development procedures could lead to more efficient use of human, animal, and material resources without compromising safety, quality, and efficacy; and (3) make recommendations of practical ways to achieve greater harmonization in the interpretation and application of technical guidelines and requirements for registration. The work products of ICH, created in working groups of experts from the regulatory agencies and industry, consist of a series of consensus guidance documents. These guidance documents, after successive ICH steps of review and acceptance, including an opportunity for public review and comment in the respective jurisdictions, are forwarded to the regulatory agencies with the expectation that they will be formally adopted by the agencies.

Officials from both CBER and CDER also participate in a consensus standard-setting activity sponsored by the Council for International Organizations of Medical Sciences that is aimed at standardizing medical definitions and adverse experience reporting.

Medical Devices and Radiation-Emitting Products The FDA's Center for Devices and Radiological Health (CDRH) has had extensive involvement with standards in its regulation of medical devices, as well as electronic products that emit radiation. The development of standards to solve problems related to medical devices involves many groups outside the FDA. The interaction between the CDRH and the manufacturing and health-care communities that frequently occurs during the standards development process provides knowledge and insight into the use of products, problems, and the effectiveness of solutions. Frequently, the public discussion of the problem that occurs in the consensus-building process results in the manufacturers and the users of the subject medical device implementing the solution before a standard is formally completed. Thus, the CDRH has encouraged participation in the development of standards as a useful adjunct to regulatory controls. CDRH's approach to use and participation in the development of consensus standards was described in a letter dated June 29, 1993, to all interested parties from the Director of CDRH. (This policy did not apply to mandatory performance standards, i.e., technical regulations, for class II medical devices as specified under the Medical Device Amendments of 1976 (Pub. L. 94-295). The Safe Medical Devices Act of 1990, SMDA (Pub. L. 101-629), puts the promulgation of mandatory standards at the discretion of the Agency.)

Over 200 completed consensus standards and selected sections of additional draft standards that are not yet complete have been incorporated into guidance documents for applications for conducting clinical trials with investigational devices and applications for permitting devices to be marketed. These guidance documents are widely disseminated by the CDRH to all interested parties. Other standards used by the CDRH, or which the CDRH has helped to develop, concern measurement or test methods, or support good manufacturing practices and quality assurance.

A new ISO Committee, Technical Committee 210 (TC-210) is developing harmonized standards in these areas. Also, the CDRH is an active participant in the Global Harmonization Task Force, in cooperation with officials from Canada, the EU, Japan, and other countries.

The CDRH has published a notice of a working draft of a final rule to revise the current good manufacturing practice regulations for medical devices (60 FR 37856, July 24, 1995), in part to ensure that they are compatible with specifications for quality systems contained in an international quality standard developed by ISO, namely, ISO 9001 "Quality Systems Part 1. Specification for Design/ Development, Production, Installation, and Servicing." This standard (ISO 9001) is becoming widely recognized by medical device regulatory authorities worldwide and is finding application in many other industry sectors as well. CDRH officials, working with counterpart foreign government officials, are pursuing in step-wise fashion the harmonization of quality system inspection procedures and enforcement.

The process of harmonizing regulatory requirements is facilitated by using an international standard as a basis. Such harmonization is not only a recognized public policy but also, for medical devices, is explicitly encouraged by provisions of SMDA (Pub. L. 101-629), which states, in part, that the FDA "... may enter into agreements with foreign countries to facilitate commerce in devices between the United States and [foreign] countries consistent with the requirements of this Act." 21 U.S.C. 383.

In a recent (April 1995) program review, the CDRH reported that, in 1994, 192 Center staff members served as primary and alternate liaison representatives on 440 committees and subcommittees in 38 standards developing organizations (domestic and foreign). The CDRH actively reviewed 286 draft standards; of these, 134 were with nine international standards organizations. The experience the CDRH has acquired over the years has provided the foundation for the standards policy it announced on June 29, 1993. The essential features of that policy are reflected in the FDA policy presented in "FDA Policy on Standards."

Regulatory Affairs   The FDA's Office of Regulatory Affairs is increasingly active in international standards activities relevant to quality control and conforming assessment, including activities relevant to ISO—9001 and laboratory regulation.

III. Response to Comments

In response to its request for comments on the draft international harmonization policy on standards, the FDA received comments from 10 organizations (standards-setting organizations, trade and professional associations, a manufacturer, and a consumer organization). A discussion of the comments received and the Agency's responses follows:

1. In general, the comments supported the Agency's proposed international harmonization policy on standards. For example, one comment stated that the policy demonstrated the Agency's commitment to the international standards development process as well as international harmonization. Another comment pointed out that the policy will better enable the Agency to establish agreements with other global regulatory bodies and ultimately permit the FDA to carry out its mandate to protect the public health in a more efficient and cost-effective manner. Other comments stated that the harmonization of regulatory requirements and supportive standards could benefit U.S. companies engaged in international trade. In addition, one of these comments pointed out that standards reflect technology and that the first priority with regard to standards should always be to develop standards that represent the best available technological solutions, adding that "harmony" and "con-

sistency" can be achieved through the general acceptance of excellent technological solutions. The FDA agrees with these comments.

A. *Potential for Lowered Standards*

2. Two comments stated that harmonization has the potential to result in lowered standards, with potential adverse effects on public health protection. One of the comments expressed concern that the FDA was subordinating the public interest in favor of voluntary standards bodies and standards developing groups in a manner that is inconsistent with the vital tasks assigned to the Agency to protect health. The second comment argued that the first priority with regard to standards should be to develop standards that represent the best available technological solutions, and that the FDA should not support international standards that reflect inferior or compromised technological solutions that become obstacles, rather than benefits, to U.S. industry. Another comment, while agreeing that international standards should be adopted as national standards whenever possible, stated that international standards may sometimes not meet the needs of our health-care community, adding that some may contain safety standards only and no performance parameters, and that the international standards may also be inconsistent with our country's codes and regulations.

The FDA wishes to reassure those who commented that the FDA's participation in international harmonization activities is intended to safeguard the U.S. public health and to assure that consumer protection standards and requirements are met. Indeed, a central principle that guides the Agency's international harmonization activities is that the activities should further the FDA's mission to protect the public health. In addition, international agreements to which the U.S. Government is a party have provisions that ensure that harmonization activities will not result in lowered standards. For example, the WTO Agreement on SPS provides that each country may determine its appropriate level of protection; therefore, the encouragement to use international standards as the basis for technical regulations will not result in "downward harmonization." Safeguards have been built into the TBT agreement and U.S. implementing legislation that protect the ability of each country to establish requirements necessary to fulfill a legitimate objective. As stated in section I.C.1. above, the implementing legislation for the new TBT agreement, which provides additional authority for the FDA's international standards activities, provides further assurance that such harmonization would not result in lowering safety or quality standards for U.S. consumers. Thus, the Agency does not agree that harmonization will result in inferior standards. Furthermore, the FDA's participation in standards development, consistent with Sec. 10.95 and OMB Circular No. A-119, and the FDA's use of standards in its regulatory programs, will be dependent not only on the substantive aspects of the standards for ensuring the safety, effectiveness, and quality of products but also on the development process for the standard. The standard itself must also comply with all applicable statutes, regulations, and policies.

B. Regulatory Issues

3. One comment stated that any time a voluntary standard is used in a regulation, the scope of that standard needs to be unambiguously determined. The comment used a hypothetical case of a voluntary standard intended to be used in the home environment being inappropriately extended to the hospital environment. The comment argued that if the regulatory need exceeds the scope of the existing voluntary standard, it may indicate the need for yet another voluntary standard that addresses the additional scope, or else provisions may need to be added to the existing voluntary standard so as to accommodate the broader scope in which the standard is to be applied.

    The Agency agrees that, when a voluntary standard is used in a regulation, the scope of that standard should be unambiguously expressed. As stated above, a basic tenet in the development and adoption of a standard is that it contributes to safer, more effective, and higher quality products. Inappropriate application of a standard (voluntary or as part of a technical regulation) would run counter to this notion.

4. Three comments questioned the need to make voluntary standards mandatory regulations. One of the comments stated that, if the Agency uses a voluntary standard as a "referee" standard, which means that the Agency uses the voluntary standard as a frame of reference for determining safety and efficacy, there should be no need for the Agency to go through the procedures required for creating a regulation. The second comment stated that, if technical standards are based on state-of-the-art science and are revised as needed to incorporate advances, they should be voluntary standards as opposed to regulatory requirements. The third comment asserted that existence of a standard does not warrant a regulation and the FDA should avoid unnecessary regulations.

    The Agency agrees that it should avoid unnecessary regulations but notes that there are times when it finds it is necessary to propose and promulgate regulations for the efficient enforcement of the laws it administers. Voluntary standards that will serve agencies' purposes and are consistent with applicable laws and regulations can be adopted and used by Federal agencies. This principle is stated in both the FDA's policy and in section 7(a) of OMB Circular No. A-119 on Reliance on Voluntary Standards. Thus, when appropriate, the FDA will adopt voluntary standards by referencing them in the regulations it promulgates. In all other instances, these standards will remain voluntary.

    As stated above, the purpose of the FDA's involvement in the development and use of standards is to assist the Agency in fulfilling its public health and regulatory missions. Thus, the Agency intends to participate in the development of domestic and international standards and to adopt or use standards, when such action will enhance its ability to protect consumers and the effectiveness or efficiency of its regulatory efforts.

C. Transparency

5. Four comments addressed the need for transparency during the development of standards, in determining "official" use of a standard or when standards are used in a regulation or adopted as regulations. The comments asserted that, if voluntary standards are incorporated into guidance documents and compliance policy guides and serves as the bases for mandatory standards and other regulations promulgated by the FDA, ample opportunity should be provided for interested parties to comment through the established procedures of notice and comment rule making. One comment further stated that the policy should include a statement of assurance that the FDA will engage potentially affected parties whenever it intends formal inclusion of a voluntary standard in an FDA document or process.

The Agency agrees that the development of standards should be conducted in an open fashion. Under Sec. 10.95, one of the criteria for FDA participation in standards-setting bodies is that the group or organization responsible for the standard-setting activity must have a procedure by which an interested person will have an opportunity to provide information and views on the activity and standards involved, and that the information and views will be considered. This is why the FDA clearly states in its policy (section IV. below) that one of the factors for the FDA's participation in standards development and use is the transparency of the process, i.e., the process must be open to public scrutiny and provide the opportunity for the consideration of views of all parties concerned.

With regard to transparency when standards are used in a regulation or adopted as regulations, under the Administrative Procedure Act, an agency that issues, amends, or revokes a regulation, whether on its own initiative or when petitioned by an interested person, must act in an open manner with adequate time provided for comment from interested parties, which will be considered before a final regulation is promulgated. The FDA's rule on promulgation of regulations, found in 21 CFR 10.40, is explicit with respect to the need for transparency of the process and opportunity for participation in the process by interested persons. Other procedural regulations govern guidelines and similar documents (21 CFR 10.90), and interested persons may use correspondence or meetings (21 CFR 10.65), petitions (21 CFR 10.30), or reviews by supervisors (21 CFR 10.75) to raise issues and present views about other nonbinding guidance documents, which provide industry with useful information about recommended or alternative ways to comply with requirements. In fact, the FDA has increasingly used public meetings to elicit and share information with regard to its guidance documents, and it currently is reviewing the procedures it uses to develop guidance documents to ensure sufficient transparency in the process.

Thus, with regard to the comment that this policy should include a statement of assurance that the FDA will engage potentially interested parties whenever it intends formal inclusion of a voluntary standard in an FDA document or process, the Agency finds that it is not necessary to do so as part of this document because there are established mechanisms under the Administrative Procedure Act and the Agency's administrative practices and procedure regulations for obtaining and considering views of interested persons. Of course, the FDA is not foreclosing future consideration of additional mechanisms toward this end.

D. Comments on Specific Issues

6. One comment suggested the alternative language, "The standard contributes to safe and effective products that meet consumers' requirements for quality," instead of "The standard contributes to safer, more effective, and higher quality products" (section III.A.1, proposed policy) and "The standard, if adhered to, would help ensure the safety, effectiveness, or quality of products" (section III.D.1, proposed policy). The alternative language was offered to simplify future negotiations and to allow the Agency to participate more fully in standards development and promulgation. The comment also questioned the use of the terms "safer" and "more effective" in section III.A.1. of the proposed policy (see above) because it is not clear what the measures for "safer" and "more effective" are. The comment further stated that the term "higher quality" is relative, leaving open to question who determines higher quality. Finally, the comment added that an international standard could conceivably result in requirements for the same degree of safety, effectiveness, and quality as those required by the FDA.

The Agency is revising the policy in a manner similar to that suggested by the comment. The FDA agrees that an international standard could indeed result in requirements for the same degree of safety, effectiveness, and quality as required by the FDA. In fact, one of the FDA's guiding principles in its international harmonization activities is that the FDA should accept, where legally permissible, equivalent standards of other countries provided such standards meet the FDA's goals to facilitate the availability of safe, effective, and properly labeled products. The Agency further agrees that the alternative language would allow the

Agency more flexibility to participate in standards development, without compromising public health, and is therefore amending the policy accordingly.

7. One comment supported the FDA's intent to develop standards on the basis of sound scientific and technical information. The comment added that the use of sound scientific and technical information will permit the development of food regulations and standards that cannot be misconstrued as unreasonable trade barriers. However, the comment cautioned that a decision on participation in standards development should be based on the purpose of the standard, not whether the standard is based on sound scientific and technical information.

   The Agency agrees that, while all standards should be based on sound scientific and technical information, not all scientifically sound standards will serve purposes justifying the Agency's participation in developing them. The FDA's regulation on participation in outside standard-setting activities states that not only will the activity be based upon consideration of sound scientific and technological information, but it also will be designed to protect the public against unsafe, ineffective, or deceptive products and [21 CFR 10.95(d)(5)(i)]. In addition, OMB Circular No. A-119 states that it is the policy of the Federal Government to participate in voluntary standards bodies when such participation is in the public interest and is compatible with agencies' missions, authorities, priorities, and budget resources. The OMB Circular adds that the providing of Agency support to a voluntary standards activity should be limited to that which is clearly in furtherance of an agency's mission and responsibility. These directives are adequately reflected in the policy.

8. One comment suggested that proposed section III.A.4, "The development of an international standard that achieves the agency's public health objectives is generally, but not always, given a higher priority than the development of a domestic standard," be deleted because it is made clear in other parts of the draft policy that the FDA complies with U.S. obligations under the GATT, other international trade agreements, and OMB Circular No. A-119.

   The Agency agrees that the draft policy document does make clear that the FDA complies with U.S. obligations under international agreements and the OMB Circular. However, the Agency does not agree that proposed section III.A.4. should be deleted. The FDA's belief that the development of an international standard that achieves the Agency's public health objectives is generally (but not always) given a higher priority than the development of a domestic standard, is an important factor on which agency participation in standards development is based and merits being clearly delineated. This is more so because proposed section III (section VI of this document), FDA Policy on Standards, is intended to stand on its own as the Agency's policy on harmonization of standards and, therefore, needs to be as complete as possible.

The FDA emphasizes that there are three routes to development of a harmonized international standard, all of which are favored under the FDA policy: (1) The U.S. voluntary standards community or an agency, such as the FDA, develops a U.S. standard and takes it to an international forum so it can be made an international standard; (2) A standard already developed in an international forum (or by another country or a regional standards body) is adopted as a U.S. voluntary or regulatory standard; or (3) A new international standard is developed, "from scratch," in an international forum. Which of these routes is followed in the particular case will vary with the facts of that case. While starting a standards activity in an international forum offers many efficiencies in avoiding duplication of effort, there will continue to be times when it makes sense first to develop a domestic standard (voluntary or regulatory) and then to take it, as appropriate, to an international forum.

9. One comment asserted that the intent of proposed factors III.A.6. and III.D.6, which state "Wherever appropriate for the product, the standard stresses product performance rather than product design, but where necessary, covers all factors required to ensure safety, effectiveness, and quality," was not clear. The comment added that inspection can be used to prevent poor quality products from being consumed but that safety cannot be inspected into a product. The comment stated further that safety must be designed into products during development, subsequent manufacturing, packaging, and transport. Further, the comment stated that product performance or product functionality issues with regard to safety are the primary focus in the development of food regulations, and therefore, the comment recommended alternative language to that in the proposed policy: "Wherever appropriate for the product, the standard stresses product safety, performance, and functionality, but where necessary, covers all factors required to ensure safety and effectiveness, including product and process design, and process performance."

The Agency believes that the suggested language is helpful in capturing the FDA's intentions in formulating these factors as the basis for participation in standards development, and use of standards in its regulatory programs. Therefore, the Agency is making editorial changes in the factors along the lines suggested in the comment.

E. Other Comments

10. One comment recommended that FDA review and revise current U.S. guidelines for toxicity testing of food additives as outlined in the Toxicological Principles for the Safety Assessment of Direct Food Additives

and Color Additives Used in Food (Redbook I), as well as the proposed guidelines set forth in the revised draft, Redbook II, and harmonize with those recommended by the OECD. The comment added that this will allow more universal acceptance of results performed throughout the world and will minimize the need to repeat expensive testing to meet different testing standards in different countries.

The Agency has stated that standards activities of organizations such as OECD are often important to the FDA and that the development of international standards and harmonization with international standards if they achieve the Agency's public health objectives will, in most instances, be given a high priority.

The Agency announced that the draft Redbook II was available (March 29, 1993, 58 FR 16536) and solicited comments on the draft revised guidelines. Redbook II is being finalized in light of comments received by the Agency, including a comment that the guidelines should be harmonized with those of the OECD; the final revised Redbook II has yet to be issued. The Agency notes that, in revising the guidelines in the Redbook, it took into account the fact that differences among guidelines can result in unnecessary duplication of effort and inefficient use of scarce testing resources. The Agency also wants to make clear that the Redbook is designed to provide guidance. Strict adherence to Redbook guidelines is not a requirement for toxicological studies conducted to establish the safety of an additive.

11. One comment indicated concern that a long-standing participation by the United States Public Health Service in the 3-A Sanitary Standards (for dairy and related food industries) is not mentioned in the text of the draft policy. The comment also stated that it is necessary that, as international agreements anticipate trade and importation of equipment, compliance with 3-A Sanitary Standards should be applied by reference to assure receipt of acceptable equipment.

The domestic and international standards-setting organizations or bodies listed under section II.B. of this document are those in which the FDA has been or is most actively involved in developing standards. The listing is not meant to be exhaustive nor is it meant to list all standards-setting bodies in which the FDA has an interest.

12. One comment urged the FDA to reference voluntary standards rather than adopt and publish standards, to maintain appropriate support for standards development. The comment argued that referencing rather than publishing the text of voluntary standards as regulations or guidance protects the standards organizations' copyrights, which provide the financial support for national and international programs.

The FDA uses standards in the manner described in OMB Circular No. A-119, which states that, while voluntary standards adopted by Federal agencies should be referenced along with their dates of issuance and sources of availability in appropriate publications, regulatory orders, and in related in-house documents, such adoption should take into account any applicable requirements of copyright law and other similar restrictions.

13. One comment advised that the value of standards is that they are the consensus product of all technology experts, not just the consensus of experts from government. Therefore, care should be exercised that government participation in voluntary standards organizations and its use of voluntary standards do not lead to an appearance that voluntary standards organizations are unduly directed or influenced by government.

The Agency is sensitive to the need for balanced participation in voluntary standards bodies and works within OMB's guidelines regarding policy to be followed by executive agencies in working with voluntary standards bodies. OMB Circular No. A-119 states that agency representatives serving as members of standard-developing groups should participate actively and on a basis of equality with private sector representatives but that, in doing so, agency representatives should not seek to dominate such groups. In addition, the number of individual agency participants in a given voluntary standards activity should be kept to the minimum required for effective presentation of the various program, technical, or other concerns of Federal agencies. Finally, while the circular encourages agency representatives to participate in the policy-making process of voluntary standards bodies, particularly in matters such as establishing priorities, developing procedures for preparing, reviewing, and approving standards, and creating standards-developing groups, it also states that, in order to maintain the private, nongovernmental nature of such bodies, agency representatives should refrain from decision-making involvement in the internal day-to-day management of such bodies.

F. Conclusion. Therefore, after considering the comments received, the FDA is issuing this statement of policy.

IV. FDA Policy on Standards[2]

It is the intent of this policy to enable the FDA to: (1) continue to participate in international standards activities that assist it in implementing statutory provisions for safeguarding the public health; (2) increase its efforts to harmonize its regulatory requirements with those of foreign governments, including setting new standards that better serve public health; and (3) respond to laws and policies such as the Trade Agreements Act and OMB Circular No. A-119

---

[2]This policy document does not create or confer any rights, privileges, or benefits for or on any person, nor does it operate to bind FDA in any way

that encourage agencies to use international standards that provide the desired degree of protection. Accordingly, it is the policy of the FDA, concerning the development and use of standards, that:

A. FDA participation in standards development will be based on the extent to which the development activity and expected standard conform to certain factors, with consideration also being given to the resources available in the FDA to devote to the effort and expected efficiencies to be gained as a result of the effort; the factors are as follows:

1. The standard stresses product safety and effectiveness and therefore contributes to safe, effective, and high quality products; when necessary, the standard also covers all factors required to ensure safety and effectiveness, including product and process design, and process performance.

2. The standard is based on sound scientific and technical information and permits revision on the basis of new information.

3. The development process for the standard is transparent (i.e., open to public scrutiny), complies with applicable statutes, regulations, and policies, specifically including Sec. 10.95 and OMB Circular A-119, and is consistent with the codes of ethics that must be followed by FDA employees.

4. The development of an international standard that achieves the Agency's public health objectives is generally but not always given a higher priority than the development of a domestic standard; and

5. The development of a horizontal standard, which applies to multiple types of products, is generally but not always given higher priority than the development of a vertical standard, which applies to a limited range of types of products.

B. The FDA is not bound to use standards developed with FDA participation. For example, the Agency will not use a standard when, in the judgment of the FDA, doing so will compromise the public health.

C. The uses of final (and selected draft or proposed) standards or selected relevant parts will include, where appropriate: (1) incorporating such standards into guidance documents for nonclinical testing, applications for conducting clinical trials with investigational products, and applications for permitting products to be marketed; (2) conducting reviews of such applications; (3) incorporating such standards into compliance policy guides; (4) conducting reviews of test protocols used by firms as part of good manufacturing practices; (5) conducting reviews of study protocols submitted by firms as required for postmarket surveillance studies or programs; (6) serving as the basis for mandatory standards or other regulations promulgated by the FDA; and (7) serving as the basis for reference (e.g., evaluation criteria) in a memorandum of understanding with other government agencies.

D. The use of a standard in the regulatory programs of the FDA is dependent upon the following factors.

1. The standard stresses product safety and effectiveness and, therefore, if adhered to, would help ensure the safety, effectiveness, or quality of products; when necessary, the standard also covers all factors required to ensure safety and effectiveness, including product and process design, and process performance.

2. The standard is based on sound scientific and technical information and is current.

3. The development process for the standard was transparent (i.e., open to public scrutiny), was consistent with the codes of ethics that must be followed by FDA employees, and the standard is not in conflict with any statute, regulation, or policy under which the FDA operates.

4. Where a relevant international standard exists or completion is imminent, it will generally be used in preference to a domestic standard, except when the international standard would be, in the FDA's judgment, insufficiently protective, ineffective, or otherwise inappropriate.

5. Where a relevant horizontal standard which applies to multiple types of products exists or its completion is imminent, it will generally be used in preference to a vertical standard, which applies to a limited range of types of products, except when such horizontal standard would be insufficiently protective, ineffective, or otherwise inappropriate.

E.   FDA employees will comply with Agency regulations (Sec. 10.95) covering participation in standard setting

INTERNATIONAL ACTIVITIES

Introduction

The growth of world trade in FDA-regulated products, such as drugs, medical devices, and foods, calls for the Agency to focus on its role in the international community. To this end, the FDA's Office of International Programs (OIP) was created to coordinate the Agency's interactions with foreign countries and regulatory counterparts, set priorities for international activities, and provide overall policy guidance on international issues. To carry out these activities, the OIP is composed of four major groups.

1. International Scientific Activities and Standards Staff
2. International Relations Staff
3. International Agreements Staff
4. International Planning and Resource Management Staff

In carrying out their responsibilities, OIP staff frequently work with scientific and technical experts from the Agency's various centers.

In a similar manner, CDER's International Activities Coordinating Committee (IACC), chaired by the Center Director, was established to lead the Center's participation in international initiatives and to coordinate and discuss these activities. IACC's activities include

- establishing and harmonizing international standards, regulations, and legislation;
- regulatory and compliance surveillance including import monitoring and foreign inspections;
- scientific collaboration;
- technical assistance, training, and education;
- hosting foreign visitors;
- monitoring trade and export issues related to health and safety;
- cooperating with foreign governments and international organizations;
- communicating with other U.S. Federal agencies on international issues; and
- supporting the FDA's international programs.

For more information on the responsibilities of IACC, please see MAPP 4160.1 (http://www.fda.gov/cder/audiences/iact/iachome.htm).

CDER also participates in discussions of scientific and technical matters with regulatory counterparts throughout the world, as well as in activities sponsored by the WHO and international trade organizations. These activities follow the mandate of the FDA Modernization Act of 1997 to establish standard regulations worldwide for the products it regulates. Among negotiators, this effort is called "international harmonization."

IACC Organization

- IACC Organization Chart
- CDER Organization Chart

Manual of Policies and Procedures (MAPP) for International Activities

MAPPs are approved practices and procedures followed by CDER staff to help standardize the new drug review process and other activities. All MAPPs are available for the public to review to get a better understanding of office policies, definitions, staff responsibilities, and procedures.

- 4160.2 Prioritizing of Requests for Training and Visits by Foreign Regulatory Agencies and International Regulatory Organization. This MAPP describes how CDER prioritizes requests for visits and training by representatives from foreign regulatory agencies and international regulatory organizations.

CDER Forum for International Regulatory Authorities

The "CDER Forum for International Regulatory Authorities" provides information about the U.S. drug regulatory processes in an organized and integrated manner. It will explain the role of CDER as well as the science, technology, regulations, and processes used to do our work.

· CDER Forum, April 14–18, 2008: Rockville, MD

ICH

ICH is the shortened name for The International Conference on Harmonisation of Technical Requirements for Registration of Pharmaceuticals for Human Use. It works to bring together government regulators and drug industry representatives from the United States, the EU, and Japan to make the international drug regulatory process more efficient and uniform. This work will help make new drugs available with minimum delays to both American consumers and those in other countries.

The drug regulatory systems in all three regions share the same fundamental concerns for the safety, efficacy, and quality of drug products. However, many time-consuming and expensive clinical trials have had to be repeated in all three regions. An ICH goal is to minimize unnecessary duplicate testing during the research and development of new drugs. Another goal is to develop guidance documents that create consistency in the requirements for new drug approval.

Some ICH projects include the following:

· Medical Dictionary for Regulatory Activities (MedDRA). MedDRA is a new international medical terminology designed to improve the electronic transmission of regulatory information and data worldwide. It will be used to collect, present, and analyze information on medical products during clinical and scientific reviews and marketing. It will be particularly critical in the electronic transmission of adverse event reporting and coding of clinical trial data. The FDA is already using MedDRA in its Adverse Events Reporting Systems.
· Common Technical Document. This document will provide an international standard format for submitting safety and efficacy information about a new drug.

For a recent summary of FDA-ICH activities, see "CDER Report to the Nation: International Activities."

ICH Guidances

The ICH process results in guidance documents that create consistency in the requirements for new drug approval. Guidance documents represent the

Agency's current thinking on a particular subject. These documents provide guidance on the processing, content, evaluation, and approval of applications. They also establish policies intended to achieve consistency in the Agency's regulatory approach and establish inspection and enforcement procedures. Because guidances are not regulations or laws, they are not enforceable, either through administrative actions or through the courts. An alternative approach may be used if such an approach satisfies the requirements of the applicable statutes, regulations, or both.

ICH guidances are developed through a five-step process: (1) consensus building, (2) start of regulatory action, (3) regulatory consultation, (4) adoption of text, and (5) implementation. For a full description of the process, please see The ICH Guidelines. When a guidance document reaches Step 2 or Step 4 in the ICH process, the FDA publishes a notice of availability in the *Federal Register*. Guidances are posted on the Internet and placed in the Docket for viewing and public comment. Notices for Step 2 guidances include a date for receipt of written comment. Because Step 2 documents are drafts, they do not conform with the Agency's Good Guidance Practices (GGP) policy. Step 4 guidances must be reformatted and edited to be consistent with the GGPs. This is because the 1997 U. S. Food, Drug and Cosmetic Act required the Agency to make GGPs the law. A proposed rule on GGPs was published in February 2000 and is in the process of being finalized.

- ICH Guidances. Steps 2 and 4 guidances grouped into four sections: (1) quality, (2) safety, (3) efficacy, and (4) multidisciplinary
- CDER ICH Guidances and Draft Guidances.
- Federal *Register* Notices of Draft and Final Guidance Availability. (7/1/00 to the present)
- ICH Q3C Maintenance Procedures for the Guidance of Industry Q3C Impurities: Residual Solvents

SPANISH LANGUAGE MATERIALS

Disclaimer: These documents have undergone review by our Spanish-speaking reviewers but not editing. The English version of the document is considered the official guidance on the topic. All CDER guidances can be found at http://www.fda.gov/cder/guidance/index.htm.

Bioavailability/Bioequivalence

- *Guía para la Industria: Procedimentos Estadisticos para Estudios de Bioequivancia Usando un Diseno Estandar Cruzado de Dos Tratamientos* (Posted April 2001)

- *Guía para la Industria: Pruebas de disolución de formas de dosificación oral sólidas de liberación inmediata.* English version: *Dissolution Testing of Immediate Release*
- *Guía para la Industria: Formas de dosificación oral de liberación prolongada: elaboración, evaluación y aplicación de correlaciones in vitro/in vivo.* English version: *Extended Release Oral Dosage Forms: Development, Evaluation, and Application of* In Vitro/In Vivo *Correlations.* (Issued September1997)
- *Exención de los estudios de biodisponibilidad y bioequivalencia in vivo para formas posológicas orales sólidas de liberación inmediata en base a un sistema de clasificación de biofarmacéuticas.* (Issued August 2000, Posted August 24, 2001). English version: *Waiver of* In Vivo *Bioavailability and Bioequivalence Studies for Immediate-Release Solid Oral Dosage Forms Based on a Biopharmaceutics Classification System.*
- *Formas posológicas orales sólidas de liberación inmediata Cambios de escala y posteriores a la aprobación: documentación química, de fabricación y controles, de pruebas de disolución in vitro y bioequivalencia in vivo.* (Issued November 1995, Posted August 24, 2001). English version: *SUPAC-IR: Immediate-Release Solid Oral Dosage Forms: Scale-Up and Post-Approval Changes: Chemistry, Manufacturing and Controls,* In Vitro *Dissolution Testing, and* In Vivo *Bioequivalence.*
- *SUPAC-MR: Formas posológicas orales sólidas de liberación modificada Cambios en escala y posteriores a la aprobación: química, fabricación y controles; pruebas de disolución in vitro y documentación de bioequivalencia in vivo.* (Issued September 1997, Posted August 24, 2001). English version: *SUPAC-MR: Modified Release Solid Oral Dosage Forms Scale-Up and Postapproval Changes: Chemistry, Manufacturing, and Controls;* In Vitro *Dissolution Testing and* In Vivo *Bioequivalence Documentation.*
- *Estudios de biodisponibilidad y bioequivalencia para productos parmacéuticos administrados oralmente—consideraciones generales.* (Issued October 2000, Posted August 24, 2001). English version: *Bioavailability and Bioequivalence Studies for Orally Administered Drug Products— General Considerations.*

Good Manufacturing Practices (GMPs)

- *Manual Del Centro Para La Evaluación Del Centro Para La Evaluación E Investigación De Fármacos E Investigación De Fármacos (Cder).* (Posted April 2001)
- *Normas de Buenas Practica Clinicas (BPC)* English version: *E6 Good Clinical Practice: Consolidated Guideline.* (Issued April 1996)
- *Guia para las Inspecciones do Fabricantes de Farmacos en Formas de Dosificacion—CGMPR.* English version: *Guide to Inspection of Dosage From Drug Manufacturers CGMPR's.*

- *Guia de Inspecciones de Sistemas de Agua de Alta Purez* English version: *Guide to Inspections of High Purity Water Systems.* (Issued July 1993)
- *Guia para Inspecciones de Laboratorios de Control de Calidad Farmaceutica. English version: Pharmaceutical Quality Control Labs.* (Issued July 1993)
- Solid Oral Dosage Forms.
- CDER Handbook Spanish Edition (April 2, 2001)

Regulatory Authority

- Exchange of Letters Between the FDA and Japan Concerning the Exchange of Certain Information on Pharmaceutical Products—Notice, Federal Register, April 24, 2001. Optional format: PDF. (Posted April 24, 2001)
- Cooperative Arrangement Between the FDA of the Department of Health and Human Services of the United States of America and the Therapeutic Goods Adminstration of the Department of Health and Aged Care of the Commonwealth of Australia Regarding the Exchange of Information on Current Good Manufacturing Practice Inspections of Human Pharmaceutical Facilities. (Issued October 11, 2000, posted October 17, 2000)
- Disclosure of Information to Foreign Regulators—Final Rule, *Federal Register*, March 7, 2000. Public Information; Communications with State and Foreign Government Officials. The rule states that the FDA may disclose confidential commercial information to international organizations only with the consent of the person who submitted the information to the FDA.
- *Federal Register:* April 10, 1998 (Volume 63, Number 69). Mutual Recognition of the FDA and European Community Member State Conformity Assessment Procedures; Pharmaceutical GMP Inspection Reports, Medical Device Quality System Evaluation Reports, and Certain Medical Device Premarket Evaluation Reports.
- United States–EC Mutual Recognition Agreement: Sectoral Annex for Pharmaceutical Good Manufacturing Practices (GMPs). Joint Procedure for the Exchange of Serious or Life-Threatening Human/Animal Pharmaceutical Product Recalls.(Issued March 23, 2000, Posted March 30, 2000). This agreement describes the procedures member countries observe to alert each other to product recalls involving drugs, biologics, and veterinary products.
- EC–U.S. MRA on Pharmaceutical Good Manufacturing Practices. After a three-year implementation period, this agreement enables the FDA to rely on our counterparts in the EU to inspect facilities in their countries that manufacture drugs for the United States market. For more

information, please see A Plan That Establishes a Framework For Achieving Mutual Recognition of Good Manufacturing Practices Inspections.

- International Memoranda of Understanding (MOU). This 1995 guidance describes how the Agency initiates, develops, and monitors MOUs with foreign government agencies. MOUs promote harmonization of laws, regulations, and enforcement activities that enhance the FDA's ability to carry out its mission.
- For more information on international agreements, please see Foreign Language and International Information.

International Partners

- globalhealth.gov. This site addresses global health, and more importantly, the link between domestic and international health issues.
- WHO. WHO's Essential Drugs and Medicines Policy provides global guidance on essential drugs and medicines, and addresses the implementation of national drug policies that ensure equal access to essential drugs, and drug quality and safety.
- ICH of Technical Requirements for Registration of Pharmaceuticals for Human Use. ICH was established in 1990 to bring together the regulatory authorities of the EU, Japan, and the United States, plus experts from pharmaceutical industries to produce common regulatory activities for the approval of new drug products. Its purpose is to eliminate unnecessary and unreasonable delay in the global development and availability of safe and effective new drugs.
- European Federation of Pharmaceutical Industries and Associations (EFPIA). The EFPIA represents the pharmaceutical industry in Europe. Its members account for approximately 98% of the pharmaceutical industry's production in the EU.
- EMEA. EMEA's mission is to contribute to the protection and promotion of public and animal health by providing high-quality evaluation of medicinal products. Its goal is to develop a single European marketing authorization controlling the safety of medicines for humans and animals.
- The International Federation of Pharmaceutical Manufacturers Associations (IFPMA). IFPMA represents the worldwide research-based pharmaceutical industry and facilitates the development of position statements on policy issues. It serves as a bridge between industry, the WHO, and other international health agencies. It also serves at the ICH secretariat.
- Ministry of Health, Labour and Welfare. This is Japan's national regulatory agency.
- Pan American Health Organization. Pan American Health Organization sponsored a series of conferences on Drug Regulatory Harmonization

related to pharmaceutical regulatory harmonization in the United States. These conferences included regulators and representatives from industry, consumer groups, and professional organizations. The Web page contains links to summaries from these conferences.

- OECD. The OECD is a 29-member international group that discusses and develops economic and social policy in such areas as trade, public management, development assistance, and financial markets.
- Trans-Atlantic Consumer Dialogue. This is a forum of U.S. and EU consumer organizations that jointly develops policy recommendations to promote the consumer interest in EU and U.S. policy making.
- Trans-Atlantic Business Dialogue. The aim of the Trans-Atlantic Business Dialogue is to boost transatlantic trade and investment opportunities between the United States. and the EU by removing excessive regulation, duplication, and differences in the EU and U.S. regulatory systems and procedures.

Topics of Special Interest to the International Community

- Information for Clinical Investigators. This Web page includes guidances, information on Institutional Review Boards, and protection of human subjects in clinical trials, along with links to clinical regulatory and compliance resources.
- Drug Application Regulatory Compliance. This Web page offers guidance documents, compliance policy programs and guidelines, and frequently asked questions about compliance activities.
- Postdrug-Approval Activities. This Web page provides descriptions of the FDA's postmarketing programs, plus the regulations, policies, and procedures for postmarketing surveillance programs.

How to Contact Us

- We ask you to take time to communicate with CDER about this Web site. What information is and is not useful to you in understanding CDER's international activities? What additional items or categories of information would you like us to add? Please use our comments form.

GLOBAL HARMONIZATION TASK FORCE, STUDY GROUP 4; FINAL DOCUMENT; AVAILABILITY

Department of Health and Human Services
Food and Drug Administration
[Docket No. FDA-2008-D-0149] (formerly Docket No. 2007D-0031)

Agency: Food and Drug Administration, HHS.
Action: Notice.

Summary

The FDA is announcing the availability of a final document that has been prepared by Study Group 4 of the Global Harmonization Task Force (GHTF). This document represents a harmonized proposal and recommendation from Study Group 4 of the GHTF that may be used by governments developing and updating its regulatory requirements for medical devices. This document is intended to provide information only and does not describe current regulatory requirements; elements of this document may not be consistent with current U.S. regulatory requirements. DATES: Submit written or electronic comments on this guidance at any time. General comments on agency guidance documents are welcome at any time.

Addresses

Submit written requests for single copies of the guidance document to the Division of Small Manufacturers, International, and Consumer Assistance (HFZ-220), Center for Devices and Radiological Health, Food and Drug Administration, 1350 Piccard Dr., Rockville, MD 20850. Send one self-addressed adhesive label to assist that office in processing your request, or fax your request to 240-276-3151. See "Supplementary Information" for information on electronic access to the guidance. Submit written comments concerning this document to the Division of Dockets Management (HFA-305), Food and Drug Administration, 5630 Fishers Lane, rm. 1061, Rockville, MD 20852. Submit electronic comments to http://frwebgate.access.gpo.gov/cgi-bin/leaving.cgi?from=leavingFR.html&log=linklog&to=http://www.regulations.gov. Identify comments with the docket number found in brackets in the heading of this document.

For further information, contact Jan Welch, GHTF, Study Group 4, Office of Compliance, Center for Devices and radiological Health (HFZ-320), Food [[Page 15760]] and Drug Administration, 2094 Gaither Rd., Rockville, MD 20850, 240-276-0115.

Supplementary Information

Background. The FDA has participated in a number of activities to promote the international harmonization of regulatory requirements. In September 1992, a meeting was held in Nice, France, by senior regulatory officials to evaluate international harmonization. This meeting led to the development of the organization now known as the Global Harmonization Task Force (GHTF) to facilitate harmonization. Subsequent meetings have been held on a yearly basis in various locations throughout the world.

The GHTF is a voluntary group of representatives from national medical device regulatory authorities and the regulated industry. Since its inception, the GHTF has been comprised of representatives from five founding members grouped into three geographical areas: Europe, Asia-Pacific, and North America, each of which actively regulates medical devices using their own unique regulatory framework.

The objective of the GHTF is to encourage convergence at the global level of regulatory systems of medical devices to facilitate trade while preserving the right of participating members to address the protection of public health by regulatory means considered most suitable. One of the ways this objective is achieved is by identifying and developing areas of international cooperation to facilitate progressive reduction of technical and regulatory differences in systems established to regulate medical devices. In an effort to accomplish these objectives, the GHTF formed five study groups to draft documents and carry on other activities designed to facilitate global harmonization. This notice is a result of a document that has been developed by one of the Study Groups (4).

Study Group 4 was initially tasked with the responsibility of developing guidance documents on quality systems auditing practices. As a result of its efforts, this group has developed document SG4/N33R16:2007. The final document (SG4/N33R16:2007) entitled *Guidelines for Regulatory Auditing of Quality Management Systems of Medical Device Manufacturers—Part 3: Regulatory Audit Reports* provides a structure for audit reports used in multiple jurisdictions, promoting consistency and uniformity and should assist the auditor in preparing a report for use by multiple regulators and/or auditing organizations. Having reports that are consistent in content should facilitate the review and exchange of audit reports. Acceptance of audit reports by multiple regulators should eventually reduce the number of audits for manufacturers. This document was announced as available for comment on February 6, 2007 (72 FR 5443). GHTF received several comments on the document proposed on February 6, 2007. In response to the comments, GHTF made changes to clarify the document.

Significance of Guidance. This document represents recommendations from the GHTF study groups and does not describe regulatory requirements. The FDA is making this document available so that industry and other members of the public may express their views and opinions.

Electronic Access. Persons interested in obtaining a copy of the guidance may do so by using the Internet. The CDRH maintains an entry on the Internet for easy access to information including text, graphics, and files that may be downloaded to a personal computer with Internet access. Updated on a regular basis, the CDRH home page includes device-safety alerts, Federal Register reprints, information on premarket submissions (including lists of approved applications and manufacturers' addresses), small manufacturers' assistance, information on videoconferencing and electronic submissions, Mammography Matters, and other device-oriented information. Information on the GHTF may be accessed at http://frwebgate.access.gpo.gov/cgi-bin/leaving.cgi?from=leavingFR.html&log=linklog&to=http://www.ghtf.org. The CDRH Web site may be accessed at http://frwebgate.access.gpo.gov/cgi-bin/leaving.cgi?from=leavingFR.html&log=linklog&to=http://www.fda.gov/cdrh.

Paperwork Reduction Act of 1995. For this final document, the FDA concludes that there are no collection of information requirements under the Paperwork Reduction Act of 1995.

Comments. Interested persons may submit to the Division of Dockets Management (see "Addresses"), written or electronic comments regarding this document. Submit a single copy of electronic comments or two paper copies of any mailed comments, except that individuals may submit one paper copy. Comments are to be identified with the docket number found in brackets in the heading of this document. Received comments may be seen in the Division of Dockets Management between 9:00 a.m. and 4:00 p.m., Monday through Friday.

Please note that on January 15, 2008, the FDA Web site transitioned to the Federal Dockets Management System (FDMS). FDMS is a Government-wide, electronic docket management system. Electronic submissions will be accepted by the FDA through FDMS only.

Dated: March 14, 2008.
Jeffrey Shuren,
Assistant Commissioner for Policy.
[FR Doc. E8-5927 Filed 3-24-08; 8:45 am]
BILLING CODE 4160-01-S

CHAPTER 10

Future Issues in Regulatory Submissions

The procedures, criteria, and issues surrounding the major U.S. (and international) drug regulatory submissions have been described in detail. These guidelines, however, are not static. They evolve erratically, sometimes unchanged for decades only to be significantly revised seemingly overnight.

The evolution is spurred by two forces. Advances in the industry, leading to improved methodologies in clinical testing, better statistical methods, and enhanced techniques for chemical composition and analysis force submission regulations to try and catch up rapidly. And emerging public demands, often goaded by media and politics, push for improved technologies and oversight methods.

Predicting the future of drug regulatory submissions therefore requires close examination of two sources of information. Emerging trends, technologies, and methods must be carefully monitored. And developing pressures affecting both the United States Food and Drug Administration (USFDA) and the industry require constant review. With these two avenues of emergence closely observed, it is possible to anticipate and plan for the next generation of submissions requirements.

EMERGING TRENDS AND TECHNOLOGIES

Electronic Submission Standards

Most submissions to the FDA are currently delivered on paper or as a combination of paper and electronic copy. Some FDA groups encourage fully electronic submissions; others seem to discourage submissions without primary or secondary paper copies. A few request hyperlinked electronic versions; others seem uncomfortable with hyperlinking. In Europe, Canada, Australia, and Japan, the situation is even more confused and confusing.

Guidebook for Drug Regulatory Submissions, by Sandy Weinberg
Copyright © 2009 John Wiley & Sons, Inc.

Slowly, as standards evolve, comfort levels increase, technology improves, and FDA guidelines [such as 21 Code of Federal Regulations (CFR) Part 11] are absorbed, the situation is gelling.

The advantages of electronic submissions are numerous and significant. Not only is there a significant savings in volume of paper, but electronic copies allow reviewers to analyze results as well, to review referenced and linked documents, and to check cross-references efficiently.

In order for these advantages to be realized, the FDA needs to assure that all reviewers are technically qualified and comfortable. This is likely to be an evolutionary process, as persons addicted to paper retire or retrain, and as new hires are thoroughly indoctrinated in the electronic reviewing process.

But comfort levels will increase more rapidly, and problems will decrease, if a single standard for electronic submissions can be agreed upon. The FDA began the process with a series of industry discussion meetings, organized and conducted by Gary Green (FDA Project Manager) in the 1980s. Significant progress was achieved only more recently, as an informal coalition of industry representatives formed Clinical Data Interchange Standards Consortium (CDISC) and developed common technical specifications.

While CDISC does not yet have official status as a common standard for submissions, it is quickly gaining widespread acceptance. Trials for IND and other submissions are currently underway, and preliminary results are very positive.

While some modifications in fine details are likely, there seems little doubt that CDISC will emerge as the de facto standard for FDA submissions over the next three to five years. While the FDA will probably officially accept a variety of submissions formats, there is little doubt that the industry will opt for the most common and acceptable format, and that CDISC will rapidly become the norm.

Good Manufacturing Practices (GMPs) Revisions

Even as the European Medicines Agency (EMEA) is introducing (GAMP5), the United States is struggling to revise the current GMPs now more than two decades old. While the CGMPs with addition of 21 CFR Part 11 (defining requirements for automated systems) incorporate most of the general principles of the GAMP guidelines, the fact remains that the FDA cannot keep abreast of technological developments in the industry and needs to periodically refine its definition of effective practices.

The effects of cGMPs on submissions are only indirect and in two areas. First, GMPs serve as the source documents for quality audits of active pharmaceutical ingredient (API) suppliers, manufacturers, and processors. The revisions under development will have little or no impact on these audits: assuming that standards in use include both the current GMPS and the automation issues addressed in 21 CFR Part 11, no changes will be required.

The second area addressed in the GMP revisions is a broad question of impurities and contaminants. Currently, the industry utilizes the general principles of the GMPS coupled with a series of guidelines and directives related to potential concerns over specific impurities—in API and in final product processing—that have caused concerns in the past. The new GMPs will likely address these concerns in specific and will call for enhanced carcinogenicity and related preclinical studies to examine the effects of all significant impurities.

The changes are, in part, a codification of current practices and, in part, a new norm for testing.

Process Analytical Technology (PAT)

PAT is an automated quality-assurance process originally developed in the petrochemical industries. It is defined by three general principles: continuous, cybernetic, and potentially remote monitoring of processes.

Traditional batch processing involves periodic monitoring of quality. A pill production line, for example, may be monitored by examining every 10 thousandth pill for integrity, coating, and stamp. If a given pill is found to be deficient, all pills produced in that batch of 10,000 would be recycled, discarded, or reexamined. The process can potentially add unnecessary expense to the production process and can lead to possible inappropriate release from quarantine (pills are stored until "passed," creating possible human error in premature shipment).

With a PAT system, the line is continuously monitored[1] and every pill is examined. The production line can then be halted and corrected immediately should the coating process require more sugar or the press pressure require adjustment.

Even better, a well-designed PAT system has built in the capability of self-correcting many kinds of problems. This cybernetic capability—much like the thermostat on a home heating system—senses the appropriate press pressure level and self-corrects if it exceeds norms. The cybernetic capability is more certain and more rapid than the notification of a human to take corrective actions.

Finally, a remote monitoring capability allows a single human monitor to oversee a number of production lines—colocated or geographically dispersed, even globally—from a central monitoring station. The capacity is cost effective, allows for fewer better-qualified quality assurance personnel, and allows the controlled invitation of outside regulatory personnel (from FDA, EMEA, etc.) to view a process to discuss possible problems or improvements.

To date, the FDA has issued general description of and guidelines for implementing PAT in manufacturing. The industry, well aware that the concepts of

---

[1] Statistically speaking, the procedure is actually one of frequent discrete monitoring rather than continuous, though the practical effect is the same.

PAT, perhaps under different names, have been integrated in pharmaceutical manufacturing in past years and are integral to new systems, has quickly adopted the terminology and the concepts. Manufacturing equipment shows are well festooned with "PAT Compatible" signs (squeezing out the "ISO 9000" signs of five years ago).

The real impact of PAT will come when the concept is expanded beyond manufacturing into automated QA monitoring of clinical studies (already in development with some contract clinical organizations) and of testing laboratories (under Good Automated Laboratory Practices, promulgated by the EPA for their contract laboratories but in general use as an interpretation of the GLPs for automated systems). As PAT is added to these environments, costs should decrease (after an initial capital investment for the monitoring equipment) and quality should improve.

All of which should lead to greater credibility in regulatory submissions [particularly in New Drug Applications (NDAs) and Abbreviated New Drug Applications (ANDAs)] and a more rapid review process of these major documents.

PRESSURES

Compounding these emerging technologies are a number of interconnected pressures that are forcing the Agency and the industry to reexamine basic assumptions about regulation, research, and the business model. Just as technological innovations—improved electronic submission approaches, automated quality assurance, etc.—reflect evolutionary changes, these pressures are affecting the essence of the submissions and review process, sometimes subtly and sometimes dramatically.

Resource Limitations

In 2007, the new FDA authorizing act, providing direction and budget, significantly expanded the responsibilities of the Agency. Postmarket monitoring was increased. Review of advertising was shifted from the Federal Trade Commission to the FDA. A new emphasis on inspection and regulation of API suppliers—particularly international suppliers—expanded the audit burden. And shifting responsibilities for vaccine liabilities placed a heavier responsibility on the government rather than the industry. Yet with all of these new and enhanced responsibilities, the FDA's budget did not significantly increase. The clear directive is to do more with less.

These resources limitations leave the FDA with some difficult choices. The Agency can, in effect, "outsource" by increasingly relying on outside expert consultants who provide client companies with reports of compliance audits, validation reviews, chemistry, manufacturing, and control analyses, and the like. The FDA can then review these reports, relying on the credibility of the outside (and, at least in part, independent) witnesses.

The Agency can decrease the frequency of field visits, inspections, and reviews. While these gaps create windows of vulnerability, the periodic (unannounced) visits can still provide some level of assurances.

The FDA can establish priorities for kinds of issues, using risk (or other) variables to define levels of priority. This strategy makes good scientific and intuitive sense but is potentially compromised by differing agendas of media, the public, and elected officials.

While there are probably other alternatives, these represent the options considered to date—all with some success and some difficulties. But all of these options and perhaps other available choices share one common thread: they result in increasing pressure on the Agency. The effects of that pressure are most likely to be seen in the review of submissions, where rationed resources result in delayed reviews, in rejections for trivial reasons, and for demands for lengthy additional studies and documents of limited value.

While it is possible to patch the problem, perhaps with stronger review guidelines, greater reliance on outside credible sources and risk-related priorities, the real issues will remain unless and until Congress couples greater FDA responsibility with balancing increases in resources.

Harmonization

In a global economy and particularly in a global sector such as the pharmaceutical industry, developed products have an international market. Yet the process of regulating and approving those drugs is at best regional (EMEA and Australia–New Zealand) and often national (United States, Japan, etc.). The effect is a disproportionate increase of regulation in the cost factors of a drug with a worldwide market.

The twin goals of reduction in the cost of regulation and enhancement of drug safety can effectively be co-met with the development of harmonized requirements, review and enforcement of standards across national borders. With a well-harmonized system, approval of a drug product in the United States would be recognized and accepted in Switzerland; EMEA approval in Europe would carry concurrent approval in the United States; and Japan would recognize and accept the approval decision of Canada Health. Companies would no longer be required to submit multiple applications for the same drug, review and testing costs could be reduced, and national agencies (such as the USFDA) would no longer need to send inspection teams to Europe, Asia, or South America.

Unfortunately, national prejudices, politics, and trade policies provide strong barriers to effective harmonization. While international associations such as The International Conference on Harmonisation (ICH) of Technical Requirements for Registration of Pharmaceuticals for Human Use have made some important progress, effective cross acceptance is still long in the future. Even with common guidelines [for example, GAMP5 (EMEA) and cGMP with Part 11 (United States) are largely compatible] the FDA continues to send investigation teams abroad; EMEA does not accept FDA registration or approval of NDA (nor does FDA accept EMEA approval), etc.

Yet the public can purchase drugs approved in other countries via the Internet, or by traveling across borders (for US citizens, to Mexico or Canada). And while the quality control images of some countries may be suspect, few, if any, Americans would object to drugs produced in Japan, Switzerland, the UK, Sweden, or Germany. The pressure to sign interagency agreements for harmonization with some of these (and other) countries is growing and is likely to influence the submission process in the next few years.

Complicating the situation is the EMEA consortium. While the United States may be willing to accept drugs approved in Germany and Sweden, the FDA may be more hesitant when the approval process was completed in Cyprus, Romania, or Turkey, where the quality reputation may be less well know and hence more suspect. Yet under European Union (EU) guidelines a quality assurance inspection by local Romanian officials is fully accepted, and the resulting drug can be exported from Germany under a local German label. While these issues are no insurmountable, they do cloud efforts.

Safety Shift

All biomedical regulation is a balancing act. On one side of the equation is public access to therapies and preventatives. With the guidance of medical professionals, the public has a fundamental and legitimate right to access to all cures and therapies—as long as those drugs have been proven to be safe and effective.

That safety issue, of course, is the other side of the equation. All drugs have some side effects, produce some allergic reactions, and negatively impact some people. For total and complete safety, all drugs should be prohibited. But, of course, that kind of total safety infringes on the right to access.

At different times the FDA has historically emphasized one side of the equation or the other. When founded, the Agency concentrated on accuracy of labeling, in effect permitting full access and leaving safety up to the public. As late as 1970 an FDA Associate Commissioner publicly argued for universal approval (with full disclosure), suggesting that physicians should be the sole arbiters of safety.

Currently, in part as a result of media attention on drug dangers, the FDA emphasizes safety over access. The result is a relatively small, generally safe pharmacopeia. Other countries have approved many drugs not available in the United States, leaning toward access over safety.

Complicating the situation is the general belief shared by the public, media, and political parties (though never fully proven) that many Americans are forced to make choices between needed drugs and other life necessities, suggesting that the cost of pharmaceuticals is in effect limiting access. And since regulation and quality assurance are significant factors in the ultimate price of drug products, presumably increased safety is impacting on availability and access.

The end result is a pressure to minimize redundant, ineffective, unnecessary, and slow regulation where they potentially add to the price of pharmaceuticals (and biological and devices). Streamlined submissions reviews, maximizing safety while minimizing unnecessary costs and delays, are the holy grail. The safety pressure, expressed in concerns over post market tracking, careful scrutiny of submissions, and review of chemical processing and API quality, is creating a dynamic tension with the pressures to maintain or lower drug prices.

Individualized Medicine

Children are more than small adults: drug models that suggest that drugs tested and approved for adults are safe and effective for children in dosages adjusted for body weight are inadequate and outdated. Similarly, testing drug only on males and extrapolating to females is inappropriate and outmoded. Today's medical models require clinical testing on males and females, and adults and children before approval for each of these subgroups.

But what is the logical limit to subgrouping? Some drugs apparently have different effects and side effects on individuals of different ethical backgrounds and races. More clearly (and less politically charged) some drugs have differential effects on persons of differing metabolisms. And seemingly all drugs have some interactions with other drugs, diseases, and genetic characteristics. Will we reach a point where all drugs are individualized?

Some would argue that we already have. If a patient and physician determine that a blood pressure medication is needed, they will examine the range of approved drugs (tested on males and females, children and adults, and perhaps persons of different races and ethnicities) and select a promising possibility. Three months later, after testing for liver effects and considering side effects, effectiveness, and other factors (perhaps including cost), another choice might be tried. Rarely is a long-term drug therapy selected without some trial and error. That trial-and-error process is, in effect, a patient–physician attempt to find the unique formulation appropriate to the specific individual patient.

The current mixture of clinical trials using a cross section of volunteers, of statistical interpretation of differences by gender and ethnicity, of extrapolation of pediatric data from preclinical and limited clinical findings, and of individual trial and error is providing a reasonably effective individualization of drug to patient matching. But as the cost of drugs becomes an increasingly dominant factor, economic theory predicts a dropout of variants within a niche: only a few drugs for any given condition will be able to be produced at cost-effective price points. The effect of this dropout—of pricing discouragement of "me too" drugs and of market consolidation—is likely to be a reversal of current individualizations. A physician may not be able to experiment with different options for a given patient either because some of those options will not be produced or because a patient's insurance carrier may not fund the more expensive choices.

The effect of this reversal of the trend toward individualization is likely to increase burdens on the clinical trial process and on the submissions of NDAs and ANDAs. If customization is not practical through physician–patient trial and error experimentation, the submission of clinical data that defines effects and side effects specific to interactive medical conditions, ethnicity, gender, age, and genetic characteristics becomes all the more important. Unless a developer is willing to settle for a high-restricted label, significantly expanded and targeted clinical trials are the most likely response to the need for customized medication.

Medical Model

The medical model represented by germ theory—that major diseases are the result of bacterial, viral (or prion) action—is slowly evolving into a more complex view of medicine.

Twenty years ago, a stomach ulcer was assumed to be the result of stress and/or poor eating habits. It was treated with recommendations for stress reduction and a diet heavy in dairy products. Today, the same condition is more likely to be diagnosed as a result of a bacterial infection and treated in part with antibiotics.

But the reality is a causality of interaction of environmental issues (stress, diet) and a bacterial trigger, further affected by a genetic predisposition or weakening of the immune system. This complexity characterizes almost all of modern medical theory and has a profound influence on future drug submissions.

Three individuals are exposed to the same virus. One becomes violently ill; a second has mild symptoms and a quick recovery; the third has no apparent effects. Yet the viral trigger exposure was identical. Clearly, there is a more complex causality than simple exposure.

Most (perhaps all) disease states are the result of that trigger (bacterial, viral, or possibly prion); some genetic weakness or predisposition; and some environmental factor or factors. So while, in a simplistic sense, your head cold is caused by a rhinovirus, that virus would not be successful without a genetic sensitivity and without environmental factors that help it to overwhelm your immune system. Your mother was at least partially right when she told you to bundle up in the winter: that scarf would not keep out the virus but might give your immune system the bump it needs to fight off the virus.

What is the impact of this more complex model on drug testing and submissions? The current causality model assumes that randomly dividing disease victims into two (or more) groups and administering a therapy in a double blind design will determine whether or not the therapy is effective. But if the victims assigned to a group are not randomly distributed—if one group has, by chance, more people whose symptoms are a result of genetic weakness while another is populated heavily by people with strong environmental influence; or if one group is a victim of viral storms while the other contains a high concentration of people with weakened immune systems, new designs may be necessary.

The argument that the random assignment to experimental and control groups should overcome these internal differences is weakened as the number of causal factors increases. Randomization will work to decrease the likelihood that an ineffective therapy will be shown to be promising. But it will also tend to suppress findings of promising therapies that work, for example, only for people with a given genetic background. Traditional designs will tend to encourage researchers to abandon promising lines of research that only help persons in specific cases and population subcategories.

Matching designs, in which patients with specific genetic markers, environmental factors, or trigger exposures are paired with control individuals with similar characteristics, will maximize the likelihood of successfully identifying positive therapies but will require new (and potentially expensive) clinical designs and submission strategies. Until the industry and the Agency are prepared to invest in these designs, we will continue to rely on a causality model known to be incomplete and on strategies known to discount promising but highly targeted treatments.

RESPONSES

The responses to these challenges fall into three general categories, each resulting in modifications in the drug submissions process. FDA responses will likely fall in the general realm of "outsourcing," industry responses will require "diversification," and the responses of the various publics will all require enhanced "information."

FDA: Outsourcing

Increasing responsibilities tied to fixed or declining budget will force the Agency to make some difficult decisions. These decisions will likely result in a further reliance on outsourcing, even in the highly sensitive area of new drug submission reviews. This is not to suggest that the Agency will form subunits in southern Asia or that the FDA will use outside commercial organizations to make fundamental submissions review decisions. But peripheral activities, supporting the submissions review process, are likely to be located outside the current FDA structure.

For example, current guidelines call for regular and period visits by the Agency to production facilities. But, if the current shift toward PAT continues, some of those visits can be made electronically. Perhaps with less objection, a single visit to a centralized PAT monitoring facility (either supporting a single company or, as in the power industry, supporting facilities of a number of organizations from a single monitoring location) can provide an FDA quality review efficiently and effectively. PAT can allow outsourcing of some quality assurance functions to electronic systems and centralized monitoring stations. As PAT is extended to clinical testing and analysis sites, the submissions process can be streamlined with remote, continuous, cybernetic monitoring or testing and statistical review.

Similarly, greater international harmonization can, in effect, outsource some drug review and approval processes to other regulatory agencies, shifting some FDA responsibility to providing a review of the procedures in those countries. While widespread cross acceptance is not on the immediate horizon, the NDA 505(b)2 process is a small step toward allowing monitored researchers in other countries (or domestically) to contribute to the submissions and review process. Over time, some agency agreements may permit more intensive cross acceptance, even as broader agreements encourage the use of some supporting data from other Agency clients. Currently, for example, medical device companies are allowed to cite precedents from non-FDA 510(k) (equivalent) submissions. Perhaps in the future, some increased cross-referencing of approvals in other countries may be formally accepted in drug submissions.

The history of the FDA is a continuous shift from direct to indirect responsibility, as testing laboratories and experimental panels have been replaced with requirements that regulated companies performing their own tests on their own subjects. It is likely that that trend will continue as the FDA shifts from regulatory of the industry (as it was originally structured) to oversight of a self-regulated industry (as it is now constituted) to oversight of a coalition of overseeing agencies, organizations, and internal departments.

Industry: Diversification

Industry response to the pressures described above—particularly the pressures for individualized medicine and for a new and more complex medical model—will be a diversification of product lines. As NDA and ANDA reviewers require more extensive testing and offer more restricted labels, industry will be forced to offer a brand extension of products. For example, look for a manufacturer of an allergy medication to introduce a variant for men, for women, for children, for older individuals, etc., much as vitamins are currently marketed.

The reason for this trend toward diversification is a potential increasing of pressure to narrow labeling. If facing an FDA demand that a label identifies a product as safe only for adult males (or for males with a certain genetic makeup), the logical action is to accept the label and target-market the product. While off-label use may enhance sales, the limited label is more valuable than a strategy of launch delay while tests are conducted on a broader market segment. And if the FDA continues to split the market with restricted labels, anticipating the submission requirements and designing clinical studies to maximize the label are alternatives of questionable success.

As the FDA succumbs to situational pressures to restrict drugs to specific categories of individuals, the industry will be indirectly pressured to respond though a market extension of brand: Pill X for Men, Pill X for Women, Pill X for Mature Adults, etc.

Public: Information

The current spate of drug advertising on television has probably gone too far, and, no doubt, new FDA guidelines will force a short-term cutback. But the real impact—providing the public with information previously available only to or filtered by the medical community—will likely be lasting and significant.

As the FDA indirectly encourages a diversification of drug options, resulting in both the brand extensions described above and in the variety of "individualized medicine" choices to be experimented with, consumers and their health-care providers will need to broaden both their information sources and the extent of that knowledge.

This increased information is likely to come from a number of sources. The popularity of web-based medical advice sites (independent, disease association sponsored, and drug manufacturer sponsored) has already been established. These sites serve both the general public directly and the medical establishment which in turn informs (often with clarification and interpretation) the public. Use of such sites is likely to increase as patients and their providers seek more and better sources of detailed information.

The controversy over genetic testing is closely tied to costs (who will pay?) and related privacy issues (if the insurance company pays, will they have access?). As drug products become increasingly customized to genetic makeup, these issues will have to be resolved. In the next 10 years, a copy of your genetic profile is likely to be as common—an as accessible—as your cholesterol score.

Television advertising is currently widespread and will increasingly be regulated. But it will continue to be a prime source of information for patients and an excellent stimulus for patient–physician discussions. While physicians will have to learn to resist patient demands when specific therapies are not needed, increased information is inevitable and probably very useful.

Finally, the technology to allow patients to carry a portable copy of personal medical history (perhaps in a wallet as a card or chip) that can be accessed by emergency medical personnel and shared with physician specialists will allow easy sharing of the information necessary to customized choices of drugs and dosage. This sharing of medical history data is likely to enhance the decision process and to allow heuristic improvement in drug selection and usage.

All of these enhanced information capabilities will allow effective response to and encouragement of more specialized drug development and utilization and, in turn, will significantly change the drug submission process. Clinical testing will become more specialized, label negotiation will become more significant, and the drug approval process will be more closely tied to the potential patient profile.

SUMMARY

The submissions process can be traumatic. Whether you are a start-up company filing your first Meeting Request or a major pharmaceutical organization with an NDA for the latest blockbuster, there is a great deal resting on the process and the result.

A good portion of that trauma flows from a perception of loss of control: the submission is delivered, and it seems to enter a black box of FDA review with no clearly predictable outcome.

But that sense of control can be regained and the result made rational and predictable through a careful Quality Assurance process that checks the submission against FDA established criteria and through the use of an internal, self-regulating review process that applies the checklist criteria used by the FDA to the submission development process.

In the future, that process is likely to evolve, in part, toward more personalized drugs requiring more targeted submissions; in part, toward a renewed and redirected focus on the submissions review process; and, in part, toward more cost-conscious regulatory processes.

But the importance of a drug regulatory submission and the need to both closely conform to stylistic requirements and to maintain the big picture view of direction, purpose, and eventual label will ream in.

Figures are indicated by *italic page numbers*, Tables by **bold numbers**, and footnotes by suffix "n"

Guidebook for Drug Regulatory Submissions, by Sandy Weinberg
Copyright © 2009 John Wiley & Sons, Inc.

Printed and bound by CPI Group (UK) Ltd, Croydon, CR0 4YY

16/04/2025

14658521-0003